# *HIV Mental Health for the 21st Century*

# *HIV Mental Health for the 21st Century*

EDITED BY

*Mark G. Winiarski*

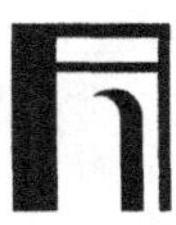

*New York University Press*

NEW YORK AND LONDON

NEW YORK UNIVERSITY PRESS
New York and London



Library of Congress Catologing-in-Publication Data
HIV mental health for the 21st century / edited by Mark G. Winiarski.
p. cm.
Includes bibliographical references and index.
ISBN 0-8147-9312-6 (cloth : alk pap). — ISBN 0-8147-9311-8 (pbk : alk pap)
1. AIDS (Disease) — Patients — Mental health. I. Winiarski, Mark G., 1950–
RC607.A26H5763 1997
362.1'969792'0019 — dc20 96-35695
CIP

New York University Press books are printed on acid-free paper, and their binding materials are chosen for strength and durability.

Manufactured in the United States of America

10 9 8 7 6 5 4 3 2 1

We have no greater responsibility than to respect the trust our clients place in us. Part of this responsibility is to safeguard confidentiality. All references to clients in this book are well and carefully disguised. Names, ages, and other identifying details have been changed. If the contents of any clinical anecdote resemble the situation of a real person, it is coincidence.

# Contents

# Foreword

*G. Stephen Bowen*

Since 1981, when the first clinical descriptions of cancers and opportunistic infections associated with what is now known as the Acquired Immune Deficiency Syndrome (AIDS) were reported, the epidemic of the causative agent, the Human Immunodeficiency Virus (HIV), has spread substantially. With that epidemic, which has substantially affected public health, have come many changes: The epidemic's epidemiology has changed, governmental responses have evolved, and systems of health financing are being transformed.

These changes now challenge mental health providers and those in training for HIV/AIDS care in the next century. Above all, providers have learned that compassion is necessary but insufficient; mental health providers must be multifaceted in their skills, creative in their program development, politically aware, and involved in governmental policy-making processes that determine, through such issues as financing, what care clients receive.

The mental health lessons of the first fifteen years of the HIV/AIDS epidemic are conveyed eloquently in this book, meant to inform the next generation of providers. The authors of the chapters have practiced during times of great uncertainty, great tragedy, and great change. They have produced a body of knowledge — in clinical practice, development of new models and programs of care, evaluation, and attention to public policy—that can be applied to mental health care generally.

To understand the context of the authors' work, it will be useful to know the epidemic's history as well as to understand its trends. This foreword notes some major issues that will confront HIV/AIDS mental health care in the next decade and suggests some responses.

## *Why HIV/AIDS Programs?*

I first want to respond to several often-asked questions: Why are there special programs for people with HIV/AIDS? Are the programs justified? Are there compelling public health reasons for them?

The answer, in each case, is an unequivocal YES! HIV infection is lifelong. People at all stages can transmit the virus to sex partners or, in the case of pregnant women, to their children. This is not true for most forms of cancer, diabetes, Alzheimer's disease, and other chronic conditions (although some have a genetic component). People do not look or act ill with HIV infection for most of the eight to fifteen years they are infected. Those with the virus and their sex or needle-sharing partners frequently don't know about the infected person's condition, thus limiting opportunities for safer behavior.

Women with HIV who receive zidovudine (ZDV, also known as AZT and Retrovir) during pregnancy and childbirth and who ensure that their newborns receive it are less likely to transmit the virus to their children. Because of reductions in levels of HIV in body fluids among those receiving mono or combination antiretroviral therapy, recently made easily demonstrable by viral load testing, people receiving these therapies may be less likely to transmit HIV to their sex partners as well. In addition, other infectious conditions associated with HIV, most notably tuberculosis and including multidrug resistant tuberculosis, present public health problems. Controlling HIV can reduce these conditions substantially.

Longevity and quality of life for those with HIV can be improved with adequate therapy. In addition, the substantial differences in health outcomes for people with HIV, depending on one's gender or race/ethnicity, as reported in the literature, can be eliminated with expert care and good access to it.

## *Changes in the Epidemic's Epidemiology*

In the early to mid-1980s the estimated number of HIV-infected people increased sharply, but by the mid-1990s stabilized. Yet, the number of people who are severely ill and in need of substantially increased care continues to grow.

Cases of AIDS in the United States are now widely dispersed geographically after initially being concentrated primarily in large urban areas in states on the East and West coasts. This dispersal increases the need for expert HIV/AIDS care in the region between the coasts and in nonurban areas, a point discussed eloquently in chapter 10.

Nationally, HIV/AIDS is now the leading cause of death for persons aged 25–44 years. By June 1996, more than half a million (548,102) persons had been diagnosed with AIDS, and 62.5 percent of those diagnosed (343,000) had died. The federal Centers for Disease Control and Prevention (CDC) estimates that 650,000 to 900,000 people in the United States are currently infected with HIV. In the coming decade, hundreds of thousands of infected Americans will become ill, and many will eventually die of HIV-related illnesses. The total number of people developing late-stage HIV-related illnesses will be much larger for the next decade than for the one past, when the magnitude of the epidemic was just becoming defined. From July 1995 through June 1996, the most recent year of AIDS case reporting, 72,416 new cases were reported. If we assume that this will be the yearly average for the next decade, then it is likely that 50 percent more people will get AIDS during the next ten years than did so during the past ten.

### *Changes in Longevity Among Persons with AIDS*

Not only will the next decade see more individuals diagnosed with AIDS, but persons with AIDS who have access to expert care will be living longer, with significant periods of severe medical problems.

This change in clinical outlook has occurred due to development and more aggressive use of improved but costly pharmacotherapeutic agents for prophylaxis and treatment of opportunistic infections; suppression of viral replication by combinations of antiviral drugs and the recently licensed protease inhibitors; and management of HIV- and treatment-related anemia, leukocytopenia, and immune suppression. Treatments now include those for opportunistic infections, antiretroviral agents, immune system enhancers, and blood cell stimulators. More clients will be taking combinations of these drugs as more people at a late stage of illness are seen more frequently by providers.

The Public Health Service now recommends prophylaxis as well as secondary treatment for many opportunistic infections, antiretroviral therapy appropriate for state of illness and previous antiretroviral experience, universal HIV counseling and testing for pregnant women, and stage-appropriate counseling and access to the AIDS Clinical Trial Group (ACTG) 076 treatment regimen to reduce the risk of perinatal HIV transmission. Combination antiviral therapies including protease inhibitors, when appropriate, appear to suppress HIV in body fluids even more than antiretrovirals do as monotherapies. It is possible that the incidence of HIV transmission to sex partners will be reduced as viral loads in semen and other body fluids are diminished. As a result the dynamics of local epidemics could be altered.

### *Demographic Changes Among AIDS Patients*

Demographic changes in the HIV/AIDS epidemic — increases in reported cases among women, children, orphan children, teenagers, injection drug users, homeless people, the chronically mentally ill, and minority populations — require changes in planning, organization and delivery of care for people and families with HIV.

Since early in the epidemic, national incidence rates of AIDS have been higher among African American and Latino populations than among whites, but the absolute numbers of those infected have always been larger in the white population, reflecting the epidemic among white gay men. In 1993 the absolute number of newly reported cases among minorities exceeded the number of newly reported cases among whites for the first time.

### *HIV and Medically Underserved Populations*

Complicating the issue of demographic changes is the fact that a significant number of persons in the newly emerging groups are medically underserved, often because they lack health insurance, and many are victims of social stigmatization.

Many people with HIV or AIDS (11 to 31 percent in one study depending on stage) do not have health insurance. Others may not be comfortable with Western health care or don't know how to access a broad range of services. Some do not speak English, are mentally retarded or have significant learning disabilities, or have numerous survival needs that are major barriers to pursuing care.

In addition, many areas around the country have shortages of health care providers and, especially, of providers expert in the care of people with HIV/AIDS. Some providers may not wish to care for people with or at high risk for HIV/AIDS, such as injection drug or crack cocaine users, sex trade workers, homeless people, previously incarcerated people, and men who have sex with men. Other providers feel they don't have the expertise to care for people with HIV. These factors have led to shortages of medical professionals in some of the areas hardest hit by the epidemic.

## *Changes in the Federal Response to HIV Care and Prevention*

Initial direct federal investments in the care of people with HIV were exceedingly modest as the precise federal role in the epidemic was debated between the executive and legislative branches of government. Federal funding for care programs began in 1986 with $15 million for service demonstration grants to develop model systems of care for adults with HIV. In 1987 $30 million for pharmaceuticals assistance, principally for AZT, and $2 million for the first AIDS education training centers for health professional training were appropriated. In 1988 the Pediatrics and Family Demonstration Grants were begun. As late as 1989 only $60 million was appropriated for categorical HIV/AIDS care programs.

Federal contributions to epidemiology, surveillance, and laboratory research in the early and mid 1980s, while substantial, were thought by community advocates and many state and local government officials to be insufficient to the size of the growing problem. Clinical trials of antiretrovirals and drugs to treat HIV-associated infections began in the mid-1980s. Federal money was first made available for prevention programs in 1985 after HIV was established as the cause of AIDS. The money was to establish "alternate test sites" where people who wished to learn whether they had HIV could go for anonymous or confidential HIV testing and counseling rather than go to blood banks to donate blood so that they could learn their HIV infection status. During the next five years the CDC budget for HIV surveillance, seroprevalence studies, case reporting, counseling and testing, minority organization funding, school education programs, prevention programs targeted to people engaging in high risk behavior, and funding of state and national public information campaigns and hotlines expanded significantly.

Unfortunately, federal prevention funding has not increased since 1990 and has never reached the levels required to bring multilevel HIV prevention programs to all communities in the United States. Prevention funding, including funds for adequate substance abuse treatment facilities and treatment "slots" for substance abusers who are not currently in treatment, continues to be small compared to the size of the problem. This has resulted in far less than adequate changes in HIV risk behaviors in critical segments of the population and slow or ineffective control of HIV transmission in many communities.

We now do know how to target interventions to specific populations, reducing the frequency of HIV-related risk behaviors and transmission. Condom use has been repeatedly shown in short-term studies to reduce or eliminate transmission. Many research-proven prevention interventions that result in lowered levels of risk behaviors have been developed and published, but none has been shown to eliminate risk behaviors for everyone over a long period.

Different interventions are required for gay men, adolescents, substance abusers, sex trade workers, heterosexual men and women, incarcerated people, serologically discordant couples, youth in school, hospital workers, and homeless people. Most approaches are labor-intensive and require at least several contacts between the prevention "intervenor/educator" and the individual or group participating in the intervention. Working proactively with and providing care for people who are already infected is an essential part of the strategy, as noted in chapter 8.

Different combinations of interventions are needed in different communities, targeted to locally important populations at high risk. These interventions can be school and street based. They can involve changing local laws to make syringes and other "works" legal to purchase and possess, setting up local hotlines, and instituting media educational efforts. The interventions must be carried out over a long period of time, with tolerance for slow success.

Prevention interventions should be planned and coordinated with CDC-funded planning bodies and Ryan White-funded community organizations. Providers of primary care in all settings, but especially in high-HIV-seroprevalence communities, should strongly encourage all adults and teens to know their HIV infection status for optimal medical management and prevention service provision.

### *Ryan White Comprehensive AIDS Resources Emergency (C.A.R.E.) Act*

A national response that provides substantial resources to community organizations and other providers of outpatient health care and support services for people with HIV/AIDS is the Ryan White Comprehensive AIDS Resources Emergency (C.A.R.E.) Act. This first categorical HIV/AIDS care program was created in 1990 by the U.S. Congress because so many people with HIV, especially in urban areas, were unable to gain access to care and were filling hospitals and emergency rooms. Such people should have been treated elsewhere and should have been diagnosed and treated at early rather than late or terminal stages of illness. The Health Resources and Services Administration of the U.S. Public Health Service has administered the Ryan White C.A.R.E. Act.

By 1995, 15 percent of the cost of care for people at all stages of HIV infection was covered by C.A.R.E. Act funds. This legislation now provides more than $700 million to cities (Title I), states (Title II), and directly to service providers (Title IIIb, IV, and Special Projects of National Significance) for outpatient health care and support services. Spending priorities for these resources are determined by locally constituted planning councils (Title I), consortia (Title II), or groups of providers (Title IIIb, IV, and SPNS). The funds are more flexible than Medicaid funds and cover people not eligible for Medicaid and Medicare. They can be used for many HIV-related outpatient services that are not covered by some other payer.

Of critical importance is the fact that the funds can be used for necessary nonmedical services, to recruit and retain providers, and to deal with problems of daily life such as transportation, day/child care, home care, housing, and hospice care.

Equally important is the legislatively mandated process requiring local assessment of gaps in care, prioritization of the uses of the funds, and preparation of a plan for coordinated, comprehensive community services for diverse populations of people with HIV/AIDS. During the first five years of the Ryan White C.A.R.E. Act, an increasing number of planning councils of major urban areas elected to use some of their federal funds for mental health services, and the Special Projects of National Significance (SPNS) program, initially funded under Title II, has supported development of new models of mental health care, some of which are described in this book. From 1994 to 1998, SPNS funds were combined with funds from the federal Substance Abuse and Mental Health Services

Administration's Center for Mental Health Services and the National Institute of Mental Health to expand mental health demonstration projects for persons with HIV/AIDS.

The coordinated outpatient programs funded by the Ryan White C.A.R.E. Act have been successful in improving access to primary care, increasing availability of diverse types of services, substantially increasing the numbers and the diversity of underserved people in outpatient primary care, and keeping people out of inappropriate care in emergency rooms and acute care hospitals. Preliminary local evaluations indicate that making outpatient services more available and funding support services such as transportation, day care, home care, and hospice care have resulted in decreased emergency room use and decreased the frequency and reduced the duration of inpatient hospitalization. The resultant cost savings are available to support the costs of outpatient services that partially substitute for inpatient care.

Since 1994 the Community Planning Initiative, a process in many ways similar to the Ryan White planning council and consortia processes, has been supported by the CDC. Local and state planning bodies plan prevention programs and prioritize the use of CDC prevention funds. In some cases the same people serve on both Ryan White consortia or planning councils and the local or statewide prevention planning body; in other cases, the planning is more formally coordinated. These linkages are critical for implementation of federal initiatives such as the universal approach to HIV testing for pregnant women recommended by the Public Health Service and the linking of women with HIV to systems of care that can offer perinatal zidovudine therapy and long-term follow-up for the women and their children, regardless of the infection status of the infant.

### *Political Advocacy*

Both of the national programs to use federal funds to plan and carry out locally responsive care and prevention programs came about because of political advocacy and the use of political power by the gay, minority, and other communities and a variety of local, regional, and national organizations working in coordination with public health and government advocates. The future of health programs targeted to specific medical conditions will depend on such organized advocacy and political action. Other efforts in political advocacy that have been at least partially successful in obtaining federal support include end-stage renal disease, hemophilia, sickle cell disease, Alzheimer's disease, and breast cancer.

### *Growing Collaboration Between Government and Communities*

During the early part of the HIV epidemic, local communities and community organizations, often from the gay community, made the most proactive and effective responses to the HIV epidemic. Prevention and care initiatives were supported by volunteers and local fund-raising. Later, local and state governments in some areas made major financial contributions to HIV prevention and care initiatives.

More communities will become involved with AIDS-related issues at school, in hospitals, in long-term care facilities, on sports teams, and in community service agencies. Mental health providers will need to play leadership roles in communities to help develop solutions based on scientific information, not on fear and myth.

## *Changes in HIV/AIDS Care Financing*

Cost remains a significant barrier to care. The direct cost of health care for people with HIV/AIDS, from the time of infection to death, has been estimated to be approximately $119,000 per patient. This estimate was made before viral load testing and combination antiviral therapy became standards of care. The monthly costs of medical care for people with AIDS who meet the pre-1993 CDC case definition (they have Kaposi's Sarcoma or some HIV-related opportunistic infection or malignancy and are not diagnosed with AIDS only on the basis of lab findings of less than 200 T-helper cells, also called CD4 or CD4+ T lymphocytes), have been estimated in 1993 — before viral load testing and combination therapies — to be $2,764. These costs, however, rise steadily during the last six months of life to more than $8,000 during the last month of life, as determined in 1994. At earlier stages the monthly costs of medical care were estimated in 1993 to be $990 for people with variable severity of illness who have fewer than 200 T-helper cells, $430 for people with 200 to 500 T-helper cells, and $282 for asymptomatic people with more than 500 T-helper cells.

In the mid-1990s there is no comprehensive way to finance access to comprehensive care for all people with HIV/AIDS who do not have health insurance. Medicaid covers 40 percent of the costs of care and therapies for people with HIV; however, this program covers some, but not all, people at late-stage illness. In addition, the financial eligibility criteria vary from one state to another, and the services covered and the levels of reimbursement to health care providers are diverse as well. To receive Medicare, one has to have been receiving Social Security disability benefits for twenty-four months, which, if one includes the five-month initial wait for those benefits, means a delay of twenty-nine months after a determination of an AIDS-related SSI disability has been made before Medicare kicks in. In other words, to get Medicare, a person with AIDS has to survive twenty-nine months after he or she is determined to be disabled. Other patients' care costs are covered by the departments of Defense and Veteran's Affairs.

### *Medicaid Changes*

Changes in Medicaid funding and administration, including the possible institution of block grants to the states, will undoubtedly significantly change eligibility and services covered for eligible Medicaid recipients, thereby increasing the pressure on the use of Ryan White funds. Some states have already reduced Medicaid reimbursement rates for providers, and many are mandating delivery through managed-care programs.

### *Managed Care*

Another major potential barrier to effective HIV/AIDS care, which includes mental health care, is the rapid movement of health care financing and service delivery systems into the diverse forms of managed care. Congressional and state action to cut spending on Medicaid and Medicare will move more clients with HIV into managed-care arrangements. Mental health service providers themselves may be part of several health plans or care networks; others may work at community organizations that bill insurers for the services provided to their clients.

Advocacy organizations and people with HIV/AIDS have expressed concern that traditional or evolving managed-care management practices will result in poorer quality of care and health outcomes for people with HIV/AIDS. These practices include allowing access only to "in-network" providers (patients can use only providers on a list provided by insurers; use of other providers results in reduced or no reimbursement of costs) or to salaried employees and facilities of the health maintenance organization

(HMO); preapproval requirements for access to specialists and specialized therapies; preapproved but possibly limited pharmacy formularies; utilization review; capitation; profit sharing for providers; limited mental health and substance abuse treatment benefits; lack of social services; and limited or no access to clinical trials.

Many managed care organizations do provide expert comprehensive HIV care with or without the use of some or all of these management techniques. The AIDS Health Care Foundation, a capitated HIV care provider in Los Angeles, uses many of these techniques and still provides excellent care.

Mental health service providers will need to be advocates for their clients to help them obtain the services they need and to alter benefits packages as needed in order to offer optimal cost-effective care to their clients and their families.

### *Carve-outs*

In some areas, HIV treatment and behavioral medicine (substance abuse treatment and mental health services) carve-outs are being developed in which managed-care clients receive specified services from a group of providers who specialize in those areas. Reimbursement may be fee for service or partially or fully capitated, with varying copayments and limits on visits or hospitalization for mental health and substance abuse treatment. It is likely that services such as behavioral medicine and care for special populations such as people with HIV, children with special health care needs or disabilities, and clients in need of rehabilitation services, will increasingly be carved out in high-population-density areas or in areas where these conditions are especially prevalent and where groups of capable and interested specialty providers are available. In rural and less population-dense areas or where conditions such as HIV are rare or of low prevalence, care will be provided by generalist physicians or regional specialists and will not be carved out.

A challenge for the future is to link service networks for people with HIV/AIDS in the private, increasingly managed sector with public-sector providers and community organizations that provide a variety of outpatient services and receive categorical federal or state subsidies or Medicaid reimbursement for the services. More comprehensive and cost-effective service networks might result.

## *What These Changes Mean to Mental Health Providers*

The trends I have described mean that many more individuals and families all over the United States will need HIV/AIDS-related mental health services but will have to seek them in an increasingly complicated care environment.

With HIV/AIDS may come a great deal of psychological suffering, including feelings of great loss and existential terror and psychiatric conditions such as depression and mania, and neurological problems, including AIDS Dementia Complex. But the role of HIV/AIDS-related mental health providers must extend way beyond coping with those issues. As people live longer with major medical, social, and health systems management problems, mental health practitioners will play an increasingly central role in their care. They will have to become broad experts on HIV/AIDS care and in advocacy.

- Clinicians will have to assist people who live in high-prevalence areas and those engaging in high-risk behaviors to learn their HIV status and must educate those infected regarding access to expert primary and specialty care. To do so, mental health providers will need to know about the local availability of specific services. They should know the local HIV-knowledgeable primary care physicians, the providers of social services, specialists in treatment during pregnancy for women with HIV infection, the hospitals prepared for providing zidovudine during delivery, and what follow-up services are available for mothers and their infected and uninfected babies. They will also need to know something about the side effects of the increasing armamentarium of HIV-related drugs both alone or in combination, since some medications have psychiatric side effects.
- Clients' depressions, anxieties, fears, and anger, their frustrations with systems of care, and many other issues will challenge the mental health provider. In many cases, family therapy, couples counseling, and/or individual mental health therapy to patients with HIV as well as to members of the nuclear and extended families will be needed. As noted by Dottie Ward-Wimmer in chapter 12 on work with children, many families include more than one person infected with HIV.
- Comprehensive, organized systems composed of linked community providers who regularly meet to solve referral and joint care

problems will be needed to facilitate the substitution of outpatient services for inpatient care. Because mental health providers, including case managers, may best know the patient's entire "system" of care, they will have to be present at those joint meetings. Much of the coordination of client services may become the responsibility of mental health service providers.

- Mental health providers who wish to work with underserved groups will need special, culturally based training. Learning how to talk with people using their own language, to build relationships with them that are based on respect, and to provide assistance in locations where they are comfortable coming for care is part of the process. Mental health professionals likely will have to spend more time with outreach workers who are members of the subculture, learning the local places where underserved groups spend time and serving them in those locations.
- To reach and keep people in HIV/AIDS care, organizations will have to provide comprehensive social services, including housing assistance, substance abuse treatment, child care and adult day care, mental health services, transportation, and emergency financial support. Services for women, children, and adult male family members may most effectively be located in the same facility so that different family members can make appointments to receive services at the same time and place. Services may have to be located in nontraditional places such as congregate living facilities, substance abuse treatment centers, homeless shelters, "storefront" operations, and mobile vans.
- New uses of technology may partially substitute for costly or logistically difficult office, hospital, or laboratory visits. Home computers, video communication, and twenty-four-hour hotlines may reassure clients and families and improve care. Mental health providers should be significantly involved in this response.
- Mental health service providers may need to be advocates for their clients to help them obtain the services they need and to alter benefits packages as needed so that their clients and their families receive optimal cost-effective care.
- As HIV/AIDS becomes more visible in communities that have not yet been significantly affected, such as suburbia, mental health practitioners must assist all to find realistic and compassionate approaches to *their* epidemic.

## *Conclusion*

The HIV epidemic and the resulting large numbers of people with AIDS are having a substantial impact on the public health of the United States, on the practice of medicine, and on mental health services. Within the epidemic, major changes are taking place in the types of clients and families with HIV/AIDS to be served, the diversity and the growing effectiveness of medical therapies, clients' longevity at later stages of infection, the types of services provided, settings for care, the organization of care systems, and the financing of care.

These changes will dramatically impact mental health providers in the upcoming decades. This book, which is about successful mental health service delivery to those affected by HIV/AIDS, presents creative and proven ideas and systems of care that can be adapted to individual and local circumstances.

The models of care described in this book emphasize at their common core a systems approach to HIV care. Comprehensive care that is planned and implemented by a partnership of all communities affected — clients, their families, providers, institutions and agencies, and others in the community — has been shown to be effective.

The contributors to this volume believe that care and prevention programs that use community resources for the betterment of all can make a transforming difference in the lives of clients and families, for the providers and for communities. Clients can be more satisfied with their care, can live and be more productive longer, and can avoid much costly emergency room and acute hospital care. Communities can more compassionately and cost-effectively live with the local reality of HIV. The authors hope that this book will contribute to improving the lives of people with HIV everywhere as much as working with people with HIV/AIDS has transformed our own.

# Introduction

*Mark G. Winiarski*

As we approach the 21st century and the third decade of the AIDS epidemic, mental health care providers must face a crucial fact: The human immunodeficiency virus (HIV) and the condition it causes, Acquired Immune Deficiency Syndrome (AIDS), threatens everyone's communities and everyone's clients. All mental health providers *must* be HIV/AIDS-knowledgeable. And the many clinicians who feel a special calling to work with HIV/AIDS-affected individuals must prepare themselves to go beyond basic training into specialized clinical work.

This book has two goals. The first is to introduce students and professional practitioners in the fields of psychology, behavioral medicine, nursing, social work, psychiatry, and counseling to the specialty of HIV/AIDS-related care. The second goal is to provide clinicians, administrators, and planners with a reference book that will not only continue to inform practice but enable them to compete more ably for governmental and foundation grants.

The area of HIV/AIDS mental health care is broad and is limited only by our creativity, perseverance, and ability to attract funding. This field extends far beyond psychotherapy and counseling and already includes mental health services delivered to the home, specialized case management, psychoeducational group work with clients with dementia, specialized care for children, and development and evaluation of new models of care, among the many aspects described in these pages.

It is the editor's hope that the chapters of this book will not only educate you but inspire you to join the growing ranks of individuals who work with HIV/AIDS-affected persons, blending the wisdom of our fields with flexibility and creativity.

Your contribution will come at a crucial time. While reports of AIDS cases have slowed in recent years, with the rate approaching a plateau, statistical calculations indicate that many individuals in their late teens through their late twenties are infected (Rosenberg, 1995). "Between the start of the epidemic and 1 January 1993, an estimated 857,000 to 1.1 million Americans had become infected with HIV but 227,000 had died of AIDS. The resulting plausible range for persons living with HIV infection as of 1 January 1993 was 630,000 to 897,000" (Rosenberg, 1995, 1374). The U.S. Public Health Service's estimate of infected persons has been slightly higher — between 800,000 and 1.2 million (Centers for Disease Control, 1990) — but is now between 650,000 and 900,000 persons (Karon et al., 1996).

The gross number of individuals affected is tragic enough. But some communities are being devastated. Rosenberg (1995) suggests that one out of every fifty black men in the United States between the ages of eighteen and fifty-nine may be infected and that slightly fewer than one of every hundred black women in that age range may be infected. Slightly more than one out of every hundred Latino men and just one in three hundred Latinas, in that age range may be infected.

Among whites ages eighteen to fifty-nine, one in two hundred men and one in two thousand women may be affected, according to Rosenberg's (1995) calculations.

The infection rates are important as we prepare to care for persons with HIV. Scientists believe that between 5 percent and slightly less than 10 percent of the population of infected persons progresses to an AIDS diagnosis each year. And we cannot leave out of this picture the many partners, family members, friends, and neighbors of HIV-infected individuals who are greatly affected by their loved ones' conditions. Clearly the challenges to care for the mental health needs of HIV/AIDS-affected and infected persons will be daunting as we enter the 21st century.

This book will introduce you to the clinical practices and the programs that not only currently assist HIV/AIDS-affected persons but that will be the foundations for the work of the next ten years. It is hoped that you will continue to turn to this volume for emotional and professional sustenance as you continue this work.

This book's design — the choosing of topics and authors — was based on the belief that although we have different personalities and participate in different communities, much more unites us than divides us. I believe this is true in the world at large; it is true as we struggle with HIV/AIDS. Too many people and communities, such as middle-class suburbs, defend psychologically against the threat of HIV/AIDS by saying, in some way, "That happens to *them. They* are not us." Labeling and compartmentalizing persons affected by HIV/AIDS, and then assigning chapters to describe the contents of each compartment, now mainly stereotypes people and serves the causes of racism, sexism, and classism. I have attempted a more inclusive approach that will confirm that the experience of HIV/AIDS is universal. Chapters describe concerns, issues, and approaches that pertain, for the most part, to all affected persons. Most of us consider our spiritual natures; we all face loss and we mourn.

At the same time, the acknowledgement of special concerns and needs is inescapable. It was important to describe therapeutic approaches to the special issues, to name a few examples, of persons who live in rural areas, HIV-negative gay men, women, and children.

I hope that readers will find this universalist stance compelling and will include themselves in the world of persons affected by HIV/AIDS. I hope too that readers will discern in this volume one therapeutic stance: caring and respect for our clients, and for ourselves.

In designing this volume, I sought authors from many areas of the United States to show readers the geographic diversity of HIV/AIDS care. I hope this will help refute the stereotypical view that HIV/AIDS affects only large urban areas on the East and West coasts. Chapters in this book originate in Pasadena, California; Oklahoma City, Oklahoma; Terre Haute, Indiana; St. Louis, Missouri; and Richmond, Virginia, among other places.

I also sought writers from a variety of disciplines, to acknowledge the gifts of all practitioners. Authors contributing to this book include psychologists, nurses, a psychiatrist, social workers, counselors, a hospital chaplain, an epidemiologist, several persons with master's degrees in public health, and a woman with a doctorate in pharmacy who has been a home care program administrator. They work in many venues: hospitals, a home nursing service, a special center that serves people facing chronic illness, a national professional organization, universities, an advocacy organization, a special center for American Indians, among others.

As I edited their chapters, my wish was that their many clinical stories and the information imparted, expressed in nonacademic style, communicate the aliveness and humanity of the HIV/AIDS-related mental health field. I asked the authors to reveal a little bit of themselves so that you can experience these clinicians as the vibrant, courageous, and consummate practitioners that I know them to be. If anything, they were too modest. But I hope that you nevertheless will gain some insight into why they do the work and the tremendous tasks they undertake.

I asked the writers to follow, at least loosely, a format that includes introductory remarks, a look at background readings, a description of their clinical work, and a list of lessons for clinical practice. In most chapters you will find these elements, although they were impractical for chapters that were not specifically clinical.

I hope you will be inspired by their work. I pray that the leaders in HIV/AIDS mental health in the 21st century are among you.

## *Organization of the Book*

The book has five parts that progress from basic concepts of care, to specialized aspects, clinical models, evaluation of care, and policy.

Part I includes eight chapters that describe basic concepts in HIV/AIDS mental health practice. Introducing this part is a description of the biopsychosocial/spiritual model, which can help you organize the many difficult and complicated pieces of knowledge about HIV/AIDS. The chapter's author writes that the process of understanding HIV/AIDS is like assembling a jigsaw puzzle: "Most of us look at the puzzle's boxtop, which depicts the finished product, before we tackle the assembly of individual pieces. This chapter is the boxtop for the HIV/AIDS puzzle. It provides a conceptual framework that will help the reader piece together the many complicated aspects of HIV. Using this template, the practitioner can skillfully integrate the many facts that he or she will gather from reading this book and from other sources." Chapter 1 is a keystone for understanding the book's contents.

Also in this part are two chapters on psychotherapy. Because the authors discussed their writings with each other, these chapters emerged as companion pieces that should be read together. In chapter 2 Thomas Eversole describes what so many HIV/AIDS-related practitioners have found — the need to "bend the frame" in order to meet the client's needs.

Chapter 3 is about countertransference — the feelings of the provider — and describes the author's careful introspection before going beyond traditional psychotherapeutic activities. I know the author, Robert Barret, Ph.D., to be a most thoughtful and kind man. The information in both these chapters is crucial to all who work with HIV-affected persons. If the reader has doubts about the theoretical "correctness" of what these two gentle men espouse, I suggest reading Mitchell (1993), who, discussing psychoanalysis, wrote, "In my view, what is most important is not what the analyst does, as long as he struggles to do what seems, at the moment, to be the right thing; what is most important is the way in which analyst and analysand come to understand what has happened. What is most crucial is that, whatever the analyst does, whether acting flexibly or standing firm, he does it with considerable self-reflection, an openness to question and reconsider, and, most important, with the patient's best interests at heart" (195). That should be the view of us all.

Much of the literature on HIV/AIDS mental health has focused on psychotherapy and counseling. For additional specific information on HIV/AIDS-related counseling and psychotherapy, I suggest you consult Kain (1989, 1996); Dilley, Pies and Helquist (1993); Boyd-Franklin, Steiner, and Boland (1995), and Winiarski (1991).

Chapter 4 is about spirituality, an issue in the minds and hearts of most persons with AIDS. Many providers, after working with HIV, also find new leanings toward spirituality. Pascal Conforti, O.S.U., a hospital chaplain and a Catholic sister, takes a stance that encompasses excellent psychological principles.

Chapter 5 describes itself in its first paragraph: "Loss and grieving echo throughout the course of HIV/AIDS. For persons infected and for those who care for them, including the mental health provider, one of the greatest challenges is the relationship we are invited to make with loss." The author, Noel Elia, M.S.W., suggests ways to meet those challenges, based in part on four years of providing therapy at a methadone clinic in the Bronx.

Chapter 6 discusses the cross-cultural issues involved in working with HIV/AIDS clients. Chapter 7 talks about the role of psychiatry, which is vital and is viewed somewhat stereotypically and, perhaps, with hostility by many other mental health providers. If all of us could work with the chapter's author, Karina Uldall, M.D., we would all have much more comfort with this medical specialty.

This part's final chapter is on secondary prevention: working with people with HIV to prevent transmission to others. It astonishes me that so little secondary prevention work is being done. Kathy Parish, Ph.D., who has worked with persons with hemophilia and their partners at Huntington Memorial Hospital, Pasadena, California, has written what may be the best article thus far on the topic.

Part II, "Specialized Aspects of HIV Clinical Care," describes work that is important but that may not be in everyone's realm of expertise or geographic practice. The specialized work described will, however, help the reader understand the scope of HIV/AIDS mental health practice.

In chapter 9 Michele Killough Nelson, Ph.D., describes her program of working in group with persons with AIDS Dementia Complex.

Chapter 10 describes rural HIV-related practice issues and is written by I. Michael Shuff, Ph.D., who has traveled widely in Indiana to teach HIV counseling. He is the director of the Heartland Care Center, Indiana State University, Terre Haute, Indiana.

In chapter 11, Ariel Shidlo, Ph.D., a psychologist who works with HIV-negative gay and bisexual men, writes, "HIV-negative gay men suffer considerably from the shadow of HIV." His chapter describes the clinical aspects of care for men in the shadow.

The final chapter in this part, chapter 12, is about working with affected children. The author is Dottie Ward-Wimmer, R.N., a pediatric nurse and the director of the children's program at St. Francis Center in Washington, D.C. She has tremendous passion for the care of children; I hope that some of this passion has escaped the editor's cursor and that you are touched by it. Her chapter made me cry.

Part III describes various models of clinical care — cutting-edge programs that will be the foundations for care in the 21st century. In chapter 13, a group of practitioners from St. Joseph's Hospital and Medical Center in Paterson, N.J., describes a mental health service that is integrated with medical care in an inner-city hospital.

Chapter 14 describes a model for delivering mental health services to the home that was tested by the Visiting Nurse Association of Los Angeles. The authors of chapter 15 tell about an organization that provides case management to Native Americans and, in doing so, provide lessons generalizable to many groups. The authors, David Barney and Betty Duran, do not say much about themselves in the chapter, but I know them to be healers who are filled with the Spirit. Chapter 16 describes a comprehensive center for women with HIV in St. Louis, Missouri, and is cowritten by a nurse and a social worker.

I included a fourth part, "How Do We Know It Works?," to communicate to clinicians and potential program developers that although we may believe that certain interventions or programs are effective, we need to evaluate our work if we want funding. Basic quantitative and qualitative evaluation issues are discussed in the chapters. Chapter 17 is written by Michael Mulvihill, Dr.P.H., a colleague who is often too generous with his assistance. Martha Ann Carey, Ph.D., R.N., wrote chapter 18.

Part V contains a single chapter, chapter 19, that provides an excellent description of the future of federal funding for mental health services. The reader of both this chapter and the Foreword will have a good grasp of public policy issues around HIV care. Doug Wirth, M.S.W., the author, patiently tracked the reauthorization of the Ryan White Comprehensive AIDS Resources Emergency (C.A.R.E.) Act for too many months.

As this book was being completed, something extraordinary occurred in the clinical care of persons with HIV/AIDS: New therapies began to suggest that improved and longer lives were possible. The Afterword, written by the editor, discusses responses to the psychosocial and spiritual implications of the new therapies.

The book concludes with two appendices: appendix A is a medical primer that provides basic HIV/AIDS-related biomedical information, and appendix B lists sources of information, with an emphasis on use of the computer and quick retrieval.

Many readers overlook the Foreword. This book's Foreword is by G. Stephen Bowen, M.D., M.P.H. As associate administrator for AIDS of the Health Resources and Services Administration, Dr. Bowen administered the Ryan White C.A.R.E. Act until his retirement in 1996. He provides an excellent review of basic psychosocial and funding policies, with a subtext of "Who will pay for the care of HIV-affected individuals?"

## *My Predictions for the Future*

This book describes practices and projects, developed in the past, that will be the foundations for the future. It takes no great insight, however, to realize that the future of mental health care for HIV-affected persons is dire. Federal funding is being transformed, as described in the Foreword and in chapter 19. Block grants and Medicaid managed care will certainly erode the quantity and quality of services, each in its own way and for different reasons. It is likely, for example, that block grants will significantly reduce opportunities to develop innovative HIV/AIDS-related mental health programs. And it is unlikely that health maintenance organizations will reduce their profits so that HIV-affected persons can receive appropriate mental health care. I doubt that medical facilities and medical practice groups, caring for HIV/AIDS patients in the context of capitation plans, will reduce their profits so that more mental health providers can be hired. It will therefore be incumbent on us to seek out whatever special funding is available and to evaluate expertly our services. More mental health services will be offered if we have evaluation data that can convince policymakers and health care administrators that mental health care is worth the investment.

If some of the changes described in chapter 19 and the Foreword come to be, then the specialty of HIV/AIDS care will certainly be threatened. If that occurs, our task will be to ensure that HIV/AIDS concerns do not become lost in the great melange of public health issues that include nutrition, smoking, heart disease, and cancer. Each of these issues is important. But so is HIV/AIDS.

## ACKNOWLEDGMENTS

I wish to express my gratitude to the authors of the chapters. They were chosen because they have made significant contributions to the field. I felt they should share their knowledge, and they responded wholeheartedly. No one approached demurred; each author contributed many weeks of work and was patient with my many inquiries. I learned much from each chapter.

This book could not have been written without the support of the Special Projects of National Significance branch of the U.S. Public Health Service's Health Resources and Services Administration (HRSA). I wish to acknowledge the leadership of G. Steven Bowen, M.D., who until his retirement in 1996 led HRSA's Office on AIDS in its administration of the Ryan White C.A.R.E. Act. He was generous enough to provide the Foreword to this book. In my work I also was supported at HRSA by Kathy Marconi, Ph.D., William Grace, Ph.D., and my project officer, George Sonsel, L.C.S.W. All understood the importance of communicating what we have accomplished in working with HIV-affected persons and encouraged the editing of the book as a component of grant number BRH 970165–02-0 from HRSA. Its contents are solely the responsibility of the author and do not necessarily represent the official views of HRSA.

I wish also to acknowledge Robert Massad, M.D., the chairman of the Department of Family Medicine, Montefiore Medical Center/Albert Einstein College of Medicine, and Kathryn Anastos, M.D., the executive director of the Montefiore Ambulatory Care Network, for their support for my work. The van Ameringen Foundation and the Ittleson Foundation have been generous in their support of my dreams to teach HIV/AIDS mental health to community providers. The members of the AIDS Mental Health and Primary Care Integration Project at Montefiore Medical Center have always pushed and prodded me. Michael Mulvihill, Dr.P.H., always a gentle man, assisted the project's survival by agreeing to conduct the evaluation. Maria Caban, M.A., Jean-Marie Rau, Ph.D., and Jennifer Pierce, M.P.H., read parts of the manuscript and provided advice, as did Kathleen Romano, Ph.D., and Michael Schroeder, Psy.D. Marc Gourevitch, M.D., the medical director of the Montefiore Medical Center Substance Abuse Treatment Program, reviewed the medical primer and offered valuable advice. Dale Ortmeyer, Ph.D., my clinical supervisor in my study of advanced psychotherapy, graciously reviewed my chapter on cross-cultural work. Anna Bolanos, my secretary, has patiently unraveled the mysteries of computers for me.

Special thanks to Timothy Bartlett of New York University Press, for his patience, encouragement, and unflagging support in the publication of this book.

Finally, I wish to express my great gratitude to my wife, Diane, and my son, Alex. In his second year of life as I was editing this, Alex left me alone for seconds on end, several times.

## REFERENCES

Boyd-Franklin, N., Steiner, G. L., & Boland, M. G. (Eds.). (1995). *Children, family and HIV/AIDS*. New York: Guilford Press.

Centers for Disease Control (1990). Estimates of HIV prevalence and projected AIDS cases: Summary of a workshop. Oct 31-Nov. 1, 1989. *Morbidity and Mortality Weekly Report, 39*, 110–112, 117–119.

Dilley, J. W., Pies, C., & Helquist, M. (1993). *Face to face: A guide to AIDS counseling* (Updated version). San Francisco: UCSF Health Project.

Kain, C. D. (Ed.). (1989). *No longer immune: A counselor's guide to AIDS*. Alexandria, VA: American Association for Counseling and Development.

Kain, C. (1996). *Positive: HIV-affirmative counseling*. Alexandria, VA: American Counseling Association.

Karon, J. M., Rosenberg, P. S., McQuillan, G., Khare, M., Gwinn, M. & Petersen, L. R. (1996). Prevalence of HIV infection in the United States, 1984 to 1992. Journal of the American Medical Association, 276, 126–131.

Mitchell, S. A. (1993). *Hope and dread in psychoanalysis.* New York: Basic Books.

Rosenberg, P. S. (1995). Scope of the AIDS epidemic in the United States. *Science, 270,* 1372–1375.

Winiarski, M. G. (1991). *AIDS-related psychotherapy.* Elmsford, NY: Pergamon Press. (Now distributed by Allyn & Bacon, Needham Heights, MA.)

# I Basic Concepts in HIV/AIDS Mental Health

# 1 | Understanding HIV/AIDS Using the Biopsychosocial/Spiritual Model

*Mark G. Winiarski*

- A woman, divorced after seven years of marriage and now in her thirties, says she refuses to date because she is afraid of AIDS.
- A fourteen-year-old high school student drinks a "40" (beer in a forty-ounce bottle) and then fails to use barriers during sexual intercourse.
- A Long Island executive, with a wife, a lively four-year-old son and a $300,000 house, dies of HIV-related illness, and the widow keeps the cause of death a secret.
- A man, proud to have stopped his habit of intravenous drug twelve years ago and having worked continuously since, is hospitalized for *pneumocystis carinii* pneumonia.

Our everyday lives are complicated enough and, too often, painful and hard to understand. Imagine, then, being faced with a condition that in the early 1980s manifested itself through a quick and unexplained illness and death. Then, within a decade and with medical progress, the condition became a long-term chronic condition, rather than a death sentence rendered quickly. Now we know this condition as Acquired Immune Deficiency Syndrome (AIDS), which is also called human immunodeficiency virus-related disease, named for the virus (HIV) that causes the disorder.

Imagine, also, as HIV/AIDS comes to public consciousness, mental health providers having to learn to respond with skill and compassion to a life-threatening situation that involves a complex constellation of personal and community considerations. As with heart disease, cancer, or a disabling injury, great emotional trauma is involved. But with HIV/AIDS, the emotional trauma is compounded by a societal reaction that judges the HIV-infected person very harshly, unlike current public reactions to those with heart disease or cancer. Often that severe reaction is internalized, creating a loathing of self.

If someone were asked to create a condition that would test our society where it was most vulnerable — on issues such as mortality and morality, compassion and judgmentalism — it is unlikely one could create anything more challenging than HIV/AIDS. Consider these issues:

- Because the human immunodeficiency virus is spread through exchange of bodily fluids — during sex, in artificial insemination, when sharing contaminated syringes during injection drug use, in transfusions and infusions of blood and blood products, and from mother to baby *in utero* and during breastfeeding — HIV and AIDS is a taboo topic for many.
- Because HIV is most often spread during sex and drug use, large portions of American society judgmentally regard persons with HIV/AIDS as moral degenerates who are to blame for their illness. The judgment is evident in the allowance made for infected children and for persons who were infected by contaminated blood products, who are viewed as "innocent" victims.
- Irrational fears of contamination have deprived many of adequate medical and other care, and even from basic human contact. As late as 1995, White House guards donned rubber gloves during a visit by a gay contingent.

Many people still believe that their communities, their family members, and they themselves are immune to HIV. The strength of this belief indicates the effects of the virus on our society. Too many claim immunity because they cannot acknowledge their fears or confront the implicit judgment, which is, "I am immune because I am not like those others."

But now, and especially for the next century, no individual and no community can afford to dismiss HIV as a condition that happens to others. HIV threatens all our communities and all our clients, in ways overt and in ways subtle, hidden, and complex.

Mental health practitioners, especially, cannot be so dismissive or unaware. Each of the clinical anecdotes that began this chapter is HIV-related, and each person described is a mental health practitioner's client. The woman who refuses to date because she fears AIDS may not be HIV-positive, but she is HIV-fear-positive, and that phobia can significantly affect her life. Or, perhaps, she may be using HIV fear as a plausible excuse that covers fears of intimacy. The secrecy that surrounded the death of the Long Island executive is fairly typical in suburban areas and is one reason that people in these communities are not aware of their incidence of HIV infection.

If a mental health practitioner believes HIV infection doesn't occur in his or her community and therefore fails to learn how to address it appropriately with clients, he or she does clients a grave disservice. In fact, many would argue that discussion of HIV issues should be a part of every mental health practice. The practitioner must be able to respond empathically and skillfully:

- Whether a client is infected with HIV or is a family member or neighbor of someone with HIV/AIDS
- When a client says a fear of HIV is preventing a desired relationship
- When a client is sexually active and doesn't fear HIV sufficiently to have safer sexual attitudes

These clients include us all.

The HIV-related tasks for mental health practitioners, then, are many and complicated. They involve constant self-scrutiny of our feelings and reactions (see chapter 3). They also involve constant learning.

Too often, however, practitioners confuse the collecting of facts with development of understanding. Certainly, the realm of HIV/AIDS knowledge is broad and can be confusing. But understanding HIV entails much more than assembling a headful of facts, be they medical or psychological, to be pronounced to oneself or to a client. Skillful practice requires, foremost, a conceptualization of HIV in which many interlocking and complicated pieces of knowledge may come together and be unified.

Think of this process as similar to assembling a jigsaw puzzle. Most of us look at the puzzle's boxtop, which depicts the finished product, before we tackle the assembly of individual pieces. This chapter is the boxtop for the HIV/AIDS puzzle. It provides a conceptual framework that will help the reader piece together the many complicated aspects of HIV. Using this template, the practitioner can skillfully integrate the many facts that he or she will gather from reading this book and from other sources.

This conceptualization enables the practitioner to make a comprehensive assessment of the HIV-affected client. The assessment findings and the model then guide the practitioner in planning care that is far-reaching. Finally, the model informs interdisciplinary practice, which will be a hallmark of the next decade of care.

## *The Biopsychosocial/Spiritual Model*

Fortunately, this author does not have to create this comprehensive view. A metamodel, which means a more comprehensive model or one that enfolds several other models, already exists that will illuminate the way. It is called the biopsychosocial model, developed by Engel and modified by this author to include spiritual aspects.

The biopsychosocial/spiritual model acknowledges that all persons have many aspects and that these aspects all interact. Figure 1.1 may help explain the model. In this figure, each circle represents an aspect of our lives. These broad, interlocking aspects have the following general definitions:

- Biological or biomedical – pertaining to flesh, blood and bone, organisms, and such entities as viruses.
- Psychological – having to do with the inner life of the individual, including emotions, self-judgments, motivations for relatedness with others, and internal reasons for behaviors, generally.
- Social – the person's participation or lack of participation in family, community and society (including the therapist), and the effects of family, community, and society on the person. One's culture resides in this realm, although one's reactions to the culture may be psychological.
- Spiritual – not necessarily an attachment to organized beliefs or religious institutions, although that certainly may be present. Spiritual aspects often include an internal belief or sense that acknowledges an "other," a reality beyond normal experience, which may be a presence or meaning that surpasses current reality. In this realm we include belief in God, "higher power," "the seed," and particular cultural expressions of spirituality.

Generally, our Western society views each of these aspects separately. When "health care" is mentioned, for example, most people think "medical care," an indication of our overemphasis on biomedical responses, to

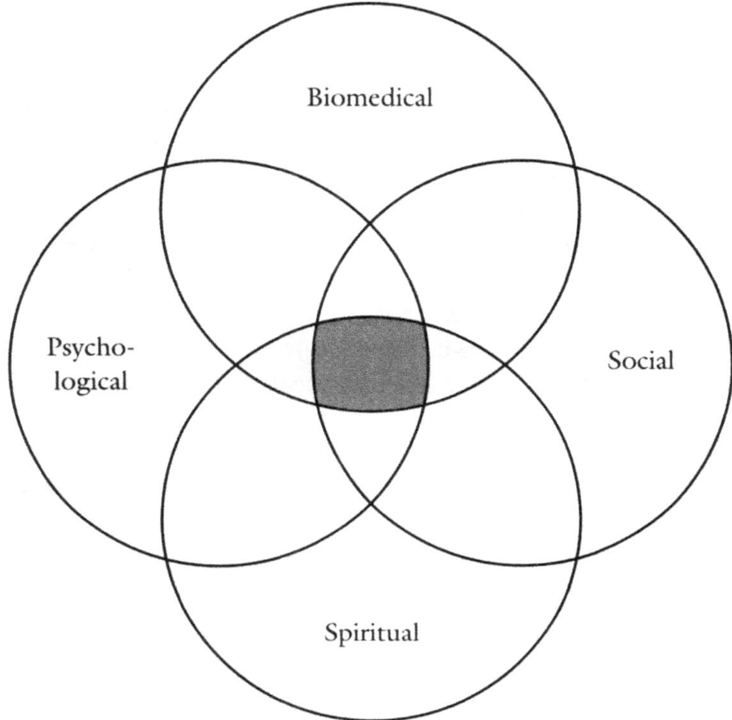


*Figure 1.1.* The Biopsychosocial/Spiritual Model

the exclusion or neglect of care of other aspects of ourselves. In the biopsychosocial/spiritual model, the different realms may be separated out for purposes of distinguishing major components and for planning our assessment and interventions. Yet, the sophisticated provider realizes that all these aspects interplay; they all affect one another.

Consider application of the model to the situation of a person who, after testing, is told that she is HIV-positive.

Since the recognition of AIDS and HIV, and in many institutions still, the person who receives a test result that indicates HIV infection is immediately drawn into a whitewater torrent of months of laboratory tests, visits with medical providers, prescriptions for prophylactic (preventative) medicines, and discussions about the newest medical interventions.

While the body may generally be well cared for, other aspects require attention, such as:

- The person's psychological reaction. Many patients, still unfamiliar with HIV, react with the belief they have been given a death sentence. (An unknowledgeable mental health provider may collude by joining in the client's hopelessness.) Even those who cognitively "know" that HIV/AIDS is chronic are likely to have a strong psychological response that may include despair, fear, dread, guilt, shame, or even relief that comes with knowledge.
- The reactions of those who love that person, who make love with the person, go to church with the person, or are estranged from the person.
- The spiritual reaction of the person, who may or may not have a system of beliefs or feelings about God, "higher power," or meanings of life. When Kubler-Ross (1969) suggested that one step in dealing with terminal illness is bargaining, she also suggested that most persons in that situation bargain with a God-type figure.

Two exercises may help you understand the interplay of our many aspects.

First, if your community has anonymous HIV testing — that is, a place where you do not have to give your name and where you will not be recognized — go and be tested. Regardless of your sexual history and your risk of having HIV, you are likely to have many emotional reactions to the experience, which will include a wait of up to two weeks for the results. Very few individuals, even those with no risks of transmission, escape the anxiety that ensues. In addition, consider telling others that you took the test. Take time to ponder your feelings and to consider what others' reactions may be. Record your thoughts and feelings in a journal. If you are anxious and have no potential for infection, then imagine the anxiety of a person who has a high risk of being infected with HIV, and imagine the courage it takes for that person to be tested. If you fear telling someone, such as a parent or sibling, about your HIV test, imagine the fear of someone with actual risk of being infected.

To this exercise I must add several important cautionary notes. If you cannot be tested anonymously or at a place where you will not be recognized, it may be better to bypass this exercise. Too often a stigma is attached even to those who are tested, regardless of the results. Furthermore, some readers may be at risk for HIV infection, and testing may yield a positive result. A counselor competent in HIV/AIDS can help you assess your risk before testing. If you believe the risk may be significant, you should be confident that you understand all the consequences of a positive result and know about the availability of competent medical and psychological care, whether anonymity or confidentiality will be preserved, and the psychological consequences for yourself. Do not conduct this exercise if you do not understand its possible consequences.

To do the second exercise, sit with a friend in a quiet place, at a time during which you won't be interrupted, and let the friend play the role of a physician or nurse who tells you something like this: "Two weeks ago, we took blood from you and sent it to a laboratory to be tested for HIV. I know you were concerned about the results because you had sex about six months ago with someone you didn't know. The results have come back, and they show that you are HIV infected." Take careful note of your emotional reactions, and imagine what the reactions of you friends, family members, and acquaintances will be. Discuss them with your friend.

Your reactions may include feeling that you should see a medical specialist, that you should pray, that you should be retested, that you should tell family members and friends or hide the fact. Your family and friends might respond with love and consolation, or they could respond with anger and shame. Personal reactions are varied — but all spring from people who are not just biological specimens but who have psychological aspects (emotions), who live in a community that has a culture (social environment), and who likely have considered the spiritual aspects of existence. Clearly, the knowledge that one is infected has significant psychological, social, and spiritual consequences.

Similarly, much that is psychological, social, and spiritual has led to behavior that carries with it the risk of introducing HIV into the body.

Take the case of the fourteen-year-old female high school student, who drank a "40," became intoxicated, and failed to negotiate the use of a condom prior to intercourse. What factors may have led up to this unfortunate situation? A biological factor may be that she had too much alcohol in her bloodstream, which may have impaired her judgment. A psychological factor, such as low self-esteem, may have contributed to her decision to drink or to have sex. Many social factors may be implicated, including her peer group's norms. A spiritual factor may also be involved: Perhaps she grew up in a traditional church and is oppositional and defiant to the church's attitudes regarding sex. Many more issues may be involved here, and a skillful mental health practitioner is likely to pursue many hypotheses regarding what is involved in the young woman's risky behaviors.

And what about the man who stopped intravenous drug use twelve years ago and has worked steadily since? His bout with *pneumocystis carinii* pneumonia, an opportunistic infection that takes advantage of a declining immune system, has serious psychological, social, and spiritual consequences. Psychological consequences may include depression and a feeling of being cheated. Social consequences may include loss of salary and of the ability to support his family, which may also affect his emotional well-being. Being sick, the man may seek a closeness to his God, or he may curse God for his situation. And what of the effects of the illness on his family, and its response? The interplay of all these aspects is what the HIV-infected person presents to the mental health practitioner, and what must be understood as such.

The biopsychosocial/spiritual model is useful because it allows us to think through what we know intuitively. Every aspect of HIV affects and is affected by others. (If we think it through, in fact, it seems that every aspect of life has biomedical, psychological, social, and spiritual components that affect one another.) But how does this awareness affect our mental health practice? It allows a sophisticated response to a client who learns that he or she is HIV-positive. The practitioner who views a client as a dynamic interaction of many different aspects assumes a professional stance that responds to each component. This response is a more comprehensive assessment that takes into account the various aspects and a treatment plan that derives from that comprehensive assessment.

## *Background Reading*

Arguments for viewing the person as a biopsychosocial system are decades old, although authors have differed in their interpretation of the concept. The addition of the spiritual element as an important part of the model is newer, and somewhat controversial.

In the medical field, Engel in 1960 articulated a "unified concept of health and disease" (459) that, he said, derived from work as early as 1951. He calls "a concept of antiquity" the view that "disease is a thing in itself, unrelated to the patient, the patient's personality, bodily constitution, and mode of life" (460). Rather, he suggests that object relations, among other factors, affect health.

In 1977 Engel used the term "biopsychosocial" and listed arguments for its adoption in medicine and psychiatry. A year later Engel (1978) alluded to an integrated model of care. He noted that the posture that science and humanism are in opposition "promotes rivalry, if not antagonism, between and among health professionals. But the care of the sick calls for collaboration and smooth interaction between professionals, with complementary roles to fulfill and tasks to perform" (173–174). This article and a later one (1980) details a biopsychosocial model based on general systems theory, taking into account culture, subculture, community, family, and intrapsychic factors, among other factors.

In the field of HIV, several persons make reference to the model, albeit from a medical vantage point. Cohen and Weisman (1986) described a biopsychosocial approach to HIV care at an urban hospital, calling it "an approach that views these individuals as deserving coordinated care and treatment with dignity" (245). In 1990 Cohen called AIDS "a paradigm of a medical illness that requires a biopsychosocial approach" (98). This viewpoint differs from what we espouse: We view HIV-related illness as a chronic, life-threatening condition with many aspects besides the medical.

The multiple-aspects model is not just theoretical and a nice way to think about humankind. It is the basis of new ways of regarding health care, as well as of studies of mind-body connections.

One example of new approaches to health care is the field of health psychology, and an example of clinical applications of research in this area is *Managing Chronic Illness: A Biopsychosocial Perspective,* edited by Nicassio and Smith (1995). In its first chapter, Smith and Nicassio (1995) outline the biopsychosocial model and provide a very helpful outline for applying the model in assessment and intervention. In subsequent chapters, the authors describe health psychology research and its applications in the interplay of the biomedical, psychological and social aspects of chronic illness.

Another example of the acknowledgement of the biopsychosocial model is the American Psychiatric Association's inclusion of a diagnosis called "psychological factors affecting physical condition" in its revised third edition of the *Diagnostic and Statistical Manual of Mental Disorders* and its revision of the diagnostic criteria in the fourth edition (American Psychiatric Association, 1987, 1994). Moreover, in the 1994 edition, known as *DSM-IV,* the American Psychiatric Association included information on culturally unique conditions.

Studies that acknowledge mind-body connections have emanated from scientific areas such as psychoneuroimmunology (Ader, 1981), behavioral medicine, and psychosocial oncology. The results are described or applied in books such as *Minding the Body, Mending the Mind* (Borysenko, 1987) and in journals such as *Health Psychology, Psychosomatic Medicine, Journal of Health and Social Behavior* and *Journal of Clinical Oncology.* More and more scientific data describe the mind-body connection. A statistical analysis of the results of many studies in psychosocial oncology, for example, led the authors to conclude that "psychosocial interventions have positive effects on emotional adjustment, functional adjustment, and treatment- and disease-related symptoms in adult cancer patients" (Meyer & Mark, 1995, 104).

Engel idealistically advised physicians to employ the biopsychosocial model in their practice. But research and experience has taught us that primary-care practitioners and, perhaps even more so, medical specialists have difficulties recognizing or finding the time to address complex psychosocial problems such as those found in HIV-positive persons. When they recognize a problem, most physicians with biopsychosocial awareness believe that the time-saving and, therefore, cost-effective move is to refer the client to a mental health specialist.

### *Addition of Spirituality to the Model*

While Engel and his successors deserve credit for uniting the biomedical, psychological, and social, those who work with HIV-affected persons soon learn that many infected clients, in the course of their illness, reveal a desire to investigate their spiritual feelings. Moreover, many professional caregivers have rediscovered their spirituality through HIV-related work.

What is it about the condition that encourages persons to look inward? In grief counseling a client often voices regret that more meaningful interactions were not experienced with the person now deceased. Similarly, a person diagnosed with a life-threatening chronic illness may come to realize that life is too short for trivialities. With crisis often comes a search for an anchoring, a deeper meaning. And many find the anchoring in a part of themselves that looks beyond this life and senses that more exists.

Fortunato (1993) notes that even those therapists who are atheistic or agnostic can respond to religious or spiritual belief by responding to "to a client's need for eschatological hope. The word *eschatological* derives from the Greek word *eschaton,* meaning end times. It alludes to what happens to us after death" (1). Fortunato (1993) suggests that counselors form no opinion about clients' belief systems. Atheistic caregivers, he says, can be helpful to clients who believe in life after death. "Perceiving a client's eschatological beliefs as illusory is fine, as long as the caregiver understands that they are useful, functional illusions (and as long as the caregiver can respect the client's perception of atheism as equally illusory)" (3).

For a more detailed inquiry into the spiritual aspects of HIV mental health care, see chapter 4.

## *Tools for Clinical Practice*

The biopsychosocial/spiritual model offers these advantages to practitioners:

- *The biopsychosocial/spiritual model provides a framework for a comprehensive assessment, which leads to sophisticated treatment and case management.*

  As the reader already has learned, the HIV-affected person's situation — both before and after infection — is complex, and the entire landscape needs to be seen and understood. To respond in a sophisticated manner, the mental health practitioner needs to survey the entire landscape by way of a complete assessment.

  The outline presented in this section groups issues in a handy way. The reader, however, now knows that each aspect is interactive with others. Although we placed sexual functioning in the psychological realm, for example, the other realms are also involved in sex. The sophisticated provider will not neglect the biomedical, psychological, social, and spiritual aspects of every issue.

Comprehensive Assessment Guidelines

I. Biomedical issues

   A. Medical Information

   - Current T-helper (also known as CD4) cell counts and other markers of immune function such as viral load assays. (See appendix A for medical information.)
   - Medical history, both HIV and non-HIV. An HIV-positive person may have other significant conditions, e.g., hypertension, diabetes, history of headaches.
   - Medications being taken and those prescribed or recommended but declined. Ask about side effects experienced.

Include drugs obtained on the street, herbal remedies given by nonmedical practitioners, and other complementary remedies.

- Other treatments, including chiropractic care, acupuncture, spiritually based healing practices.
- Self-care practices, including nutrition and exercise.
- Names of all caregivers, medical and nonmedical, including dentist, ophthalmologist, occupational therapist, physical therapist, visiting nurse, nutritionist, Christian Scientist practitioner, and clergy. Understand their roles and the client's choices. Are these persons well chosen, do they know about each other, do they work well together?
- Response to treatment, generally.
- Understanding of HIV-related conditions and his or her own condition. If the client is not knowledgeable or forthcoming about these issues, what might be the barriers?

B. Neurological condition

1. Because HIV, like certain medications, has a neurotoxic effect that affects the client's quality of life, please consider:
   - Client's baseline cognitive functioning
   - Symptoms of central nervous system involvement, such as cognitive slowing, memory loss
   - Client use of compensatory strategies, such as note taking or a reminder system
   - Peripheral nervous system involvement, indicated by pain, numbness or other symptoms in arms, hands, legs, or feet

II. Psychological issues

A. Mental state

- How has client's pre-HIV psychological functioning changed with knowledge of infection and progression of illness?
- Client's emotional response to HIV issues.
- Acute psychological symptoms that the client attributes to HIV status or to other stressors, e.g., anxiety, unhappiness, depression, despair.
- Longstanding psychological presentation. Neglect of personality disorders severely undermines any mental health intervention and can lead practitioners to feelings of inade-

quacy. The personality disorders of clients must be taken into account.

- History of, and attitudes regarding, current or past experiences with mental health professionals, who may include substance abuse program counselors; past or current participation in twelve-step programs, such as Narcotics Anonymous, Positives Anonymous.
- Use of psychiatric medications and psychoactive substances, either prescribed or obtained from street dealers. Do not overlook abuse of prescriptions and the possibilities of substance abuse in persons who do not meet your stereotype of drug abusers. The very respectable-appearing actor River Phoenix died in 1993 with cocaine, heroin, diazepam, marijuana, and an over-the-counter cold remedy in his bloodstream. When inquiring about substance use, use both street names and brand names. I usually ask, "Have you ever taken Librium . . . Valium . . . (etc.)? Have you ever done speedball . . . (etc.)?"

B. Sexual Functioning

- Assess history and current sexual functioning.
- Does the client practice safer sex?
- Type of sex preferred — anal, oral, receptive?
- What has changed since diagnosis or appearance of symptoms?
- Unwanted sexual occurrences?
- If gay, lesbian, or bisexual, the client's comfort with his or her sexual preference.

III. Social issues

- For sophisticated and deeper understanding of the HIV-affected individual, strive to understand his or her culture. The client's cultural affiliations may be multiple. How does the client identify himself or herself culturally? Ask the client to explain his or her cultural identification(s). (For more cultural issues, see chapter 6.)
- Consider the individual's socioeconomic place in society; his or her vulnerability to racism, classism, heterosexism, and sexism; and the educational and economic opportunities denied or afforded this individual.
- Do not overlook one very important social aspect — the cli-

ent's relationship with you, who becomes part of his or her social network. Note the client's ability to have a relationship with you, to accept your empathy, and to open up to you. The person's style of interaction with you is likely to mirror his or her style with similar figures outside the therapeutic relationship.

- Who are the caregivers? Does the client have two families—one of blood relatives and another of affiliation, such as friends and a partner? A genogram, or a visual display of the family, is always helpful (see McGoldrick & Gerson, 1985).
- What has been the response of "family"? Consider long-time family patterns of care and current support. Are any family members likely to flee during a crisis?
- Are others in the support system HIV-positive?
- Whom does the client designate to make treatment decisions if incapacitation occurs? Are the proper documents signed and filed with physicians and others? Whom should you contact in an emergency?
- Are children involved? What is their biopsychosocial status?
- What does the client want you to do if he or she misses an appointment and has no telephone or doesn't answer?

IV. Spiritual Issues

- History of religious observance and current attitudes.
- Client's definition, explanation, and practice of spirituality.
- Are these beliefs comforting or a source of discomfort? Do the beliefs facilitate patient's dealing with his or her HIV status or hinder it?
- With whom does the client discuss spirituality?
- What are the client's spiritual concerns?

This is by no means a comprehensive list of information that should be obtained. (For a broader list, see Winiarski, 1991). The information gathered should be expanded to encompass the client's specific circumstances. On the basis of the information obtained through this process and your knowledge of HIV/AIDS, enter into a realistic therapeutic contract that anticipates, as well as reacts to, biopsychosocial and spiritual issues.

- *The mental health practitioner who uses the biopsychosocial/spiritual model acknowledges and responds to a client's many aspects.*

  Many years of experience providing mental health services to

HIV-affected persons have convinced providers that rigid frames of practice do not adequately serve clients. The inadequacy has several causes, including these:

- Much current practice is based on Western European models, that is, white majority-culture models, of providing psychotherapy. These models are foreign to and perhaps inappropriate for minority-culture clients and fail to meet their needs.
- Current psychotherapeutic models fail to account for the diverse and complex needs of medically involved patients.

This author emphasizes the need to be therapeutically flexible (Winiarski, 1991, 1993) and to use a style of practice called "bending the frame" (explained further in chapter 2).

While much is said about culturally sensitive or culturally competent practice, in fact it is so complicated that mental health practitioners largely ignore its implementation. Practitioners must realize that acceptance of, or sensitivity to, a client's culture is insufficient; they need to be well versed in the culture, to understand it, and to accept its role in the client's life. The therapist must create a therapeutic relationship and make interventions that are culturally consonant for the client. Obviously, cultural competence requires a great deal of study and experience.

- *The model provides a metamodel under which many disciplines can interact.*

Many contributors to this book practice as part of interdisciplinary teams. They realize that just being around the same table doesn't make for a team. Full teamwork — what many of us call integrated care — comes when people talk with each other and regard each other with respect. But, often, teamwork is hindered by a lack of a common way of thinking.

Because practitioners in this country all speak English, we fail to recognize that disciplines have different professional cultures and that these differences create some of the greatest barriers to integrated patient care. Physicians, nurses, psychologists, and social workers generally emerge from training with different worldviews, including etiological presumptions, treatment strategies, and decision-making styles. Even within specific disciplines, persons have different assumptions. A person who provides cognitive-behavioral psychotherapy, for example, likely has different assumptions about behaviors than a psychodynamically trained psychotherapist.

The biopsychosocial/spiritual model does not require practitioners to change their worldviews. Rather, it facilitates a consensual treatment plan based on a common understanding that a person has biomedical, psychological, social, and spiritual aspects. On the basis of that common acceptance of the model, practitioners of diverse views can sit together, view the patient in many different ways, and blend their different views into a biopsychosocial/spiritual treatment plan. Thus, the entire patient is acknowledged, and different team members competencies to deal with the different aspects are validated.

One clinical example involves an anxious patient who sought benzodiazepines (a family of drugs that includes Valium and Xanax) to quell his symptoms. A physician wanted to write a prescription for what he viewed as a biomedical phenomenon. Psychosocial providers suggested that underlying psychological causes of the anxiety would not be addressed if the symptoms were medicated. The treatment plan that evolved from a multidisciplinary discussion included a prescription of medication that would be contingent upon significant participation in psychotherapy.

- *The biopsychosocial/spiritual model assists us in incorporating knowledge from other disciplines.*

The blending of knowledge within a system as just described also has to occur within each practitioner.

What occurs when the client tells his social worker that his T-helper cell count has dropped below 200? Will the worker understand the implications and respond appropriately? Similarly, if the patient tells his physician that he takes pleasure in nothing, will the practitioner recognize a symptom of depression?

Too often, we become prisoners of our training. A social worker may limit himself or herself to the social work aspects of care. But with the many aspects of HIV, this limitation is now insufficient for practice. To respond fully to the HIV-affected person, providers have to learn some of other disciplines' knowledge (see figure 1.2).

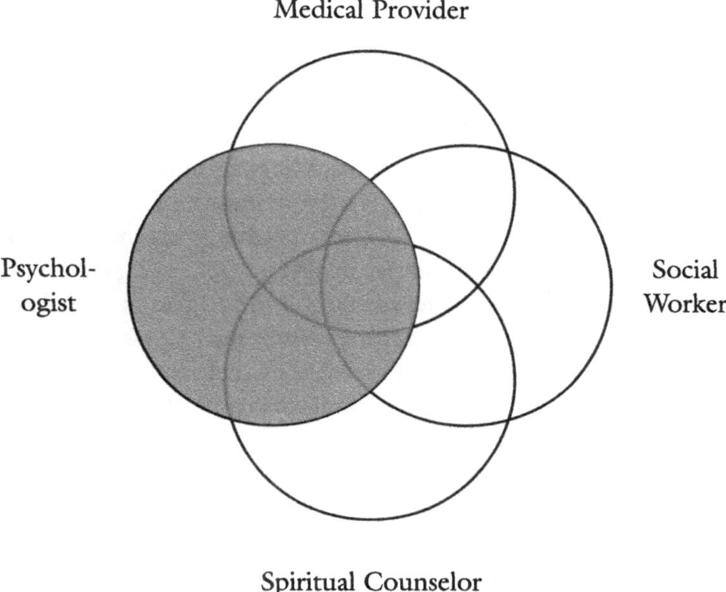


*Figure 1.2.* Incorporation of Expertise from Different Disciplines

The darkened area in figure 1.2 represents the realm of knowledge owned by a well-rounded psychologist doing effective HIV work. This psychologist not only knows the knowledge of his discipline but has incorporated knowledge from the biomedical, social, and spiritual realms as well.

This incorporation of new knowledge allows the practitioner to understand the implications of information of different aspects, such as T-helper cell counts and case management issues, and to respond in a sophisticated manner. The psychologist will never have the training of a physician, a social worker, or a member of the clergy. But he or she must be able to understand the HIV-affected client's concerns, no matter the aspect from which they come. Having a sense of other providers' knowledge allows the psychologist to work better with colleagues and extends his or her professional reach.

## *Barriers*

Barriers to the implementation of a biopsychosocial/spiritual model include the following:

- Being entrapped in one own's discipline and unwilling to extend one's breadth of knowledge. The greatest asset of a mental health provider is an open mind. If one's mind is made up, one ceases to grow professionally and personally.
- Adaptation of a simplistic, cartoonish view of what is meant by biopsychosocial/spiritual factors. While many practitioners use the term, few allow the concept to guide their practices. The term implies sophisticated, multifactorial conceptualization that should lead to multifactorial assessment and treatment.
- Current reimbursement systems for health care, both medical and mental health. These now pressure providers to be more productive, that is, to see more clients, and therefore allow less time for interdisciplinary meetings and discussions.
- Skepticism among patients. People who seek assistance in medical facilities generally believe that assistance comes in the form of medication. This belief requires mental health professionals in multidisciplinary programs to persuade clients of the worth of psychosocial, nonmedical services.

## *Conclusion*

HIV/AIDS has been presented as a biopsychosocial/spiritual condition that requires a sophisticated, knowledgeable response that incorporates all its aspects. The biopsychosocial/spiritual model has been presented as a guide not only to understanding the condition but to assisting health care providers in structuring assessment and guiding intervention. The metamodel also informs multidisciplinary practice and encourages providers of HIV-related services to extend their knowledge beyond their disciplines. Understanding the model leads to a mental health practice that addresses all aspects of the person. This type of practice is often one in which we "bend the frame" of our theories. That is the topic of chapter 2.

## REFERENCES

This chapter was made possible by grant number BRH 970165-02-0 from the Health Resources and Services Administration. Its contents are solely the responsibility of the author and do not necessarily represent the official views of HRSA.

Ader, R. (1981). *Psychoneuroimmunology.* San Diego, CA: Academic Press.

American Psychiatric Association (1987). *Diagnostic and statistical manual of mental disorders* (3rd Ed., rev.). Washington, DC: Author.

American Psychiatric Association (1994). *Diagnostic and statistical manual of mental disorders* (4th Ed.). Washington, DC: Author.

Borysenko, J. (1987). *Minding the body, mending the mind.* Reading, MA: Addison-Wesley Publishing Company, Inc.

Cohen, M. A. A. (1990). Biopsychosocial approach to the human immunodeficiency virus epidemic: A clinician's primer. *General Hospital Psychiatry, 12,* 98–123.

Cohen, M. A., & Weisman, H. W. (1986). A biopsychosocial approach to AIDS. *Psychosomatics, 27,* 245–249.

Engel, G. L. (1960). A unified concept of health and disease. *Perspectives in Biology and Medicine, 3,* 459–485.

Engel, G. L. (1977). The need for a new medical model: a challenge for biomedicine. *Science, 196,* 129–136.

Engel, G. L. (1978). The biopsychosocial model and the education of health professionals. *Annals of the New York Academy of Sciences, 310,* 169–181.

Engel, G. L. (1980). The clinical application of the biopsychosocial model. *American Journal of Psychiatry, 137,* 535–544.

Fortunato, J. E. (1993, June). A framework for hope. *Focus: A Guide to AIDS Research and Counseling, 8(2),* 1–4.

Hepworth, J., & Doherty, W. J. (1992). *Medical family therapy: A biopsychosocial approach to families with health problems.* New York: Basic Books.

Kubler-Ross, E. (1969). *On death and dying.* New York: Macmillan.

McDaniel, S. H. (1995). Collaboration between psychologists and family physicians: Implementing the biopsychosocial model. *Professional Psychology: Research and Practice, 26,* 117–122.

McGoldrick, M., & Gerson, R. (1985). *Genograms in family assessment.* New York: W. W. Norton.

Meyer, T. J., & Mark, M. M. (1995). Effects of psychosocial interventions with adult cancer patients: A meta-analysis of randomized experiments. *Health Psychology, 14,* 101–108.

Nicassio, M., & Smith, T. W. (Eds.). (1995). *Managing chronic illness: A biopsychosocial perspective.* Washington, DC: American Psychological Association.

Smith, T. W., & Nicassio, M. (1995). Psychological practice: Clinical application of the biopsychosocial model. In M. Nicassio & T. W. Smith (Eds.), *Managing chronic illness: A biopsychosocial perspective* (1–32). Washington, DC: American Psychological Association.

Winiarski, M.G. (1991). *AIDS-related psychotherapy.* Elmsford, NY: Pergamon Press. (Now distributed by Allyn & Bacon, Needham Heights, MA.)

Winiarski, M. G. (1993). Integrating mental health services with HIV primary care: The Bronx experience. *AIDS Patient Care, 7,* 322–326.

# 2 | Psychotherapy and Counseling: Bending the Frame

*Thomas Eversole*

Human immunodeficiency virus and AIDS are established among the general population, and traditional notions of counseling, psychotherapy, and case management are being tested as never before.

Mental health practitioners have responded to the challenges presented by the medical, psychological, social, and spiritual aspects of HIV/AIDS by expanding their range of services and by combining professional roles, thus "bending the frame" of psychotherapeutic practice. In addition to making home visits (see chapter 14) and counseling clients on spiritual issues (see chapter 4) and safer sexual practices (see chapter 8), some practitioners speak at memorial services, serve as client advocates, and facilitate decisions about advanced directives or suicide. New for many therapists is the role of accompanying their clients to the ends of their lives, being one of few if any significant *friends* at the client's deathbed. Challenging, frightening, and rewarding, AIDS-related mental health care pushes the limits of traditional practice as we enter the 21st century.

Traditional psychotherapy roles are delineated by what are called "frames" of practice, dictated largely by the theory—such as psychodynamic or cognitive—that guides one's work. Bending the frame suggests that mental health providers not limit themselves to traditional roles but, as necessity demands, go beyond the ordinary limits and established

TABLE 2.1.
*Comparison of Traditional Mental Health Services and "Bending the Frame"*

| Topic | Traditional | Bending the frame |
|---|---|---|
| Home visit request | Decline visit | Consider visiting |
| Case management | Refer to case manager | May do varying degrees of case management, making contacts for client, etc. |
| Spiritual/religious issues | Refer to clergy | Sharing, disclosure, discussion |
| Self-disclosure | Usually very limited | Often more disclosive, mentoring, modeling |
| Medical information | Usually refer to medical worker | Often provide basic HIV information, educate and facilitate client's medical decision making |
| Advance directives | Explore meaning of directives in context of therapy | Often educate and facilitate client's decision process |
| Contact with family, partner, friends | Minimal or none | At client's request: joint sessions, other meetings, grief work |

boundaries. (For comparison of traditional and "bending the frame" responses, see table 2.1.) This requires:

- Development of a large repertoire of skills and resources with which to serve clients. Provider roles now encompass a field of skills as diverse as advocacy, case management, and existential psychotherapy.
- Deliberate, ethical, and theoretically sound selection of therapeutic responses to client needs. Bending the frame brings with it responsibilities. Its practice demands that professionals reexamine the legal and ethical aspects of their work, their real and therapeutic relationships, and the sources of personal authority from which they practice.

Winiarski (1991, 1993a, 1993b, 1995) conceptualizes the range of psychotherapeutic styles along a continuum of paradigms. At one extreme are therapists who maintain a friendship-like relationship with their clients. At the other are those whose therapy is not a dialogue and who are always neutral. Winiarski (1991) maintains that no single, unbending therapeutic frame can serve the HIV-positive client's changing needs through the course of illness. Immediately after diagnosis, the client may require shoring up, crisis intervention, and family intervention for support. Through the asymptomatic period, the patient may benefit from attention to preexisting problems and to short-term goals that reflect meaning in life. Toward the end of life, the client may require case management and assistance in obtaining services.

The preceding chapter noted that the issues relating to HIV/AIDS do not clearly sort into biological, social, psychological and spiritual components. Similarly, the mental health service needs of people with HIV/AIDS do not fall into well-circumscribed domains of counseling, psychotherapy, and case management. Many issues are addressed in service areas where all three disciplines overlap, a psychosocial Bermuda Triangle of sorts, where professional distinctions disappear. Still more work falls outside the traditional boundaries of *all three* fields. Mental health workers of the next century must develop the skills and the support networks to move in all three domains and beyond.

## *Background Reading*

Winiarski (1991) initiated the concept of flexible therapeutic frames and the need to move along a continuum of roles and therapeutic styles in accordance with a client's changing circumstances. The term *bending the frame* appeared first in his description of integrated medical and mental health care for people living with HIV (Winiarski, 1993a). The American Psychological Association's AIDS training curriculum appropriated the term to reinforce the necessity of using a flexible therapeutic frame in this work (Winiarski, 1993b).

Other authors have mentioned the concept of work beyond the traditional limits of their professions. When describing psychoanalysis with poor, urban clients, Altman (1993) emphasizes the multiple roles that therapists are called on to fill and notes that diverse worldviews challenge practitioners to differentiate pathology from cultural diversity. Blechner (1993) similarly observes that therapists with clients who have AIDS sometimes abandon their roles and become involved in their patient's lives. When discussing the helplessness therapists feel, Farber (1994) acknowledges the biopsychosocial complexity of HIV/AIDS as well as the necessity for case management of HIV-related needs.

Of course, these stances have not been without criticism. In their review of Winiarski (1991), Wagner and Schell (1992) wrote, "It is generally believed that meeting the client's 'needs and desires' is not the role of the psychotherapist" (183). Rosica (1995) observes that the emotional aspects of HIV-related therapy are strong and that practitioners may avoid experiencing the pain that accompanies accurate empathy. This avoidance may be manifest as either emotional distance (excessive boundaries) or overidentification (loss of boundaries). Learning to sustain a balance between the two requires supervision and ongoing emotional support. Thus, practitioners need to be deliberate when tailoring and maintaining boundaries that are appropriate to each client's needs. Still, as Curtis and Hodge (1995) note, AIDS work requires "new kinds of helping relationships for which traditional clinical boundaries provide little specific guidance" (5).

## *My Clinical Work*

As a psychotherapist working with people with HIV at a large, inner-city medical center, I was frequently challenged by personal, professional, and ethical situations not addressed in my graduate studies. Almost daily I experienced anxiety about "bending the frame." Later, as training director of the American Psychological Association's HIV-related training program (the HOPE Program), I heard a secret held by most of the faculty experts: To practice effectively, these practitioners "bent" the frames of psychotherapy theory.

The faculty reported making home visits, bartering for services, eulogizing clients at memorials, facilitating decisions about suicide, and accompanying clients to AA meetings. These senior therapists reported a sense of relief once the group had shared its common "secret," and a new sense of enthusiasm for the work ensued. The telling of our unorthodox stories was so powerful that we built it into the seven HOPE Program curricula.

## *Barriers to Bending the Frame*

Those who choose to bend the frame of professional practice face at least four types of challenges: personal barriers, professional/ethical barriers, legal barriers, and systemic barriers.

### *Personal Barriers*

The personal barriers are perhaps the most challenging and rewarding to overcome. Serving people with HIV, we are called on to confront our own attitudes, values, beliefs, traditions, habits and fears about our clients, ourselves, and the ways we practice. A client once asked me: "Why do you think AIDS is here?" I responded that I thought it was "to show us where we need to love more." Over the course of therapy, he taught me a great deal about the FFA (Fist Fuckers of America), and I had an opportunity to test my hypothesis. In supervision I learned techniques to notice but "bracket" or set aside my own feelings as a therapist. In my own therapy, I worked on those bracketed issues and explored my barriers to regarding clients positively.

### *Professional/Ethical Barriers*

Many professional codes of ethics are general and difficult to apply to individual HIV-related cases. Even specific HIV-related policy statements yield conflicting interpretations. Practitioners may encounter codes of ethics that do not accommodate the nontraditional aspects of practice necessary to serve HIV-affected clients effectively.

Furthermore, professional codes of ethics and policies based in the dominant culture may be irrelevant to the worldviews of some clients. If a client's culture holds that the only possession over which one has dominion is one's body and that suicide, therefore, is acceptable, then requirements to prevent suicide may counter ethical principles such as autonomy.

### *Legal Barriers*

Laws may pose real challenges, especially if they or their interpretations are unjust or unclear. Laws regarding suicide, duty to warn, right to know, and partner notification may prescribe practitioner behavior. Given the social-political climate in the United States in the 1990s, future laws or work place policies may contradict the therapist's and the client's personal values and beliefs about life, freedom, and justice.

### *Systemic Barriers*

Many providers work within systems that do not espouse a biopsycho-social/spiritual outlook on HIV/AIDS. AIDS work requires an interdisciplinary effort by the health, mental health, community, and social service members of a care team. Each discipline brings its own culture, values, rules, assumptions, and ethical practices to bear on the person with HIV and on other members of the team. The values of providers may, for example, conflict with those of administrators regarding teaching safer sex negotiation skills to seriously mentally ill persons and making condoms available to them. It is doubtful that all interacting disciplines and personalities will arrive at the same solutions in response to the AIDS pandemic, and practitioners must learn to negotiate the differences.

## *Recommendations for Future Practice*

Given the demands of working with HIV/AIDS clients, I offer the following recommendations to practitioners:

- It is important to develop a theoretical basis for practice that accommodates bending the frame. Unresolved role conflicts, limiting practice to a narrowly defined role, and focusing on knowledge, facts, and philosophical issues impede effective work with clients who have HIV/AIDS (Namir & Sherman, 1989). AIDS work has called on many of us to reassess the paradigms from which we practice in order to serve effectively the needs of our clients as they move across the spectrum of HIV/AIDS. A contemporary theoretical foundation forms the basis of one's discernment and helps prevent making capricious decisions about when to bend the frame. It also demands continuing assessment of the implicit and explicit guidelines for practice.
- Ongoing supervision must be an integral part of HIV-related practice. Trying to do too much alone puts practitioners at high risk for unskillful practice and burnout. Many larger urban facilities provide supervision and peer consultation. Rural practitioners who work in relative isolation should find periodic supervision at metropolitan AIDS facilities. Telephone consultation, teleconferences and e-mail consultation are also advisable.
- Often mental health service workers are the only members of institutional staff who understand the full scope of issues facing the HIV-positive client and his or her feelings about them. With the client's permission, practitioners can serve as advocates for disenfranchised clients within complex medical-social service systems.

## *Tools for Clinical Practice*

The following are my observations on critical aspects of working with HIV/AIDS clients:

- *HIV/AIDS work requires a broad repertoire of professional role responses, skills, and therapeutic styles that allow practitioners to function in psychotherapist, counselor, and case manager roles.*

  The therapist must understand that to work with an HIV-positive client requires a broad range of professional skills. He or she must actively undertake to learn those skills, rather than work unknowledgeably and, likely, unethically with HIV-affected clients. Psychotherapists need to be knowledgeable about clients' current and future likely situations and to enter into a contract based on the abilities of both parties to sustain this relationship. The practitioner must honor the therapeutic goals of the client, which may not be the goals the therapist would choose. Effective AIDS mental health work requires that practitioners be client-centered and serve the whole person.
- *HIV work involves education and case management. Therapists who bend the frame find therapeutic moments while performing those services.*

  AIDS has disproportionately affected marginalized and stigmatized people in the United States. Reliable case management is necessary for most people with HIV/AIDS, because most will require a number of social services throughout their illnesses.

  After the client undergoes HIV testing, part of the therapist's work will entail educating the client about available resources as well as about HIV/AIDS itself. Adherence to medical recommendations may be an issue, and the clinician can explore what it means to the client to have so much time consumed by medical and social service appointments.

  An issue that often arises in HIV-related therapy is the client's frustration when negotiating the welfare system. People with AIDS need to make decisions about ceasing to work, getting Social Security benefits, and being designated "disabled." Furthermore, clients receiving public assistance cannot move in and out of the wage-earning work force as their health fluctuates without losing medical coverage for the future when they may be sick again.

  These case management issues have a therapeutic component. Consider such a disenfranchised client in therapy who needs to access social services. This is a client who lacks the social skills, emotional stability, and physical stamina to negotiate the social service system independently. There may be a temptation to provide the client with appropriate phone numbers or to refer him or her to a case manager with whom he or she will have to establish yet another relationship.

Generally, a therapist who bends the frame might determine with the client what part of the task the client can perform successfully, such as obtaining initial information over the phone, and what therapeutic goals that might achieve. The therapist might assume an advocacy role, placing a call, negotiating with the social service worker, and putting the client on the phone all during the therapy session. The remainder of the therapy session might center around processing the interaction. Here the therapist has worn several hats: counselor, case manager, advocate, teacher, mentor, and therapist.

One barrier to bending the frame is the risk of "enabling" clients to maintain their pathology if the therapist performs duties outside the traditional role. The practitioner does not need to discontinue therapy in order to facilitate case management tasks; however, continued therapy might not be possible if such tasks are not performed. Effective clinicians will evaluate what they and their client feel is most helpful.

- *HIV-related psychotherapy involves exploring a range of themes.*

Adjustment to seropositive status is a process of integrating new information about oneself into one's existing identity. It is nearly a developmental process of redefining oneself, ***and it takes time.*** The change involves a true grief/loss/rage response in many people. For some, dealing with guilt is an issue.

Other clients may have experienced a lifetime of discrimination and abuse as a result of their sexual orientation. Many gay men have considered or attempted suicide prior to acquiring the virus in part as a result of their own internalized heterosexism. Therapists do well to explore issues of unresolved childhood emotional, physical, and sexual abuse as well as rejection by school and family. Many clients have been disenfranchised from their families and have left home. When forced to return to their families due to their nursing needs, some find themselves in a reconstructed childhood role, and a host of unresolved family issues may come to the surface again.

For more psychotherapy themes, see Winiarski (1991) and Kalichman (1995).

- *Legal and ethical dilemmas abound in AIDS-related work.*

  Practitioners need some framework or model for making ethical decisions that will sustain them even when some other parties are not pleased with it. They should rely heavily on consultation and documentation as necessary. Kitchener (1984, 1988, in press), Melton (1988), Reamer (1991, 1993, 1994, 1995) and Burris (in press) have written extensively about ethical and legal issues. The American Psychological Association's Office on AIDS has developed a training curriculum (Jue & Eversole, 1996) to help practitioners apply a model for making ethical decisions related to HIV/AIDS.

  When confronted with an ethical dilemma, it is important to pause and deliberately identify one's personal responses to the case (Jue & Eversole, 1996). The practitioner's countertransference can greatly influence the decision-making process. It is helpful, then, to review the facts of the case and to conceptualize an initial plan on the basis of the clinical issues involved. While codes of ethics for the practitioner's professional association may give additional guidance, evaluating the initial plan according to five ethical principles (i.e., autonomy, beneficence, do no harm, fidelity, and justice) provide a better understanding of the codes and how best to apply them. Practitioners may need to consult an attorney to identify the legal issues and risks in order to assess the options. In addition to considering all the personal, clinical, legal, and ethical perspectives, workplace policies and consultation with supervisors influence the decision. With careful consultation and documentation, practitioners can then choose a course of action and move forward with it.
- *AIDS work brings practitioners into the arena of sex, drugs, and death.*

  The traditional role that psychotherapists or counselors play doesn't include demonstrating the use of a condom with a dildo. Consequently, few professional programs prepare students to deal with their own countertransference around sex and diverse sexual orientations. Practitioners of the 21st century must be able to talk freely with clients about sex. They must possess the information, skills, and language to teach safer sex techniques and especially the negotiation of safer sex. They must be comfortable taking a thorough, explicit sexual history with *all* clients in order to make accurate HIV risk assessments. Workshops and professional training should include experiences that normalize conversation to acquire explicit sexual information. Practitioners must be sensitive to any discomfort they experience with these issues and address them in supervision and in their own therapy.

AIDS work requires providers to be grounded in a framework for dealing with addicted clients and to be very aware of their feelings about individuals who continue to use substances. They must be competent to take a drug use history, to identify substance abuse, and to address its treatment. They must make decisions about treating clients who continue to use drugs or occasionally relapse. Since one policy may not serve all clients equally well, practitioners should decide whether therapy under such conditions helps move the client toward a healthier state and, if so, whether the situation is abusive to the therapist.

In addition, practitioners must understand their own issues around loss, grief, and bereavement. Many clients need to grieve the death of their partners, children, and many of their friends in rapid succession. Therapists should be cognizant of disenfranchised grief (mourning that cannot be publicly displayed and supported by the client's family and friends, such as the loss of one's lover). Often the therapist's office is the only place the client has the opportunity to grieve, and the therapist is the only person trusted to witness and validate the client's loss. Clients may need to grieve the loss of the healthy persons they used to be. They may need to grieve the loss of their dreams and aspirations. AIDS is a disease of loss after loss after loss, and it challenges good therapists to uncover sources of hope with the client.

Clients may want to talk about death and what they perceive it will be like. They may want to make preparations for death, including completing relationships with significant people in their lives. Practitioners must be prepared to facilitate clients' decisions about wills, living wills, do-not-resuscitate orders, durable powers of attorney, guardianship of children, suicide, and funeral arrangements.

Practitioners also need to know their own "trigger issues" related to grief and loss and to learn techniques such as "bracketing" or putting their own issues on hold in order to remain faithfully present for their clients. It is incumbent on helping professionals to do their own work on grief issues once they identify them. Grief work can involve identifying one's own losses, relating them to the tasks of grieving (Worden, 1982), and taking steps to move toward completion of those tasks. Finally, they must actively attend to their own methods for effectively grieving new losses associated with their work. Grieving requires some way of externalizing the emotion and the pain of loss (see chapter 5).

- *Bending the frame requires practitioners to reevaluate their notions about "compliance."*

  Many clients move in and out of therapy over the course of their illnesses, not wanting to be reminded about their disease when they feel well. Therapists may find themselves angry with clients who only come for therapy when things are not going well. Clients who are very ill may not be able to come to therapy sessions at all but may need it most at that time. First and most of all, the therapist should try to help the client understand the meaning of the "noncompliant" actions. With understanding, a client has more freedom to make choices rather than being limited by reflexive, unconscious responses.

  In response to the client's inability to attend sessions, bending the frame might include making home or hospital visits and conducting therapy sessions at the client's bedside in a semiprivate room or literally spoon-feeding the client throughout a session.

- *Counselors can help clients deal with issues of disclosing their HIV status.*

  Clients must make decisions about informing sexual partners and people with whom they may have shared injection equipment. Disclosure may involve considerable risk for clients. It may entail disclosing their sexuality, adulteries, or addictions as well as notifying significant others that they may be infected with the virus. Clients may risk physical harm, death, eviction, rejection, and loss of children or jobs by disclosing their serostatus to others. Counselors and therapists can assist clients in assessing the real and perceived dangers of disclosure.

- *Bending the frame sometimes involves an untraditional degree of self-disclosure and mentoring.*

  The real relationship may be therapeutic. Once, when a long-term client told me that he had been diagnosed with a terminal cancer, an involuntary tear rolled down my face. My client asked, "Why are you crying?," and I answered him honestly: "Because you told me you have cancer, and I am feeling sad." Practicing a relationship of fidelity and honesty had been a therapeutic goal, so it was important for me to be congruent when asked about our real relationship.

Clients with AIDS may ask therapists directly about their sexual orientation. Some sexual minority clients, lacking role models and mentors, ask their lesbian or gay therapists how they manage certain aspects of their lives. Here again the real relationship is called on to be therapeutic. Therapists need to understand their own internalized oppression and to make choices that benefit the client. In bending the frame, the boundaries between client and therapist may shift, but a sound rationale for how and why the frame is bent can keep providers from falling into an unhelpful relationship. Boundaries may be more flexible at the therapist's discretion; however, the therapist is no less aware of or responsible for them.

- *AIDS work lends itself to a transpersonal approach.*

  Perhaps one of the greatest honors for therapists is the journey they take with a client up to and through the client's death. Therapists may notice themselves becoming more transpersonal in their approach as the roles of learner and teacher change over the course of therapy. In essence, the therapeutic relationship becomes one of two partners in a shared covenant (Driscoll, 1992; May, 1983). The counselor agrees to serve as a guide whose faithful presence, honesty and boundaries will be therapeutic. For practitioners who bend the frame, that agreement includes a commitment to continue with a patient through death or cure. A mental health professional may be the only *friend* the client expects to outlive him or her, and the therapeutic relationship may be the only trustworthy relationship in the client's life. Kain (1996) observes:

> We must become good guides. We must be willing to ride the rapids of our HIV-positive clients' lives without complaining about the cold temperature of the water or the heat of the sun. We must remain present at our clients' side from the time they first set into the water until the time they are lifted out. (xxvi)

- A *practitioner is only one player in the client's larger physical-spiritual phenomenon and comes to understand his or her own life-death transition differently.*

In some theories, the client is expected to internalize the healthy aspects of the therapist, and there may be an implicit (or explicit) assumption that the therapist will remain unchanged. The therapeutic covenant, however, is created in a closed vessel, a crucible, in which both the therapist and the client are exposed to the energy of living and growth. As the client transitions from an incarnate being to a spiritual being, the therapist is exposed to a changing life energy and perspective that is operationalized in the client's behavior, emotion, and insight.

Many therapeutic frames are based on ego and healthy differentiation of self. While the therapist usually does not die during the covenant, the HIV-positive client usually does. In the later stages of the client's life, there may be an unspoken conflict in therapy if the therapist tries to strengthen ego and differentiation while the client, who is moving from an incarnate being to a spiritual oneness, is attempting to lose it.

As clients move toward death, some constrict their circle of relationships, and the counselor or therapist may be terminated before he or she is ready. Ordinarily, one might explore the client's reasons for terminating, but dying people move to another set of priorities and may not "process" this change with their therapists. Practitioners may experience a feeling of being left behind. We cannot repeatedly walk this transitional path from body to spirit with clients and remain unchanged.

- *Effective AIDS-related practitioners clarify their spiritual beliefs.*

  If mental health service providers are not comfortable bringing the genuine and spiritual aspects of themselves into therapy, they may not serve clients fully. Therapists must be willing to sit with a client through conversations about spiritual issues and experiences. Discomfort with the topic and quick referral to a cleric or medical practitioner can betray the fidelity of the relationship. The practitioner's spiritual beliefs often expand and strengthen as a result of doing AIDS work, and these beliefs can serve as a true resource when cases seem confusing or overwhelming (see chapter 4).

- *HIV/AIDS creates more need than any one person can supply, and practitioners need actively to address their own tendencies to burn out.*

  Garfield (1982) notes that some of the factors promoting burnout include isolation, lack of support, unrealistic self-expectations, lack of self-monitored time out, and excessive responsibilities. Furthermore, the stigma associated with AIDS and dying compounds all other stressors and denies caregivers external reinforcement. Mental health service providers, in systems unsympathetic to substance users and HIV-affected persons, often are caught in the middle of conflicts, negotiating the dilemmas between client rights and the needs of clients, their families, significant others, staff, and self. Practitioners need to develop strategies in their personal lives and at work to address the exhaustion and disenchantment common in HIV/AIDS work. These ways include:

— Appreciating all the successes or "wins" practitioners can find in their work, such as facilitating a decision about treatment so that a client lives long enough and well enough to complete an unresolved relationship or goal.
— Clarifying those things in which we have faith. Faith isn't discussed much as a therapeutic tool in graduate and professional training. It can be extremely sustaining to know that the ordinary and unspectacular moments in sessions serve a purpose. A client, who I feared was benefiting little from our work, once told me before he died that the insights he'd gained in therapy were instrumental in reconciling his relationship with his family. The value of our efforts may not always be made clear to us, but we need to have faith that they are worthwhile.
— Reviewing our motivations for doing AIDS work and making sure we get those needs met. Practitioners should monitor their tendencies toward work addiction and routinely evaluate whether they want to continue doing this work. A hallmark of "AIDS burnout" is the belief that leaving this work is not acceptable.

## *Conclusion*

Providing mental health services to people with HIV requires practitioners to bend the frame. Bending the frame is a paradigm shift from traditional service delivery ("doing to") toward facilitating empowerment of clients ("doing with") as successful consumers of mental health services. To make the shift, practitioners need a wide range of psychotherapeutic, counseling, and case management skills and the ability to move easily from one mode to another as the client's situation requires. In addition, the work requires us to be very deliberate in managing our professional relationships with clients and to value our real relationships with them as well. As for our clients, AIDS calls on us to reexamine the sources of authority in our professional and personal lives and to respond in a way that is true for us. AIDS work compels us to look at our own issues and to grow as professionals. It reminds us to live fully. It shows us where we need to love more.

## REFERENCES

Altman, N. (1993). Psychoanalysis and the urban poor. *Psychoanalytic Dialogues, 3,* 29–49.

Blechner, M. J. (1993). Psychoanalysis and HIV disease. *Contemporary Psychoanalysis, 29,* 61–80.

Burris, S. (In press). The law and its limits regarding HIV/AIDS issues. In J. R. Anderson (Ed.), *Resource manual on ethical issues in HIV-related mental health service delivery.* Washington, DC: American Psychological Association.

Curtis, C. C., and Hodge, M. (1995). Boundaries and HIV-related case management. *Focus: A Guide to AIDS Research and Counseling, 10(2),* 5–6.

Driscoll, J. M. (1992). Keeping covenants and confidence sacred: One point of view. *Journal of Counseling and Development, 70,* 704–708.

Farber, E. W. (1994). Psychotherapy with HIV and AIDS patients: The phenomenon of helplessness in therapists. *Psychotherapy, 31,* 715–724.

Garfield, C. (1982). Stress and coping of volunteers counseling the dying and the bereaved. *Omega Journal of Death and Dying, 12,* 1–13.

Jue, S., & Eversole, T. (1996). *Ethical issues and HIV/AIDS mental health services.* Washington, DC: American Psychological Association.

Kain, C. D. (1996). *Positive: HIV affirmative counseling.* Alexandria, VA: American Counseling Association.

Kalichman, S. C. (1995). *Understanding AIDS: A guide for mental health professionals.* Washington, DC: American Psychological Association.

Kitchener, K. S. (1984). Intuition, critical evaluation and ethical principles: The foundation for ethical decisions in counseling psychology. *The Counseling Psychologist, 12,* 43–55.

Kitchener, K. S. (1988). Dual relationships: what makes them so problematic? *Journal of Counseling and Development, 67,* 217–221.

Kitchener, K. S. (in press). Thinking well about doing good in HIV-related practice: a model of ethical analysis. In J. R. Anderson (Ed.), *Resource manual on ethical issues in mental health service delivery.* Washington, DC: American Psychological Association.

May, W. (1983). *The physician's covenant: Images of healer in medical ethics.* Philadelphia: Westminster Press.

Melton, G. B. (1988). Ethical and legal issues in AIDS-related practice. *American Psychologist, 43,* 941–947.

Namir, S., & Sherman, S. (1989). Coping with countertransference. In C. D. Kain (Ed.), *No longer immune: A counselor's guide to AIDS* (263–280). Alexandria, VA: American Association for Counseling and Development.

Reamer, F. G. (1991). AIDS, social work and the "duty to protect." *Social Work, 36,* 56–60.

Reamer, F. G. (1993). AIDS and social work: The ethics and civil liberties agenda. *Social Work, 38,* 412–419.

Reamer, F. G. (1994). *Social work malpractice and liability.* New York: Columbia University Press.

Reamer, F. G. (1995). *Social work values and ethics.* New York: Columbia University Press.

Rosica, T. C. (1995). AIDS and boundaries: Instinct vs. empathy. *Focus: A Guide to AIDS Research and Counseling, 10(2),* 1–4.

Wagner, M. K., & Schell, E. K. (1992). Book and film reviews. *AIDS Education and Prevention, 4,* 183–184.

Winiarski, M. G. (1991). *AIDS-related psychotherapy.* Elmsford, NY: Pergamon Press. (Now distributed by Allyn & Bacon, Needham Heights, MA.)

Winiarski, M. G. (1993a). Integrating mental health services with HIV primary care: The Bronx experience. *AIDS Patient Care, 7,* 322–326.

Winiarski, M. G. (1993b). Substance abuse and HIV disease. In T. Eversole and J. R. Anderson (Eds.), *HIV, psychology and persons with chemical dependency* (93–100). Washington, DC: American Psychological Association.

Winiarski, M. G. (1995). HIV and AIDS. In A. M. Washton (Ed.), *Psychotherapy and substance abuse: A practitioner's handbook* (428–450). New York: Guilford Press.

Worden, J. W. (1982). *Grief counseling and grief therapy: A handbook for the mental health practitioner.* New York: Springer Publishing Co.

# 3 | Countertransference Issues in HIV-Related Psychotherapy

*Robert L. Barret*

Since Freud (1910/1959) first suggested the ideas of transference and countertransference, clinicians have learned to be especially aware of the ways their own emotional issues may influence the course of psychotherapy. While the debate about the validity and the application of these two concepts will never be completely resolved, contemporary practitioners are using terms such as boundaries (Rosica, 1995), overidentification (Caldwell, 1994), and compassion (Winiarski, 1995) to describe what is at least a similar phenomenon.

As the incidence of HIV infection has increased, mental health workers and researchers have reported the highly complex issues that force the practitioner to step beyond the traditional boundaries of the client/clinician relationship. This "stepping beyond" requires a creativity in treatment that can increase the likelihood of a dangerous countertransference (Macks, 1988; Shernoff, 1991).

Eversole, in the preceding chapter, writes about the necessity of "bending the frame" in HIV/AIDS-related psychotherapy. Stepping beyond the limits of the traditional psychotherapist's role is demanded by the need for home and hospital visits and the often close relationship that can develop between the clinician and the client, as well as the client's support system. Eversole explores specific behaviors such as attending funerals or becoming involved in a client's support system as examples of tasks that most would not include in a description of psychotherapy or counseling. Nevertheless, these behaviors are often justified as the clinician faces the stigma, rejection, and political debate that surround HIV treatment. Working with clients who may have been rejected by their families or who have no medical, financial, or social support systems brings the practitioner face to face with human needs that demand attention.

Consider the situation of an HIV-infected mother of three young children who has no money for basic needs. During a home visit the counselor discovers that there is no food in the house and the mother is too sick to go to the grocery. Obtaining some food for this family might take precedence over becoming involved in interpersonal exploration. Similarly, agreeing to take responsibility for planning a client's memorial service puts the mental health professional in an entirely new role, one that is likely to involve significant emotional responses. The clinician "bends the frame" when direct involvement in such activities takes place; the emotional responses to needs such as these constitute potential countertransference. Countertransference is a more internal process and can certainly be positive or negative. Some clinicians react angrily to injection drug users who present with HIV or refuse to step beyond their traditional role because of internal emotional responses that reflect unresolved personal issues as opposed to appropriate clinical assessments.

This chapter reviews contemporary views of countertransference as seen in HIV-related psychotherapy, summarizes a case that clearly reveals the potential emotional difficulty that some practitioners experience, and gives suggestions for ways to address the dangers posed by this phenomenon. Let's begin by looking at what the literature tells us about countertransference.

## *Background Reading*

Freud (1910/1959) provides the generative material on countertransference, and more contemporary writers, using other terms, expand this concept. Freud defined countertransference as the projection by the analyst of his or her feelings, attitudes, or desires onto the patient. These projections can take positive or negative forms but represent an unconscious desire to satisfy the analyst's internal need. If left unaddressed, this process will impede the analysis. Countertransference calls on the analyst to examine internal material to understand self more completely. It can pull us more fully into the patient's life or push us away, but it also can provide an opportunity for much personal growth and increased appreciation for the richness of each person's life experience.

In the case of the HIV-infected, issues such as death at an early age, family rejection, stigma, the often intense political debate, a reliance on experimental treatment, and other very complex issues, countertransference is likely to occur in the form of intense overinvolvement or distancing.

Genevay (1990) suggests that in working with elderly dying clients, many practitioners remain detached because of their own fear of helplessness and loss of control. The helplessness that many professionals report as they encounter the dying can generate fears of one's own death that are intense enough to lead to denial and distancing. This denial can take the form of telling clients how well they look, encouraging them to consider participating in future events that clearly will occur after their deaths, and even staying away in the belief that there is no crisis.

Examining feelings like these can lead the psychotherapist to the realization that the real fear is of his or her own death and suffering. When the unconscious motivation for such behaviors is realized, there is the potential for a kind of honesty and realness that is rarely found in the workplace. Engaging such fears leads to a kind of personal development that enriches life. According to Genevay (1990), being helpless with the client empowers the client as well as the practitioner, but she warns that keeping clear the distinction between being a professional and being a friend is essential. This means that while the clinician may become more involved, limits must be clear between the client and the helper, and a constant eye must be kept on the ethical parameters of the relationship. Appropriate caring takes place within these limits. The trick is to learn to be present, to let the patient lead, but to also be clear about the limits of the relationship.

Federn (1952) was among the first to liken countertransference to boundaries. According to Federn, ego boundaries are flexible and serve to mark the limits of the ego and the outside world. When the therapist loses ego boundaries, he or she merges with the client and experiences a conflict between being empathic and preserving self. The potential loss of self increases the threat of countertransference in all psychotherapy, but especially in HIV-related psychotherapy. According to Rosica (1995), such blurring of boundaries leads to suffering by both the therapist and the client: "The therapist loses his or her identity as clinician, objectivity and distance from the client, and the ability to keep reality in perspective" (1). Such loss of boundary can lead to feelings of guilt, rejection, abandonment, helplessness, loss, sadness, and grief and a struggle among empathic identification, overidentification, and loss of self. Gabriel (1991) sees the bereavement reported by therapists who work with the HIV-infected in group settings as an example of countertransference. As they struggle with a wide range of internal emotional responses, helpers are called on simultaneously to help surviving group members live with these deaths and to face the threat of their own deaths.

Winiarski (1995) points out that HIV may elicit unsettling issues and feelings, such as "moral judgments regarding sex and substance use; psychological discomfort regarding alternative sexual practices and substance use, including but not limited to injection drug use; judgments regarding women, their sexual activity and childbearing responsibilities; racism and classism that include anger at disadvantaged urban minority-culture members; feelings of helplessness, and seeming inevitable loss" (429). He points out that in HIV-related psychotherapy, provider attitudes often interfere with skillful practice. The effective use of compassion can become blocked by the practitioner's seeing clients as stereotypes and by his or her emotional reactions to the situation, ranging from viewing HIV-infected substance abusers as poor candidates for help because of perceived character deficiencies to the need for emotional distance because of fears of helplessness or death. Reactions like these are common for all professional groups involved in the treatment of persons with HIV disease (Silverman, 1993).

Caldwell (1994) uses the term "overidentification" to describe similar phenomena and sees gay psychotherapists as especially vulnerable. McKusick (1988) identifies common countertransference issues as fear of the unknown, fear of contagion, fear of dying and of death, denial of helplessness, fear of homosexuality, overidentification, anger, and need for professional omnipotence.

Other examples of potential countertransference include viewing HIV-infected children and hemophiliacs as most deserving of treatment because they are "truly innocent victims," to refusing to work with an HIV-infected drug user until the substance abuse is under control, to becoming overinvolved in one of the HIV-infected communities to the exclusion of others who are suffering. The problem posed in countertransference is not necessarily the action that one takes but the often unconscious personal issue that is serving as the disguised motivator. Certainly the practitioner who greets his or her emotional responses as an opportunity for further self-understanding will encounter the kind of growth that can lead to more competent practice.

Countertransference is thus a potentially powerful event that seems to permeate HIV-related psychotherapy and that can serve as a signal to the therapist that personal issues are present. While some, like Genevay (1990), may see this awareness as a call for growth and a potential enhancement for both the therapist and the client, others, such as Winiarski (1995), point out potential negative influences. In either event, the presence of countertransference demands that the practitioner proceed carefully. Before we examine ways to address this issue, let's look at a case to get a feel for what might happen.

## *The Case of Mike*

Mike was a twenty-nine-year-old gay man who had been rejected by his family and who had few friends. He initially consulted me because of depression related to chronic fatigue syndrome. As months passed he presented with symptoms of HIV disease but insisted that his physician had assured him that the proper diagnosis was chronic fatigue syndrome. Eventually at my urging he consulted another physician who diagnosed him with AIDS. I quickly became part of his primary support system, for his friends knew little about medical care and Mike's resources were limited. Although I encouraged him to contact our local AIDS service organization, his social skills were such that he remained alone and agonized about being rejected by his family, who lived in another state. Without my knowledge he approached a fundamentalist church, hoping for acceptance and assistance but finding judgment and rejection. When he spoke to me about this, I was very distressed, and I quickly sought out a minister who agreed to visit him and simply listen to what he had to say.

Perhaps this "overidentification" seems to have been executed easily and without thought. Each step I took was a troubling one. Aware of my own struggle with my father, now deceased, who failed to value me, I knew that some of my motivation was to show Mike that he was a person of worth and deserving of dignity and love. At the same time I carefully weighed the "cost" of moving beyond the traditional psychotherapy relationship into more of a nurturing friendship. Rarely did I step forward without hesitation and often intense internal debate. Knowing I could not do as much for each of my clients, I attempted to identify the specifics that drew me to Mike. I tried to keep my focus on what might help him through each crisis and held on to a philosophical belief that all humans deserve to die surrounded by people who care for them. Unfortunately, Mike had virtually no one who understood his need for reassurance and love.

As his medical condition worsened, he was frequently alone for long periods of time, and I was one of the few who visited him. These visits began in his home but soon took place in hospital rooms and intensive care units. He spoke frequently about his fear of dying alone and his enormous sense of abandonment by his family. As he weakened, I assured him that someone would be present at his death. I spoke with his two friends about the importance of being there, and I instructed his nurses to call me if they failed to show up. The call came in the middle of a night marked by severe storms. Phone lines were down in various parts of the city, and his friends could not be notified. I went to the hospital and sat holding Mike's hand while he died. He was in a coma and unable to talk, so I spoke to him about his life and how much I had appreciated knowing him and told him it was OK to go, that he had finished his time with us. After some time he squeezed my hand twice and simply quit breathing.

When I left the room, his two friends appeared, and we shared some time together. Mike had not wanted to be buried in the local pauper's field. I was fortunate to be able to find a funeral home that donated services and a church to purchase a burial site for him. I gave his friends directions on what to do and tried to put them in charge, but they did not have a clue about how to make arrangements, and I found myself in an unexpected role as the key person in planning a funeral. I was amazed that people stepped forward with offers to help. A minister volunteered, Mike's former boss provided flowers, and, at the very end of the service, his family piled out of their car to attend the burial. On request, I made some comments at the grave.

What I had done was "bend the frame," maybe even twist the frame completely out of shape. At the same time, I was struggling internally, trying to figure out if I had totally lost my professional self and worrying that what I was doing was very wrong. For days I puzzled over my actions: Did I sit with him through the night for him or for me? Was this really a selfless act or was I reassuring myself that I would not be alone at my death? Was I in some twisted way trying to bank compassion so that I could draw on it from others when I was in need? Did his helplessness and death in some strange way reassure me about my own power and future? Was I needing to witness his death so I could live more fully? What was I to do with all this sadness? Questions like these haunted me, and I felt very alone. To label these emotions as countertransference seemed at once appropriate and also demeaning.

As I struggled with these issues, I turned to colleagues for assistance. Most said to me, "What difference does it make? Mike had a companion when he died and that is what he wanted, and maybe you had an opportunity to work on one of your issues." While reassuring, these supportive comments did not end my self-examination.

Like most practitioners, my professional training was very traditional. The psychologist is supposed to be somewhat detached, should not reveal much personal information, and certainly is not supposed to have physical contact with the client. Psychoanalytic concepts such as transference and countertransference seemed of little use in my cognitive-behavioral world. Of course, over the years there have been those clients that I did not like and some who evoked intense compassion in me. And I would run across the occasional client who seemed unduly attached to me and curious about my personal life. But rarely did I conceptualize the dynamic in psychoanalytic terms. My training taught me to be a professional and to keep my personal feelings separate. I had accepted the role of a distant and personally uninvolved clinician without much question. That orientation began to change when I became a volunteer counselor with cancer patients. Suddenly I was in close contact with my client's family members and a regular visitor in their homes. Helping a client tell his sons how sad he was that he would not live to see them graduate from high school evoked many emotions in me. My yearning for such a loving and courageous father and my sense of rejection by my own father was obviously present in that moment. Once I became involved in HIV work I knew quickly that my own feelings were going to a significant part of this experience.

As I have spoken with other professionals who work with HIV-infected clients, I have asked what draws them into this difficult work. A usual reply is that in the work they find a kind of honesty and love that is rarely encountered. They speak of being moved by courage and commitment and of developing a keen awareness of the preciousness of life. They talk about the strength of family and support systems and of their growing spirituality. They report not fearing death so much and even discovering increased confidence about being alone.

Another group of professionals reports being angry all the time. They talk about the lack of resources and even the undependability of many of their clients. Their lives have become dominated by an insidious anger that destroys virtually all of their enjoyment of normal life activities. They are not just burned out; they are totally depleted and feel trapped in the work because "there's no one else to do this if I give it up." They have become professional and chronic victims. It is not hard for me to see that some have been drawn to the work because of previous feelings of anger and victimization and that they remain in the work in a futile attempt to deny their own issues with negative emotions. If their attachment to the work is pathological, what do I make of the more positive experiences I am having?

Naturally, the answers to questions like these are complex and are usually not readily apparent. The bottom line for me is whether I can defend my actions and find a sense of internal understanding and peace about what I am doing. For me, that is the crux of using my countertransference issues productively. And I have learned that I cannot reach such tranquility alone. Working with HIV-infected clients demands that I be willing to engage my emotional responses more fully and be alert to the ways that my own issues create potential pitfalls.

Not all countertransference is in the direction of compassion. One of the first HIV-positive injection drug users I treated had been brought to the clinic by his girlfriend. She had reported to her physician several horror stories about his suicide threats, disappearances, and abusive rages. She took his abuse and arranged for him to come to the clinic to talk to me. After waiting for him for twenty minutes, I was surprised to see his girlfriend open the door to my office. Startled because he was not there with me, she dashed about the clinic and found him in a restroom shooting up his drug. When she brought him to me he was high and unable to speak coherently, and I found myself thinking of ways I could terminate the case before it had even gotten started.

In supervision I learned that my resistance to working with him was created by my fear that I had nothing to offer that would help him control his drug habit. Once I recognized my reaction as my problem, I was able to interact with him more successfully.

The conflicts that arise in HIV-related psychotherapy or counseling demand careful attention. Often the clinician cannot resolve these issues alone. And sometimes there are few in our communities who understand the unique quality of this work. If unaddressed, countertransference can lead to ineffective treatment. Fortunately there are ways to "turn up the volume" on these issues to guard against negative outcomes.

## *Tools for Clinical Practice: Resolving Countertransference*

Clinicians working with HIV/AIDS clients may benefit from following these suggestions:

- *Don't just do something; stand there.*

  Recently I co-led a workshop on living with a chronic illness. My colleague spoke about the kind of professional helplessness he often felt when faced with a dying client. He reported that he gained comfort in realizing that the old adage "Don't just stand there; do something" could be changed to "Don't just do something; stand there!" This change helped him understand that in being present, he was offering something very precious — his willingness to feel his own helplessness and not run away. In our outcome-oriented culture, it is difficult for many to continue to be involved in such difficult work when there are not always mileposts of progress to give reassurance of effectiveness.
- *Engage in case management.*

  Case management (Curtis & Hodge, 1995) is one of the means of dealing with countertransference. Learning about community resources and knowing when and where to refer clients can reduce the sense of helplessness reported by many practitioners. AIDS service organizations, social service departments, food banks, emergency housing, and the family and support systems that surround the client can be valuable resources. Getting to know the medical and social support systems reduces the sense of isolation that many clinicians experience. Such a "team approach" allows for consultation in a crisis and pools the talent for the protection of the client.
- *Form peer supervision groups.*

  Some practitioners report forming peer supervision groups to address individual situations and to allow for the ventilation of emotion. These groups can meet weekly or monthly and serve as a major source for emotional exploration and support. Delgado and Rose (1994) encourage the use of informal helping networks like peer groups to help caregivers cope with the stress.

Gabriel (1991) outlines a model of group supervision that focuses on therapists' unconscious communications, defensive functioning, and resistances, as well as on countertransference issues. Her model helps the counselor develop an increased intellectual and emotional comfort with issues like facing a deteriorating illness, accepting death, and dealing with survivors. She believes that such groups reduce the likelihood that helpers will be overwhelmed by feelings of helplessness, anger, and loss, especially the pain of multiple loss.

- *Get a buddy.*

  Some practitioners contract with a professional colleague to create a peer supervision team. Whenever either of the pair determines the need to process what is going on in a particular case, the other partner agrees to meet, listen to the dilemma, and suggest possible alternatives. With such an ongoing relationship, partners can check each other on possible countertransference issues. Such conversations also serve as checkpoints when bending the frame and help ensure more competent care. They also help reduce some of the isolation and helplessness that characterize this work. Arrangements with a buddy can last the duration of one case or extend over several years.

- *Schedule regular clinical supervision.*

  Another way to surface countertransference issues is through regular clinical supervision. Contracting with an HIV-wise clinician who understands the complexities can help practitioners provide more competent treatment. Several authors stress the importance of clinical supervision in dealing with countertransference issues. When the supervisor is competent and unafraid to confront the practitioner with instances where attitudes and values are interfering with competent treatment, there is an immense opportunity for personal growth and improved service delivery.

  Winiarski (1995) suggests that the supervision must deal with rescue fantasies ("A cure is just around the corner"), instill a belief in the effectiveness of ongoing treatment, encourage more direct intervention when the practitioner is withdrawing, and reduce feelings of despair and demoralization. The supervisor needs to be particularly alert to unexposed and unexpressed anger. Further issues of burnout prevention are essential if the helper is to continue to provide competent treatment. Bell (1992) believes this is especially true when working with substance-abusing clients.

- *Be in psychotherapy.*

  Perhaps the most powerful means of understanding individual countertransference issues is for the practitioner to enter psychotherapy. Facing one's fears of death, helplessness, anger, rejection, lack of confidence in treatment skill, and the many other emotional responses that accompany HIV-related psychotherapy may demand more individual attention than can occur in group or individual supervision. Individual psychotherapy suggests that the clinician is taking responsibility for his or her professional and personal growth and development and may be the best arena for conflict resolution.

- *Pursue additional training and balance in life.*

  Other approaches include clinical training and continuing education, use of the professional literature, and common burnout prevention techniques such as exercise, journal writing, reflection on meaning, and the pursuit of personal interests and hobbies (Imhof, 1995). Above all, the maintenance of predictable life structure will help the clinician retain balance in life. Unfortunately, all too often, this is the first quality-of-life component to go when faced with the overwhelming needs presented by persons with HIV.

## *Conclusion*

Perhaps the most difficult issue in determining whether countertransference is present, in either positive or negative form, is that many of our responses to suffering reflect a deep human compassion that is not pathological. Caring for the sick and dying does offer the opportunity for increased meaning in life and often an enormous sense of fulfillment. When Mike died, I went through days and weeks of turmoil. While his death was easy, his dying was difficult, and I believe that my presence made some slight difference to him. I also know that my presence reflected in part some of my own fears of abandonment and death. Under supervision and in psychotherapy I have learned more about my personal issues. That has been Mike's gift to me. As I bent the frame and worked through some of my fears, I can now work with human suffering by being more fully present. And when I find myself distancing from a difficult situation, I know to start examining what is going on inside me, to see if there are personal issues that are getting in my way, to lean into the discomfort these issues generate, and to learn, once again, that both positive and negative emotional responses can serve as reminders of my own frailty and incompleteness as a human being. Through engaging my own suffering I can more fully understand the struggles of my clients. I can "just stand there" and recognize that my willingness to be present may be the most significant and helpful action.

## REFERENCES

Bell, J. (1992). Treatment dependence: Preliminary description of yet another syndrome. *British Journal of Addiction, 87,* 1049–1054.

Caldwell, S. A. (1994). Over-identification with HIV clients. *Journal of Gay and Lesbian Psychotherapy, 2(2),* 77–99.

Curtis, C., & Hodge, M. (1995). Boundaries and HIV-related case management. *Focus: A Guide to AIDS Research and Counseling, 10(2),* 5–6.

Delgado, J., & Rose, M. (1994). Caregiver constellations: Caring for persons with AIDS. *Journal of Gay and Lesbian Social Services, 1(1),* 1–14.

Federn, P. (1952). *Ego psychology and the psychoses.* New York: Basic Books.

Freud, S. (1959). The future prospects of psychoanalytic psychotherapy. In E. Jones (Ed.), *Collected papers of Sigmund Freud* (Vol. 2) (285–296). New York: Basic Books. (Original work published 1910.)

Gabriel, M. A. (1991). Group therapists' countertransference reactions to multiple deaths from AIDS. *Clinical Social Work Journal, 19,* 279–292.

Genevay, B. (1990). Creating a more humanistic dying. In B. Genevay & R. Katz (Eds.), *Countertransference and older clients* (27–39). Newbury Park, CA: Sage.

Imhof, J. (1995). Overcoming countertransference and other attitudinal barriers in the treatment of substance abuse. In A. M. Washton (Ed.), *Psychotherapy and substance abuse: A practitioner's handbook* (3–22). New York: Guilford Press.

Macks, J. (1988). Women and AIDS: Countertransference issues. *Social Casework, 69,* 340–347.

McKusick, L. (1988). The impact of AIDS on practitioner and client. *American Psychologist, 43,* 935–940.

Rosica, T. (1995). AIDS and boundaries: Instinct versus empathy. *Focus: A Guide to AIDS Research and Counseling, 10(2),* 1–4.

Shernoff, M. (1991). Eight years of working with people with HIV: The impact upon a therapist. *Gays, lesbians, and their therapists: Studies in psychotherapy.* New York: W. W. Norton.

Silverman, D. (1993). Psychosocial impact of HIV-related caregiving health providers: A review and recommendation for the role of psychiatry. *American Journal of Psychiatry, 150*, 705–712.

Winiarski, M. G. (1995). HIV and AIDS. In A. M. Washton (Ed.), *Psychotherapy and substance abuse: A practitioner's handbook* (428–450). New York: Guilford Press.

# 4 | Spirituality

*Pascal Conforti*

In the early years of my practice with HIV-infected patients in an acute-care hospital, I met Edwin. Ed, who died several years ago, was an Hispanic man in his early forties, born a Roman Catholic in New York City. He had spent most of his adult life in and out of prison, and for most of the time I knew him, he remained an inmate in the New York State correctional system.

One day Ed was musing on his life. "You know," he told me, "when I was growing up, I was sure that I wasn't lovable, that I wasn't good enough, that somehow I didn't meet the mark or the standard. I kept trying to be macho, to earn my way, to be recognized in the crowd." With a gentle smile, he continued: "What I've learned is that eventually you have to outgrow your ego. And what I finally discovered is that who you really are ain't so bad after all."

Edwin did not have a college education. He had not studied Jung's theory of individuation or his theory of the emergence of the self and transformation, nor had he been connected beyond his childhood with any institutional religion, Roman Catholic or otherwise. Yet, he had one of the most thoughtful and developed spiritualities of anyone I have ever met. There was a peace about him — a kind of spaciousness of spirit — that remained with him even as his body weakened and his mental faculties deteriorated. How might we describe that inner process that was so apparent in Ed's case? And what might it tell us about the holistic care of persons who are living and dying with HIV-related illness?

It is undoubtedly a truism that it is persons who get sick, not just bodies. It follows, then, that care needs to be directed to the whole person, not simply to a set of physical symptoms. Occasionally, I have been asked as a chaplain/pastoral counselor how I deal with persons who are not religious or "spiritual." I have long since ceased to offer any elaborate explanations about practice in this regard. I simply note that I have yet to meet anyone who regards himself or herself simply as the sum of his or her body parts.

More often, it seems to me, it is the physically healthy person — the counselor or therapist — who is uncomfortable or unfamiliar with the spiritual, both in him- or herself and in others. In professional practice, this discomfort can show itself in any number of ways. A therapist may think, "I'm not a believer, so I cannot help anyone when he or she starts talking about God." An even more subtle barrier to effective work may be found in this statement: "He's talking about God and how God will help him. But I'm not so sure of that. My God is a different God. I'm religious, but he's not talking my kind of religion."

In either case, the caregiver starts with predispositions or assumptions — about him- or herself and about the client — that are barriers to skillful care. The therapist's task in this work is not to make judgments about the client's expressions of spirituality. Rather, the therapist needs to appreciate the client's revelation of something deeply personal. The client's statement begins to communicate how the transcendent presents itself to that client. It is an opening to consideration of eternal questions. Now the task is to listen for and to work with the client's images, views and expressions of spirituality. All that is required of the clinician is to remain open to these expressions.

With this in mind, this chapter deals with the area of spirituality as it is experienced in the world of HIV-related illness. Following some introductory comments on what we mean by spirituality and on the distinction between spirituality and formal religious practice as it is generally understood, the chapter is divided into three sections:

1. HIV-related illness as an opening into the deeper levels of human life and consciousness, that is, into the area of spirituality. What is it about

the illness and its surrounding circumstances that seem to evoke—one might even say require—the journey inward?

2. HIV-related illness as requiring us to look more fully and directly at death, not only as the inevitable outcome of the course of HIV-related illness but much more as a teaching about life. How can we be with the client whose life span is considerably foreshortened in a way that will be genuinely skillful, helpful, and, most of all, loving and compassionate?

3. HIV-related illness as inviting us as caregivers in the field to a consideration of our own lives and spirituality. Is there a gift for us in the work? Is there an opening for us, an invitation into the deeper levels of human life and consciousness? What are some of the intrapersonal and interpersonal dynamics involved in this process?

## *Spirituality and Religion*

The term *spirituality* as I use it here is to be understood in its broadest and most basic sense. Spirituality encompasses the relationship between a person and the transcendent, however it is that the transcendent is imaged, experienced, or named by that person—God, life with a capital "L," Jesus, one's Higher Power, Enlightenment, Unconditional Love. It embraces one's entire life as felt, imagined, and understood in relationship to the transcendent, the metarational, or the profoundly immanent—an imaging and an approach that might be more characteristic of persons who come out of an Eastern rather than a Western worldview.

Religious practice is an expression of this relationship, offering in its healthier forms a loving and consistent community of support and encouragement in the journey toward wholeness and communion that represents the best of the human spirit. Religious practice also includes a host of symbolic and ritual expressions of the relationship between the human person and the transcendent.

While formal religious practice is not synonymous with spirituality, it is important for the mental health practitioner or pastoral caregiver to be aware of the client's religious and cultural background, even if the person has long since left behind any formal church or congregational affiliation. This is so simply because particular symbols will carry (or fail to carry) for particular persons the experience of the transcendent or unconditioned, depending primarily on the person's background, personal history, and culture.

Just as the caregiver needs to be cognizant of the person's religious and cultural history, it is also essential that he or she remain open to how that person's religious or spiritual journey has unfolded over the years. We need to be wary of making unwarranted or rigid assumptions — for example, that Pentecostals always respond in a particular way, or that persons out of Jewish tradition would never respond to this or that practice. The skillful practitioner always takes his or her lead from the patient, open to the unexpected as it presents itself. In the area of spirituality, as with so many other dimensions of life, Stephen Levine's (1987) observation that the mind can be a wonderful servant though it makes a terrible master is especially appropriate.

## *HIV/AIDS as an Opening into Deeper Life and Consciousness*

What is it about HIV-related illness that seems to evoke or even require a deeper exploration of life in all its dimensions? Is there something distinctive in this regard with respect to the world of HIV/AIDS care, something that distinguishes it from practice with persons suffering from other serious or life-threatening illnesses?

There is no doubt that HIV-related illness and its surrounding psychosocial context present a distinctive challenge and opportunity. The following realities shape and describe the world of HIV-infected person. They need to be kept in mind, since they provide the backdrop or context within which we do our work:

- The relative youth of persons who are HIV-infected. Somehow, our worldview, particularly in the West, suggests that people ought to become ill and die in some sort of chronological order. To put it another way, we assume that it is natural or normal for older persons to get sick and die, but not so for younger persons. There is an assumption, often unspoken but nevertheless communicated at a nonverbal level, that the value of a life is measured in terms of the number of years a person has passed on earth rather than in terms of the quality that has characterized these years. This is not so, for example, in an American Indian culture, where one is seen not in a linear way but rather as a circle that becomes complete at about puberty with the rites of passage. From that time on, one is seen as a wholeness that continues to expand outward. Once the circle has formed, anytime one dies, one dies in wholeness. And wholeness, in American Indian wisdom and spirituality, is seen not as the duration one has lived but rather as the fullness with which one enters each complete moment (see Levine, 1982, 4–5).

- The enormous loss connected with HIV-related illness. A diagnosis of HIV-positivity and the course of the illness as one becomes sicker carry with them a series of losses that can be genuinely devastating. The person is dealing not only with the loss of good health and the loss of a sense of physical well-being but, more profoundly, with the loss of work, productivity, economic independence, normal social life, and, in some cases, family relationships. Given some of the enduring fears and prejudices in our society regarding HIV-related illness, there can also be a sense of loss of respectability, with a concomitant need for secrecy and a pervading sense of embarrassment and shame. This, of course, can impact the person spiritually or at the deeper levels of human consciousness by eroding his or her sense of self as worthy or lovable and of the diminished life as worthwhile or "useful" at all.
- The reality of death as coming sooner rather than later. Although there has been substantial progress in the treatment of the opportunistic infections related to HIV-positivity, and although patients generally live longer from the time of diagnosis than they did ten years ago, there is still no proven way that the virus can be removed from the body once it is there. In that sense, HIV-related illness remains incurable and ultimately uncontrollable by our present advanced medical technology and knowledge. It is a life-threatening condition, a fatal illness. It brings one face to face with the reality of impermanence and death. At one level, it is a terrible blow; at another level, it is a precious gift that can uncover aspects of the person and his or her most precious values, values that have been hitherto unacknowledged or unexplored.

Randy was a black man in his early thirties. When I first met him, he was hospitalized with a serious HIV-related pneumonia. Randy was gay, articulate, well educated, and successful. He came from a socioeconomically poor urban background, and his parents had worked hard to educate him and his six siblings. He grew up in a Baptist tradition, but when we met he was not connected with any church or congregation.

When he was well enough to chat, Randy spoke with simplicity and candor about his situation. He was clear that his physical condition was terrible. "I certainly do not want to suggest that this illness is a good thing," he told me. "At the same time," he continued, "something has really happened to me since I was diagnosed and particularly as I have grown sicker. I was really on the fast track. I was ambitious, doing well in my career, making a lot of money, and enjoying a very active and not always wise social life. But this illness stopped me in my tracks. So many of the things that seemed important to me didn't matter that much any more. I got back in touch with my family in a way that was wonderful for me. I've slowed down, and I've discovered deeper levels of myself and of life, dimensions of love and relationship and values that I had somehow lost track of when I was well and active in the business world. In that sense, the illness has brought its own gift."

Randy's story, though it may not always be so well articulated, is repeated over and over again in the world of AIDS care. Randy came in touch with the distinction between healing and cure. His HIV illness was never cured, and he died a relatively young man. But Randy experienced healing in the sense that he felt more and more whole as his illness progressed. His spirit was intact, even as his body was assaulted by the illness.

I believe that it is our task as practitioners simply to provide a context or caring environment within which such stories can be told and within which that deeply instinctive exploration of both inner and outer space can take place.

To facilitate this process, I suggest three attitudes or stances on the part of the practitioner (therapist, case manager, chaplain, counselor) that are central to providing such an environment or context: attentiveness, acceptance, and compassion. These stances are undoubtedly essential to any therapeutic relationship. But in the area of spirituality they take on an added dimension, since they represent, communicate, or symbolize that which is, in all the classic religious or deeply humanistic traditions, most characteristic of the mystery we call God, Unconditional Love, or ultimate Union.

### *Attentiveness*

Listening carefully is undoubtedly at the heart of our work. In the area of spirituality, it requires a centeredness on our part, an in-touchness with our own inner worlds. This is not so much a rational thing — a habit of mind, so to speak, that keeps us aware of what we think. Actually, what we think often changes, so what is important is that while we remain aware of that changing mental scene, we stay rooted in the Mystery of Life which goes far beyond any verbalization of how things are or ought to be. In that sense, we need to be wary of any facile attempts to explain the meaning of life, the meaning of illness, a "theology of suffering," or some other such approach. If that mental apparatus is churning away in us, we will be distracted and not really able to hear the openings into the transcendent, into the metarational, that are always there in the patient or client.

We do not need to work hard at this. The content that we deal with in this area is deep within the person. We do not have to "bring it up" or produce it. What we need to listen for are clues to the person's larger sense of himself or herself, questions related to why this is happening, who the person is in the midst of all this physical limitation and illness, what will become of him or her as this process continues on what is apparently an inexorable course.

### *Acceptance*

As mental health practitioners, we are present to our patients or clients at some level simply to receive them where they are in their journeys and to hear what they have to say. It is not necessary or helpful, particularly initially, to "do something." We have neither to agree or disagree, approve or disapprove. I have from time to time seen brochures offering what is termed "nonjudgmental" pastoral care. Is there any other kind? And what does it say about the field, about churches and religious congregations, or about the society in general, that we feel compelled to assure our sick brothers and sisters that we offer them "nonjudgmental" care?

At the same time that we offer our clients an accepting and hospitable space in which to tell their stories, there are ways — through conversation, through our manner (particularly in what is communicated nonverbally), through the skillful use of ritual — in which we can assist the person to come more in touch with what is, in any sound religious or humanistic tradition, a more genuine and helpful spiritual belief and practice.

In the world of HIV-infection, we have more than our fair share of clients whose personal histories have been defined by physical and mental abuse, low self-esteem, and a kind of affective deprivation in their formative years that is astounding and deeply distressing. In many cases, they have experienced the world from their earliest years as a hostile and unloving environment. And it is often out of this early experience that an equally hostile and unloving deity emerges. This may be either a deity who is busy punishing so-called wrongdoing by inflicting illness and general reversal of fortune, or one who stands by idly in some remote and distant way when he (or she) could be doing something useful to alleviate the situation. Either way, it is not a perspective that is in keeping with healthy religious and spiritual tradition, nor is it helpful in the process of healing and wholeness that is at the heart of the human journey.

Where we are dealing with clients whose religious or spiritual belief and practice torture and constrict them, or if the person is obsessed or consumed by religious images and concepts that are clearly not loving or peace-giving, it might be wise to refer the person, if he or she is open to it, to a more specialized practitioner such as a skillful clergyperson or pastoral counselor. That clergyperson or counselor might assist the client, through conversation, instruction in prayer and meditation, ritual (sacramental confession, the anointing of the sick, special blessings, affiliation with a congregation or spiritual support group), or a combination of these things. In any event, the assistance of a spacious, gentle, accepting mental health practitioner remains an important modality in filling out the spiritual dimension in HIV mental health care.

### *Compassion*

No quality, affection, or feeling comes closer to the heart of spirituality — both belief and practice — than compassion. Compassion is an emotion or quality of connection, rather than separation. It recognizes that, at the deepest level, we are all one as participants in a common humanity. It is clearly distinguishable from pity, which arises primarily out of our fear and which is characterized always by a sense of distance.

Despite the differences that may exist between ourselves and our clients by reason of personal history, lifestyle, education, culture, and other factors, it becomes obvious with any kind of openness and attentiveness that all of us have the same essential needs and seek the same things in life: love, acceptance, and some help when we are in need. We share the same fundamental desire to be happy and to avoid suffering. We experience the same loneliness, the same fear of the unknown, the same secret areas of sadness, the same half-acknowledged feelings of helplessness (see Rinpoche, 1992, 175). In the long run, the transcendent is reflected in our lives most by the longing in our hearts for love — for a love that goes beyond our so-called worthiness or unworthiness, for a love that in some mysterious and inexplicable manner lives on without limit. There is a sense in which a single lifetime, no matter its extent chronologically, does not seem capable of holding and completing the longings of the human heart. The very impermanence of everything we experience as human beings on this earth or on this plane of existence seems to point toward something else, toward something beyond what is immediately tangible.

Offering to our clients who are affected by HIV-related illness our compassionate, connected, loving presence is perhaps the greatest therapeutic gift we can give them, since it most nearly reflects the transcendent dimension of human existence and, as such, provides a context or environment for the healing of spirit that is always available to us in the human situation.

## *Looking More Fully and Directly at Death*

HIV-related illness remains incurable at this point in history. As indicated earlier in this chapter, it is a life-threatening condition, a fatal illness, and, as such, it brings one face to face with the reality of impermanence and death. In one sense, it is the ultimate invitation to spiritual reflection. Difficult as facing this reality may seem at one level, it is also at another level a "window of opportunity," an invitation to deeper reflection on values and on what really matters in the course of a human lifetime.

In Tolstoy's masterful short novel, *The Death of Ivan Ilych* (1886/1981), Ivan Ilych is close to death and struggling mightily with the meaning of his life. Ivan has lived a superficial, self-satisfied, proper, ordered, somewhat mean, externally successful life; yet, he finds himself deeply depressed, angry, tortured, and isolated as his illness proceeds on its relentless course. His life seems to him at this point to have had no meaning at all. Ivan muses: "Yes, all of it was simply *not the real thing*. But no matter. I can still make it *the real thing* — I can. But what *is* the real thing? Ivan Ilych asked himself and suddenly grew quiet" (132; italics are the author's).

Perhaps that is the central question of everyone's life. What is the real thing? What is really of enduring value? What or whom do I care about most? These are the questions for all of us, and we can offer no better service to our clients with HIV-related illness as they grow sicker and come closer to death than to be with them in a skillful, gentle, and compassionate way as these questions present themselves.

There was a short film produced several years ago in one of our state correctional systems. It was a skillful piece of film making, and it was designed, I am sure, with the good intention of raising inmates' awareness of risk behaviors that could lead to HIV infection. However, it had an unfortunate title: *AIDS: A Bad Way to Die.* HIV infection is undoubtedly a "bad thing" to get, but dying from the complications of AIDS is not necessarily a "bad" way to die any more than is cancer, heart disease, or kidney failure. When all is said and done, a good way to die is the same as a good way to live: in love and connection.

In the day-to-day world of HIV mental health care, what are some of the ways in which we can be of assistance as illness becomes more serious and death becomes more imminent? I suggest the following as essential in care and support of our clients at this stage of their illness:

- *Deal with the fear of death*

  Underlying all spiritual care of the dying is our view of the relationship between life and death, between living and dying. Particularly in our Western mentality and worldview, we tend to separate living and dying too sharply. Actually, death is not the opposite of life, but rather an aspect of life. It is an event in that process we call being or becoming. Joseph Campbell suggests that one can experience an unconditional affirmation of life only when one has accepted death not as contrary to life but as an aspect of life. He goes on to suggest that dealing with the fear of death can be the recovery of life's joy (see Campbell, 1988, 152). If this is so — and my experience of working with hundreds of terminally ill AIDS patients over the past decade tells me that it is — then, paradoxically, looking directly at the prospect of death often allows for a better, fuller, happier life. One terminally ill patient is said to have commented during the course of her illness that she had never been so fully alive as since she was told that she had a terminal illness. And another quipped: "I think that survival has been vastly overrated." One of my own patients, Dan, told me on his thirty-seventh birthday, an occasion that he celebrated in the hospital in the last stages of his illness, how happy he was. "I don't have to prove myself any more," he said. "All I have to do is love."
- *Be truthful.*

  It follows from the first point that we need to be truthful. Truthfulness does not mean insensitivity, or a kind of awkward, self-conscious bluntness that is ill attuned to the sick person's timing and inner space. But it does mean that we recognize and acknowledge what the patient usually knows already: That there are limits to medical knowledge and technology, that he or she is not getting better, that the body is weakening, and that he or she will die sooner rather than later. Again, Tolstoy describes the sick person's predicament:

> Ivan Ilych suffered most of all from the lie, the lie which, for some reason, everyone accepted: that he was not dying but was simply ill, and that if he stayed calm and underwent treatment he could expect good results. . . . And he was tortured by this lie, tortured by the fact that they refused to acknowledge what he and everyone else knew, that they wanted to lie about his horrible condition and to force him to become a party to that lie. (Tolstoy, 1886/1981, 102–103)

In this context, too, I suggest that it is generally not helpful to suggest to persons, particularly at this stage of the illness, that they "fight." "You can beat this thing," some well-intentioned friend, relative, or caregiver might say. But the truth of the matter is that this is a battle that, ultimately, we cannot win and are not meant to win. Suggesting, therefore, that the patient put his or her already limited energy into fighting death can exhaust the patient and make him or her feel like a failure or disappointment in our eyes. Finally, there is often a direct correlation between fighting life and fighting death. It is time to put the battle to rest and to encourage our loved ones and clients to use the energy saved to live fully and attentively and to love deeply and extravagantly.

- *Counsel to live in the present.*

  The best preparation for death, the best "spiritual practice" for living and dying, is to live in the present moment and to embrace whatever is happening. It is resistance to the moment—in a sense, it is resistance to life—that can cause suffering as death approaches and that seems to evoke such tightness and fear in all of us when death is mentioned. Whatever we can do to assist the very ill person to live in the present, to be free of the endless cycle of guilt and regret over the past or fear and apprehension over what will happen in the future, is all to the good. Practical matters—such things as advance medical directives, guardianship of minor children, and financial concerns—are best taken care of earlier rather than later when the person becomes very ill. The task at the end is primarily a task of the heart and of the spirit. As far as possible, we need to encourage our clients to leave themselves space for that task by taking care of the rest earlier along the way.

- *Provide an atmosphere of love.*

  Finally, it is important in the care of the terminally ill and dying to provide an atmosphere of love and encouragement, rather than one of agitation, fear, regret, and excessive "busyness." We need to remind the person verbally and nonverbally that we are more than bodies and that who we are is far greater than what is happening physically. I have sometimes said to patients along the entire course of their HIV illness: Remember — you have the illness. The illness doesn't have you.

  Ultimately, our true nature — our most essential identifying characteristic as human persons — is the ability and desire to love and to be loved. To remind a person at the end he or she is loved is perhaps the greatest service we can offer. Ivan Ilych discovered this in the midst of his anguished question, "But what *is* the real thing?" Tolstoy tells us:

> This took place . . . an hour before his death. Just then his son crept quietly into the room and went up to his bed. The dying man was still screaming desperately and flailing his arms. One hand fell on the boy's head. The boy grasped it, pressed it to his lips and began to cry. At that moment Ivan Ilych fell through and saw a light, and it was revealed to him that his life had not been what it should have but that he could still rectify the situation. "But what *is* the real thing?" he asked himself and grew quiet, listening. Just then he felt someone kissing his hand. He opened his eyes and looked at this son. . . . (Tolstoy, 1886/1981, 132)

## *An Invitation to Caregivers*

There is a wonderful vignette in the Franciscan tradition that recounts a conversion story of Francis, that great medieval romantic and founder from whom sprang a number of religious communities that survive even to the present. It is a story that is significant in the context of this chapter, since it is particularly germane, I believe, to how we go about our work in the field of HIV/AIDS mental health care and to the gift that the work might conceivably hold for us.

The historical sources tell us that Francis, the son of a wealthy Italian merchant, gradually was drawn to leave his worldly position, of which he was quite fond, to follow Jesus and to explore more deeply his own religious and spiritual journey even as he served the poor of his day. One day, so the story goes, Francis was on the road between Assisi and Lazzaro, the location of the hospital that cared for those suffering from leprosy, an illness that in Francis's time was viewed with fear and aversion. In the course of his journey, Francis met one of the patients from that hospital, and, in spite of the man's appearance, he found himself deeply moved and drawn to him. Francis bent down and kissed the sick man, and, in so doing, he finally came in touch with himself—with himself as he was: limited, lovable and loved, capable of loving.

In the Franciscan tradition, this event is regarded as a key moment in Francis's conversion, as a kind of turning point in his spiritual journey. It is noteworthy, too, that some of the hagiographers over the centuries attempted to "clean up" the story by changing the original account to read that Francis saw Jesus in the leper—and that's what led him to embrace the man. But subsequent Franciscan scholarship has confirmed the original version: The story—and the teaching it reveals—remains as written.

Perhaps this vignette reflects the central reality of the connection between our professional work as practitioners in the world of HIV mental health and our own human and spiritual journey. There is a gift for us in the work that is real, mysterious, and at some level priceless. Essentially, we are in service to our brothers and sisters with HIV-related illness not as some sort of distant benefactors but as fellow human beings on the same human journey. There is only a single work, really: The work with ourselves and the work with our patients or clients are one and the same.

Working with HIV-related illness, particularly in its later stages, encourages us to learn, ourselves, to live fully in the present moment, to let go of our strong need and desire to control, and to embrace the reality of impermanence and death. The work invites us to an awareness that carries with it a simultaneous mindfulness of what is going on in the person who is ill as well as what is going on in the inner world of the clinician. We become aware of our own fears, yearnings, doubts, and hopes. In short, we become aware of our own search for "the real thing." Joseph Campbell (1988), the teacher and scholar who did such important work in the exploration of myth, suggests that the only really inexcusable sin is inattention, and Stephen Levine (1987) regularly reminds us that anything that is not brought to awareness cannot be healed.

In the Christian spiritual tradition, there is a way of reading some of Jesus's stories, particularly the parables of the kingdom, on an intrapersonal level, and this is undoubtedly true of stories in other traditions. The familiar lost sheep and the lost coin, for example, represent those pieces of our experience and of ourselves that we have marginated, denied, or exiled. Failure to come back in touch with them, failure to acknowledge them and to invite them back in can close us to healing and can block the further growth to which we are called all along the way. Working with those whom the society has frequently marginated invites us not to perpetuate that mode either with ourselves or with others. As we encourage our clients to wholeness, we are reminded to seek such wholeness for ourselves. Conversely, continuing to marginate or deny parts of ourselves and of our experience inevitably allows us, both individually and as a society, to continue to shut out from our embrace and our care those who are most in need and who often have the most to teach us.

Finally, attentive work with persons with AIDS teaches us compassion, a sense of profound connectedness and benevolence, what a Buddhist tradition might term "nonduality" and what is expressed in the Judaeo-Christian tradition as "loving one's neighbor as oneself." In a very real sense, our neighbor is ourself, and as we befriend him or her we befriend ourselves. As the work continues to invite us to reclaim or recall those parts of ourselves and of our experience that we reject or disallow, inevitably we come to realize, as Edwin did, that who we really are "ain't so bad after all."

## REFERENCES

Campbell, J. (with Moyers, B.) (1988). *The power of myth.* New York: Doubleday.

Levine, S. (1982). *Who dies? An investigation of conscious living and conscious dying.* New York: Doubleday.

Levine, S. (1987). *Healing into life and death.* New York: Doubleday.

Rinpoche, S. (1992). *The Tibetan book of living and dying.* San Francisco: Harper.

Tolstoy, L. (1981). *The death of Ivan Ilych.* (L. Solotaroff, Trans.) New York: Bantam Classic Edition. (Original work published 1886.)

## READINGS ON SPIRITUAL ISSUES

In my experience of nearly ten years of working exclusively with persons suffering from HIV-related diseases, many of them in the last stages of their illness, I am particularly indebted to the work of Stephen Levine. Three of his books provide an excellent source of both theory and practice:

- *Who Dies? An Exploration of Conscious Living and Conscious Dying* (New York: Doubleday, 1982)
- *Meetings at the Edge* (New York: Doubleday, 1984)
- *Healing into Life and Death* (New York: Doubleday, 1987)

Levine has also written a more recent book that includes some excellent material that can be adapted to a wide spectrum of patients or clients at various stages of their illness: *Guided Meditation, Explorations, and Healings* (New York: Doubleday, 1991).

For those who would like to explore more deeply and thoroughly some of the connections between mental health practice and spirituality, there is a fine work by a psychiatrist, Gerald May, titled *Will and Spirit: A Contemplative Psychology* (San Francisco: Harper and Row, 1982). The chapter titled "On Being a Pilgrim and a Helper" is particularly pertinent to our work in the field of AIDS. Also, Jon Kabat-Zinn's most recent book, *Wherever You Go There You Are* (New York: Hyperion, 1994), is a good practical guide in the area of spiritual practice.

Finally, there is a collection of excellent interviews in *Timeless Visions, Healing Voices* by Stephan Bodian (Freedom, CA: Crossing Press, 1991). The book comprises a series of conversations with persons Bodian describes as "men and women of the spirit." The interviews with Arnold Mindell, Joan Borysenko, David Steindl-Rast, and Stephen Levine are especially relevant to the subject matter that we have been considering in this chapter on spirituality.

# 5 | Grief and Loss in HIV/AIDS Work

*Noel Elia*

Loss and grieving echo throughout the course of HIV/AIDS. For persons infected and for those who care for them, including the mental health provider, one of the greatest challenges is the relationship we are invited to make with loss.

The instant the client receives test results showing infection, the client becomes a participant in an ongoing grieving process. This individual immediately grieves the loss of his or her HIV-negative status. Now he or she is living with HIV, and the future, as previously imagined, is changed forever. Concurrently, the individual has to begin the process of integrating the new status—"HIV-positive"—into his or her psychological world.

As the illness progresses, there is a loss of the previous, healthier identity. Each new set of symptoms forces adaptation to the new identity—"symptomatic," "AIDS patient."

For the provider, too, the feelings of loss begin when we first meet the HIV-positive client. During the course of the therapeutic relationship, we shall always be aware that the client has a chronic, life-threatening illness. The awareness of potential loss will, consciously or unconsciously, prompt memories of our own earlier losses, and sometimes we may act out of these unconscious reverberations. We may offer the client health education, for example, instead of working toward processing his or her feelings, or we may neglect to follow up with a very sick patient who misses sessions, hiding (perhaps even from ourselves) our feeling of relief that we do not need to be with the person's pain. Later in the client's life, we may avoid hospital visits, rationalizing that we are "too busy."

Our work with loss and grieving in the area of HIV/AIDS is further complicated by our society's unwillingness to respect feelings of loss and bereavement.

The work described in this chapter is revolutionary to the dominant culture, which focuses on the here and now and denies the reality of death. In the last half of this century Americans have become less familiar with the dying process because it has been removed from their direct experience.

In the first half of the 20th century dying was a family affair. Large extended families helped care for dying family members, relatives bathed the corpse, and wakes were conducted in homes. Technological "advances" and family mobility, however, have changed this. Just as childbirth has been relegated to medical staff in hospital settings, so has dying. Only those who are proactive in their choice to experience birth or death in their homes, or in special care centers set up for these purposes, have access to the full emotional experience that these transitional events can evoke.

Now, from hospital to burial, the dying process is essentially controlled by professional specialists who "spare" those closest to the dying person the pain of attending to him or her in intimate surroundings. Physicians sometimes prescribe tranquilizers to assist family members in coping with the dying and death of their loved ones. Bodies are neatly packaged in funeral homes. Society which deems death an "event," expects mourners to resolve their feelings quickly and return to normal home and work lives within days or, at most, weeks. (See Nuland [1993] and Mitford [1963] for description and comment on dying and death.)

While we hand over dying-related responsibilities to the medical profession, physicians and other medical providers often mirror society's death anxiety.

Deidre had signed a Living Will specific to persons with AIDS that included her directive not to be kept alive by machines. When she was brought to an emergency room dying of AIDS and with a collapsed lung, she was immediately intubated because the physician did not read her chart, which was available to him and clearly specified her wishes.

Unfortunately, Deidre's situation is common. In medicine, as in society, death is considered the enemy. "I've lost the patient" is medical jargon that personalizes the death, implying unrealistic control over life. One reason medical providers are uncomfortable with AIDS care is that all clients eventually "don't make it," in doctors' language.

While these practices have evolved from the exigencies of modern life, we pay an emotional price for them. Essential grief work facilitated by active participation in the dying and mourning process is now neglected and lost. When grieving is suppressed or interrupted, the losses are likely to go unmourned, complicating bereavement. More will be said about this later.

## *Background Reading*

Many of the pioneers of psychotherapy have considered issues of loss and their effect on personality development.

Freud's paper *Mourning and Melancholia* (1917/1959) considers the fundamental process in melancholia (depression) to be loss of the early love object and the failure of the person to establish the lost loved object within its ego. Bowlby's attachment theory (1969) explains that attachments are formed from a need for security and safety. His (1970/1979) work on separation and loss within the family informs us that "many of the troubles we are called upon to treat in our patients are to be traced, at least in part, to a separation or a loss that occurred either recently or at some earlier period in life" (81). Melanie Klein (1934/1948b) considers the infant's loss of the breast to be "the first fundamental external loss of a real love object" (307), and she states that the infant mourns this loss. In her writings on mourning and depression (1940/1948a) Klein further hypothesizes that "this early mourning is revived whenever grief is experienced in later life" (311).

*The Denial of Death* (1973) describes Becker's thesis that "the idea of death, the fear of it, haunts the human animal like nothing else; it is a mainspring of human activity—activity designed largely to avoid the fatality of death, to overcome it by denying in some way that it is the final destiny for man" (ix). It is suggested that readers follow Becker's book with Yalom's *Existential Psychotherapy* (1980), which discusses a dynamic approach to focusing on patient's concerns about existence.

To educate health care professionals to become more familiar with the needs, concerns, and anxieties of individuals who face the end of their lives, Kubler-Ross wrote *On Death and Dying* (1969). Her five stages of mourning — denial, anger, bargaining, depression and acceptance — were originally thought to be linear, but it is now recognized that people loop around and in and out of these stages as the grief process unfolds. The stages serve as a guide; it is not clinically sound to expect a client to follow any theoretical grief pattern in a predetermined fashion.

Worden (1982) outlines four tasks of mourning: accepting the reality of the loss, experiencing the pain of grief, adjusting to an environment from which the deceased is missing, and withdrawing emotional energy from the person or object of loss in order to reinvest in life.

Rando (1984) describes three psychological reactions to normal grief: avoidance, confrontation, and reestablishment. She states that these reactions are typical yet not universal and that the griever will probably move back and forth among them.

In *Life Is Goodbye, Life Is Hello: Grieving Well Through All Kinds of Loss* (1982), Bozarth-Campbell identifies three stages in the processing of loss: shock, the feeling stages (fear, guilt, rage, sadness), and well-being. While we are typically not taught to grieve well, either by word or example, Bozarth-Campbell's work normalizes what has become for many the very foreign, frightening work of grieving. She also recognizes that people have different styles of grieving and that some use several styles in different stages of the mourning process.

Lindemann (1944) identified grief as work, describing the emotional and physical energy required to do it. My experience has been that the most emotional presence and investment is in the middle "stages" of grief. Kubler-Ross's (1969) depression, Worden's (1982) experiencing the pain of the loss, Rando's (1984) confrontation, and Bozarth-Campbell's (1982) feeling stages all make heavy physical, psychological, and spiritual demands. There is a natural tendency for clients and providers to skip over this portion of the grief work, either consciously or unconsciously. Providers must be equipped to notice when this is happening and make the client aware. When the client is experiencing the pain, we need mostly to "just stand there," as Robert Barret so eloquently describes in his chapter on countertransference.

## *My Clinical Work*

For the past four years, I have provided psychotherapy to HIV-infected and affected persons who are clients at a methadone maintenance program at Montefiore Medical Center in the Bronx. Primary care and mental health services are integrated into the program, on site. The majority of my clients are Latino and African American, and all have histories of injection drug use. Some continue using substances such as alcohol, cocaine, or pills while on methadone.

My work with colleagues in this setting inspired the creation of a comprehensive assessment and treatment model called the Model of Multiple Oppression (Millan & Elia, in press). The model acknowledges the themes of loss, grief, and rage that are predominant in our clients' lives. Multiply oppressed persons with HIV/AIDS have suffered traumatic and abusive childhoods; they are people of color, living in poverty, addicted to drugs, struggling with gender roles and often with their sexual orientations in culturally and familially hostile settings. Most are suffering from chronic posttraumatic stress.

These multiple oppressions render the client multiply stigmatized, which causes self-hatred, pervasive secret keeping, and, often, despair from all of the unexpressed loss. Many clients hide parts of themselves from their families, others are ostracized from them, and some even choose to disassociate from those they love. One of the most therapeutic aspects of group treatment for the multiply oppressed person with HIV/AIDS is the opportunity it offers for the individual to expose all of his or her "labels" and to be whole in a "family" that does not impose judgment.

When Rhonda died of AIDS, several members of her HIV support group attended her funeral. There they were confronted by Rhonda's siblings, who accused them of drawing their sister into the street life and of killing her.

Harold, an African-American bisexual man, never used needles. He knew that when his wife discovered he had AIDS she would also learn about his "double life."

Jose instructed his teenage sons not to tell their friends that their father has AIDS for fear that those friends will abandon them.

These anecdotes, and virtually every story I have heard from my Bronx clients, are about loss and grief, be it expressed or unexpressed.

The provider working with the multiply oppressed person with HIV/AIDS must envision the client's illness within the context of the person's whole life situation. At times the client may not be able to focus on the loss issues relevant to HIV/AIDS because he or she is attending to other life and death concerns, such as a welfare snag, recovery from addiction, or violence in his or her neighborhood or home. The practitioner who wants to "work on the AIDS issues" may become frustrated. But I have learned that work in one area affects the whole person. The most therapeutic thing we can offer the multiply oppressed person is love and respect. Even the most difficult clients respond favorably to this.

## *Tools for Clinical Practice*

I offer these observations on loss and grief in HIV/AIDS clients:

- *The social isolation of our HIV/AIDS clients, which stems mostly from stigma, is a psychological death experience that precedes the physical death.*

  A colleague was explaining our work with HIV-infected injecting drug users to a medical doctor who remarked, "It would be wonderful if these skillful interventions could be used with cancer patients, who would really benefit from them." The implication of this remark, and other versions of it, is that our patients are unresponsive to and undeserving of quality care. No such judgments are made regarding patients, even those terminally ill, with other conditions, such as cancer. So the remark about AIDS patients reveals unspoken stigmatization: that they come from an underclass or brought the illness upon themselves, that they do not deserve or do not want help with their suffering, and that they are content to have less than meaningful lives or deaths. The truth is that most people welcome compassionate care, and many are open to learning about the benefits of dealing with death more candidly.

  Another stigmatizing factor is fear of contagion, despite knowledge of routes of transmission. Karen had a close relationship with her two nieces, ages three and five, until she told her brother she is HIV-positive. Since then she has been able to talk with them only on the phone. Herbie notices that his mother keeps separate dishes for his HIV-infected cousin when he comes to eat there. These behaviors stigmatize clients even more because their own families seem to be rejecting them.

  Once the feeling of stigma becomes internalized, patients may isolate themselves from others, leaving their apartments only to complete the bare minimum of chores. One patient described feeling like one big germ when she is around family members, who have stopped touching her since learning she is HIV-positive.

Another man, who has ten siblings and dozens of nieces and nephews, spent five days in his apartment without hearing from anyone. He emerged only to express his despair upon realizing he could have been dead and no one would have known.

- *Facing death, clients' behavior varies greatly, ranging from denial or avoidance to direct confrontation and acceptance.*

Most people admit that they do not really know how they would react if suddenly faced with a terminal diagnosis. While much has been written about normal and pathological grief patterns, it is clear that no two people grieve exactly alike. Some clients remain in denial until they are in end-stage AIDS, when they are almost forced to acknowledge directly their approaching deaths. Others talk openly about their fears from the time they first discover they are HIV-positive.

It is necessary for the provider to respect the client's defenses while at the same time helping the person to face the reality of his or her condition in the moment. A client's ability to handle the situation varies considerably, and it is influenced by several factors. These include but are not limited to the client's general coping abilities, sobriety, mental status, developmental stage, sense of shame, and belief system.

Related to this is the subject of disclosure. My experience has been that it is most helpful for clients to disclose their status as early as possible to immediate family members for two main reasons: First, for some clients the diagnosis becomes real only when they share it. Second, it affords everyone involved, including the client, the opportunity to begin the process of anticipatory grieving (see Fulton & Fulton, 1971). Anticipatory grieving offers people the chance to work out unfinished business. While it does not eliminate grief later, it can soften the blow because the process of integrating the loss has occurred gradually.

While the client struggles with whom to tell, the provider's anxiety can be great. Clients in some form of denial about their illnesses may be unable to tell lovers that they have tested positive. While it is tempting to rebuke clients for not being honest about their illnesses, it is not therapeutic. It is, however, imperative to work with the reluctance.

- *The client's religious or spiritual belief system is an important influence on outlook about death.*

  Some clients fear death and even punishment for their perceived transgressions against God and humankind. Others may believe in reincarnation, while some practice religions that proclaim the presence of evil spirits within them.

  There are many variations on these themes, and we must be open to learning about the client's family belief system from a somewhat historical perspective. It is just as important, though, to assess current "spiritual status" (Elia & Cherry, 1996). An assessment should include these questions:

  - What is the client's current view of God, or the transcendent?
  - If the childhood religion has been abandoned, how does the client feel about that?
  - Has being HIV-positive or having AIDS affected the client's spiritual development? If so, how?

  For our part, we must ask how comfortable we are talking about all of this. What effect do our own beliefs have on client care? My experience is that there is a natural gravitation to the spiritual dimension of life for those infected and affected by HIV/AIDS. Providers must be open to exploring this dimension with clients throughout their journey with AIDS. In fact, it is sometimes necessary to raise the topic when clients do not because the clients may believe it is something the provider would not understand. This is especially true when the provider is from a different culture. See the preceding chapter for more information on spirituality.
- *Mourning is the outward expression of grieving, and mourning practices are heavily influenced by culture and class.*

  The practitioner must remain open to different mourning patterns and must recognize the validity of different grieving styles. This is especially important for those working cross-culturally. Jacqueline Kennedy was admired for the reserved manner she displayed during the funeral of her assassinated husband. Her Anglo ethnicity and her socioeconomic class helped define this mourning pattern. If she had thrown herself on top of the coffin, sobbing, people would have felt she was "falling apart" or "having a breakdown." In most Latin cultures, however, a more demonstrative display of emotion would have been totally understood and fully expected. In some African countries mourners wear white in celebration of the deceased person passing over into a better world, while Italians may wear black for a year to show respect for their dead. A part of mourning is ritual, and people creatively develop rituals as a means of coping. The Bronx has many graffiti-style memorial walls, poignantly expressing the grief of youth who have lost their peers to AIDS and to the streets. Like the AIDS Memorial Quilt or the Vietnam Memorial, these walls are their attempt to display publicly their otherwise disenfranchised grief (Doka, 1989), as society does not really care about the body count of so many young people of color in the inner cities.

- *AIDS-related grief is disenfranchised grief.*

  Disenfranchised grief (Doka, 1989) is grief that is not openly acknowledged by the griever, is not socially sanctioned, and is not publicly mourned. When a gay man loses his lover to AIDS, he cannot always talk openly about the loss because society does not recognize gay and lesbian relationships as valid. If the person has not "come out" to those close to him, such as coworkers or even family members, there is no opportunity to mourn openly. Many in the gay community have described feeling as if they are living in their own private hells, burying friend upon friend, while society at large appears to be oblivious to their holocaust. Similarly, in communities where there is a high percentage of the multiply oppressed infected, whole families are being eliminated by the virus.

  The case of Matilda both illustrates the way to avoid disenfranchised grief in an institutional setting and reveals the role of the practitioner in actually promoting disenfranchised grief.

  Matilda is HIV-positive and is the mother of two daughters, ages one and eight years. I had met with her about a half dozen times when I learned she had become pregnant by her abusive alcoholic boyfriend from whom she was trying to separate. Matilda stopped coming to see me, despite my efforts to contact her, and she decided to keep the baby.

  At five months she went into labor and gave birth to a boy, whom she named Joey, after his father. The baby died within a few minutes after delivery. A week after the baby's funeral Matilda called for an appointment.

  Upon her arrival, Matilda immediately began to tell her story.

She described having had the opportunity to hold her baby, to baptize her baby, to name her baby, and to bury her baby in a formal funeral service, which she attended alone. She also explained the loss to her older daughter and brought her to visit the gravesite. Fortunately for Matilda, the hospital staff where she delivered her baby was sensitive to the loss that she was experiencing as a mother. The rituals they performed with her from birth to death prevented the loss from becoming disenfranchised. Matilda was encouraged to acknowledge the loss and to mourn it publicly.

I asked Matilda what had kept her away from therapy during the pregnancy. She stated that she felt ashamed and thought that I was disappointed that she became pregnant. She did not want to think about an abortion, and she felt that if we met she would be encouraged to weigh all of her options. Although she said that she didn't think I would judge her, I believe she knew intuitively that I did not sanction her relationship with her boyfriend or her pregnancy, since she is HIV-positive. As a therapist, it is my job to monitor constantly my feelings toward my clients and to discuss countertransference with a supervisor. Matilda had sensed my judgment, which subtly caused her grief experience with me to become disenfranchised.

- *Unmourned loss complicates bereavement.*

Old losses that have gone unmourned have an effect on the current grief process of the client. While no one can completely mourn all of his or her losses, bereavement is most apt to become complicated when major losses have not been addressed.

The case of Angela demonstrates the powerful effect that unmourned losses can have on the client's life choices and establishes the need to document the client's loss history. At twenty-seven years of age, Angela has been HIV-positive for four years. Though she was raised in foster homes, Angela is certain that she became infected by her biological mother, who died two years ago, since they shared needles. Angela's two children have been taken away from her, though she is currently working hard at recovery to get them back. Three months ago her sister Maria — "she was like a real mother to me" — died from AIDS.

Angela lives with her boyfriend, Robert, whom she has not told her HIV status, but she thinks "he must know." Angela tells me they are thinking about having a child. For the first time she also reveals the existence of a daughter, taken from her at birth twelve years ago and not seen since. Moreover, Angela's childhood was fraught with early losses that led to substance abuse by the age of nine. Her ability to grieve adequately now is severely limited by this psychosocial history.

My task is to help Angela prioritize her grief work. At the very least she has not mourned her relationship with her mother or the loss of her oldest child. In our sessions she cries often for her younger children in foster care and for her sister Maria. While it will not be possible for Angela to grieve all of her losses completely, it may not be necessary. Her relationship with her mother is the seedbed for much of her pain. My focus will be to help Angela to come to terms with this relationship and to help her make sense out of her seemingly chaotic life choices. Early in the work Angela announced, "Gee, I wonder if the reason I want a baby now is to make up for the one I lost twelve years ago."

- *Because grief work is so hard, many people use and abuse substances in order to self-medicate the feelings that are associated with loss.*

It is my belief that the psychological etiology of much drug addiction is unmourned loss. Substance use complicates bereavement because the person's psychological, emotional, and spiritual development is arrested. Sometimes people are prescribed drugs during the week leading up to and including the funeral of a loved one. This puts the necessary emotional tasks on hold, but it does not eliminate them.

The case of Leslie demonstrates how clients often learn to self-medicate from their families, by observing as children the way painful feelings such as grief are handled.

Leslie was a methadone patient who died from AIDS at age thirty-three, leaving behind a live-in boyfriend who "didn't know why she was always sick" and two children, a boy, ten, and a girl, eight. Leslie had two brothers and a sister, all of whom had died from AIDS, and she felt unable to tell her children that she was dying. Even when in the hospital bed, having wasted away to eighty pounds, she insisted on telling them that she would be home soon. Having done some work with the family, I was invited to the funeral, where I encountered Leslie's father, outside drinking beer with Leslie's uncles. Inside, her mother explained that her husband "was taking the death hard."

- *Bereavement overload is an issue for those infected and affected by HIV/AIDS.*

Johnny has AIDS and lives in a residential hotel in New York City. It is typical of those facilities that a city agency fills with persons with AIDS. Johnny describes the difficulty of seeing bodies carried out of his hotel on a weekly basis.

Neil is a fifty-year-old Vietnam veteran, who lost many of his friends in the Vietnam War. He is now losing many to the virus. When his cousin Rosie died last month, Neil stated that he simply could not attend any more funerals, including hers.

Irma comes into the clinic looking exhausted and very sad. Three of her four adult children have died of AIDS. She states that she is having trouble sleeping and that she is feeling depressed.

Thomas is a forty-five-year-old gay man who has lost almost his entire friendship circle to AIDS. He is HIV-negative.

All these people are coping with bereavement overload (Kastenbaum, 1969), a term originally coined to describe the plight of the elderly person whose loved ones all die and leave (usually) her behind. AIDS has made the concept applicable to people of all ages. In communities where the epidemic is rampant, infected and affected people have been traumatized by the way AIDS has ravaged their lives. When there is a steady onslaught of fresh loss, the grieving process is constantly interrupted, and it is not possible to grieve each loss completely.

The grieving process requires the client to work on many levels concurrently. In the case of an HIV-infected man who loses his wife to AIDS, his main tasks are to deal with the guilt he has from infecting his wife, to mourn the loss of his wife in order to reestablish himself as a single man, and to organize his emotions around his own terminal condition. There are also myriad secondary losses that will require attention. The person with AIDS is often juggling more than one major life loss simultaneously, and he or she may not understand that the work is naturally overwhelming. Especially in cases like this, I have found it helpful to provide the client with information about the normalcy of what he or she is feeling. This is not false reassurance but instead an effort to help the client to feel "less crazy."

While some unresolved loss is inevitable, it appears that, with treatment, "healthy enough" resolution is generally possible. In working with clients who are faced with massive bereavement, practitioners can use some of the same clinical skills they apply to survivors of trauma in general: Give clients the opportunity to talk about their feelings in a way that gives them some control of the process, because the profundity of the loss makes them feel so out of control; offer clients therapy sessions more than once a week when necessary; use psychoeducation to normalize the grief process, helping clients who may think they are "losing their minds" because they are overwhelmed with grief; and encourage group therapy since the hard work of grieving always seems lighter when it is shared.

- *The caregiver is also subject to bereavement overload.*

  To remain effective, we must learn to deal with the accumulated grief. Competent work with the terminally ill requires the clinician to come to terms with his or her own mortality and with death in general. Because the work is so demanding emotionally, spiritually, and psychologically, it is essential for the caregiver to have ongoing supervision. Staff support groups that are offered in a politically safe atmosphere also prevent the negative effects of massive bereavement. Memorial services provide much-needed ritual for provider and client alike.

- *The provider working with PWAs must ultimately be capable of talking about death in a direct manner.*

  When I first began working with people with HIV/AIDS, I was fearful and anxious as I grappled with constant change and complete loss of control. I was dragged kicking and screaming, by supervisors and colleagues, through the myriad emotions that the work elicits. This labor of love has changed my life.

  It is a very unique and powerful experience to be invited into a person's life when he or she is HIV-positive or has AIDS. The relationship makes both client and provider very vulnerable, as a real connection is encouraged despite the ever-present knowledge that death is near. This connection that we feel with our clients, and they with us, is not explainable solely in psychological terms but instead feels spiritual to me. The provider and client are on equal footing, both human, both mortal.

  Working with people with AIDS has allowed me to become comfortable "enough" with death to talk about it in a direct way.

This may be what clients most appreciate about our presence in their lives. The ramifications of being involved with clients on this level are really quite enormous, and the work has afforded me the opportunity to grow right alongside them. Together we have faced our anger, fears, doubts, and insecurities about how to handle the real stuff of life. Through loss and grief, I feel we have experienced genuine healing.

## REFERENCES

This chapter was made possible by grant number BRH 970165–02-0 from the Health Resources and Services Administration. Its contents are solely the responsibility of the author and do not necessarily represent the official views of HRSA.

Becker, E. (1973). *The denial of death.* New York: Free Press.

Bowlby, J. (1969). *Attachment and loss* (Vol. 1). New York: Basic Books.

Bowlby, J. (1979). Separation and loss within the family. In *The making and breaking of affectional bonds.* London: Tavistock. (Original work published 1970.)

Bozarth-Campbell, A. (1982). *Life is goodbye, life is hello: Grieving well through all kinds of loss.* Minneapolis, MN: CompCare Publishers.

Doka, K. J. (Ed.) (1989). *Disenfranchised grief: Recognizing hidden sorrow.* Lexington, MA: Lexington Books.

Elia, N., & Cherry, J. (1996, May). *Assessing the spiritual status of the person with AIDS.* Paper presented at HIV/AIDS '96: The Social Work Response, Eighth Annual Conference on Social Work and HIV/AIDS. Atlanta, GA.

Freud, S. (1959). Mourning and melancholia. *Collected papers.* New York: Basic Books. (Original work published 1917.)

Fulton, R., & Fulton, J. (1971). A psychosocial aspect of terminal care: Anticipatory grief. *Omega, 2,* 91–99.

Kastenbaum, R. J. (1969). Death and bereavement in later life. In A. H. Kutscher (Ed.), *Death and bereavement* (28–51). Springfield, IL: Charles C. Thomas.

Klein, M. (1948a). Mourning and its relation to manic depressive states. In *Contributions to psycho-analysis 1921–1945.* London: McGraw-Hill. (Original work published 1940.)

Klein, M. (1948b). The psychogenesis of manic depressive states. In *Contributions to psycho-analysis 1921–1945.* London: McGraw-Hill. (Original work published 1934.)

Kubler-Ross, E. (1969). *On death and dying.* New York: Macmillan.

Lindemann, E. (1944). Symptomatology and management of acute grief. *American Journal of Psychiatry, 101,* 141–148.

Millan, F., & Elia, N. (In press). Model of Multiple Opression in psychotherapy with HIV-infected injecting drug users. *Journal of Chemical Dependency Treatment.*

Mitford, J. (1963). *The American way of death.* New York: Simon & Schuster.

Nuland, S. B. (1993). *How we die: Reflections on life's final chapter.* New York: Alfred A. Knopf.

Rando, T. A. (1984). *Grief, dying and death: Clinical interventions for caregivers.* Chicago: Research Press.

Worden, J. W. (1982). *Grief counseling and grief therapy. A handbook for the mental health practitioner.* New York: W. W. Norton.

Yalom, I. D. (1980). *Existential psychotherapy.* New York: Basic Books.

# 6 | Cross-Cultural Mental Health Care

*Mark G. Winiarski*

> Culture-free service delivery is nonexistent (Navarro, 1980). The differences between client and practitioner in values, norms, beliefs, lifestyles, and life opportunities extend to every aspect of the health, mental health, and social services delivery system, which is itself a cultural phenomenon.
>
> — Pinderhughes (1989, 13)

Most of us would readily admit that our society is multicultural, encompassing many complex differences in values, beliefs, and perceptions of self and others, not to mention idiom and language. And most of us would say we are sensitive to the cultural difference of our clients.

Why, then, is mental health training and practice so devoid of multicultural influence? It reflects not the multicultural society we acknowledge but rather European-American white male middle-class heterosexual values (see, for example, Sue & Sue, 1987; Tyler, Sussewell, & Williams-McCoy, 1985).

Too often mental health practitioners regard a client from a different culture as many do a great and complex painting in a gallery: They acknowledge it as complex and demanding and may even voice an opinion such as, "It moves me." But rarely does the gallery goer seek to understand in any depth the context of the work, such as the culture in which the artist lived and the experiences from which the painting emerged. Likewise, rarely do mental health practitioners seek to move beyond being "culturally sensitive" — acknowledging that differences exist — to being "culturally competent" — understanding the cultural contexts and experiences of each client.

Current psychotherapy and counseling practice seems unable to divest itself of historical practices that placed a premium on verbal intelligence expressed in English, compliance, and ability to tolerate the clinician's anonymity and neutrality without "acting out." Client issues are seen through theories that are social-class- and culture-clad (see Altman, 1993).

These criticisms are hardly new. Fromm (1980) wrote that Freud "identif[ied] the social structure of his class and its problems with the problems inherent in human existence" (24). Unfortunately, many practitioners, while adopting different theoretical orientations, still make, albeit unconsciously, the same social class/human existence correlation. When members of minority groups avoided psychotherapy or "terminated prematurely," many providers blamed the clients rather than questioning their own practices. Even now, many practitioners are unwilling to bend their rules for persons from cultures and in situations that were not considered when the "rules" were created.

HIV/AIDS, which in so many ways holds a mirror to the face of America and is not concerned about flattery, confronts mental health practitioners with the necessity of investigating their practice and attitudes, acknowledging their shortcomings, and working diligently not only to be sensitive to clients but to soak themselves with the clients' experience. How can one begin to enter into a relationship with someone without the intense desire to understand all there is about that person?

The practice of HIV/AIDS mental health demands the intense desire to understand individuals. HIV/AIDS has compelled many persons, otherwise unfamiliar or uncomfortable with mental health care, to seek assistance for themselves and family members. This is especially true in the inner city, where quality culturally appropriate care has been scarce.

From the outset, HIV mostly affected members of minority groups that were considered outcasts and stigmatized by members of the majority culture even before the epidemic. First affected by HIV was the gay community, an embodiment of culture based on sexual preference. Almost concurrently, HIV was found to be spreading in communities of injection drug users. Mostly in the inner cities, these communities are intersections of many diverse cultures, including:

- That of drug use, which has its own idioms, hierarchies, and belief systems. There also is a culture of drug abstinence, with its own beliefs, embodied in various twelve-step programs.
- Those of different racial backgrounds and, within the category of race, diverse ethnic groups.

- Cultures based on geography: urban, rural, suburban, for example. Even within New York City, there are cultural differences in different neighborhoods when race and ethnicity are not factors.
- Cultures based on sexual preference. Many argue that American culture is heterosexist, with the gay and lesbian cultures given attention only because of their contrast with the majority norm.

Psychologically speaking, our HIV-affected clients raise all the issues that come from cultural differences, including dissimilar ways of experiencing the exterior world and interpreting inner experience (Gomez & Caban, 1992; Cancelmo, Millan, & Vazquez, 1990); different perceptions regarding power and control over one's life and oppression experienced at the hands of others (Millan & Elia, in press), and different ways of interpreting phenomena that majority-culture clinicians may view as pathological (see, for example, Eaton, 1986; Erikson, 1962; Grusky & Pollner, 1981; and Scheff, 1974).

The practice of cross-cultural mental health care is complicated even further by several other factors:

- Even if an individual is born into a specific ethnic or racial group, his or her identification with that group may fall at any point on the continuum from complete identification to complete rejection of that culture.
- Probably because of the strictures of research, we still know little about the psychotherapeutic effects of matching client and therapist on ethnicity and language (Flaskerud, 1990).

We do know that clients stay longer with therapists who speak their languages and are of their cultural/ethnic backgrounds (Flaskerud, 1986). And while gay and lesbian clients increasingly seek therapists of the same sexual preference, many do not have easy access to such people or are comfortable with heterosexual practitioners.

Clients in the inner city have even a narrower choice of mental health practitioners, and it is often difficult to match clients with therapists of the same culture/ethnicity. But even ethnic/racial matches do not guarantee therapeutic success.

Mental health practitioners are faced with a basic and crucial issue: Can a majority-culture psychotherapist really understand the inner life of a client from a minority culture? If we are not so sure of the answer, then we should understand the reluctance of a member of a minority group to expose himself or herself to a majority-culture therapist.

This chapter does not offer a cookbook of cultural differences and the "proper" responses. The process of cultural sensitivity and competence only partially involves gaining information. The more difficult task, by far, is the majority-culture provider's self-examination of heart and psyche for racism, prejudgments, stereotypical thinking, and anger. This chapter will assist in the beginning of self-examination.

## *My Clinical Practice*

The author is a white heterosexual man with almost a decade's experience in HIV/AIDS-related mental health. In the beginning I worked at a hospital, in the Manhattan borough of New York City, that specialized in HIV-related care, and my clients there were gay men, gay men of color, and men and women of color infected through injection drug use and/or heterosexual sex. In 1990 I moved to Montefiore Medical Center in the Bronx, working in a program that integrated substance abuse treatment with primary care, in clinics where 43 percent of the clients were HIV-positive. I subsequently received federal funding for an HIV mental health service integrated with primary care at community health sites operated by the Department of Family Medicine. In this project I was confronted daily with issues of race and culture — both by clients and by a project team of psychologists and social workers who included lesbians and gays, blacks and Latinos.

The Bronx experience convinced me that the reason traditional psychotherapy was so poorly received by minority culture clients was that it was culturally inappropriate in so many respects and failed to meet clients' immediate needs. New praxis was required, and initiated, using a "bending the frame" format (Winiarski, 1993; see also chapter 2).

Many experiences have convinced me that the process of becoming culturally sensitive and competent entails painful and continuous analysis of cultural holdings. A story, about a famous event, illustrates this.

Like most whites, I was aghast when a Los Angeles jury declared O. J. Simpson not guilty of murdering his former wife and her friend. Later that day, a Latina colleague, who is brilliant and whose understandings I admire, told me that the evidence had failed to persuade her of Simpson's guilt. As I listened to her reasons, I realized that issues of justice are more complex and more shrouded in the mysteries of racial experience than I had ever imagined. I realized also that my incomprehension of the deepest feelings of minority community members in matters of justice is repeated constantly as I deal with issues of power, justice, oppression, and just about every other topic that emerges in my work. Wrote Gates (1995), "As blacks exulted at Simpson's acquittal, horrified whites had a fleeting sense that this race thing was knottier than they'd ever supposed — that, when all the pieties were cleared away, blacks really were strangers in their midst" (56). For mental health practitioners, the sense cannot be merely fleeting. There is much to do.

## *Background Reading*

Many exceptional books and articles argue that we should be culturally competent. The American Psychological Association (1991), among other groups, has issued guidelines for services to "ethnic, linguistic, and culturally diverse populations."

Too often, students and practitioners think the literature that espouses cultural competence (that is, a full understanding of the client's culture) is peripheral at best to the body of mental health practice. Some students and practitioners of psychodynamic psychotherapy believe that a person's culture is only intrapsychic and should receive no special attention as an external influence.

In fact, a large and rich appreciation of culture in psychoanalysis immediately followed the Freudian emphasis on drives. The "interpersonalists" were a group of eminent psychoanalysts who broke from Freud and emerged in the early 20th century. This group included Harry Stack Sullivan, Erich Fromm, Clara Thompson, and Sandor Ferenczi. Karen Horney, not generally considered an interpersonalist, also emphasized the role of culture (Ortmeyer, 1995). These individuals "were firmly convinced that cultural and economic realities contribute to character formation, as well as to psychopathology, and they emphasized that knowledge of the individual's cultural and environmental realities, past and present, is required for understanding people's strengths and weaknesses" (Ortmeyer, 1995, 11). Their appreciation of the role of culture can be understood by reading Ortmeyer (1995) and Hegeman (1995) and, if interest is piqued, picking and choosing among the many other chapters in the *Handbook of Interpersonal Psychoanalysis* (Lionells, Fiscalini, Mann, & Stern, 1995).

The works of the interpersonalists and of Horney deserve reading to learn how the role of culture was appreciated more than half a century ago. For example, Horney (1939) emphasized culture and wrote that "Although it is true that childhood experiences vary not only in individual families but also with respect to each child in the same family, nevertheless most experiences are the result of the entire cultural situation and are not incidental" (170).

The field of family therapy is perhaps the greatest proponent of consideration of cultural issues in therapy. Monica McGoldrick's works should be read. *Ethnicity and Family Therapy* (McGoldrick, Giordano, & Pearce, 1996) is a classic text.

An expert on working with black families is Nancy Boyd-Franklin. In addition to doing a literature search for her current work, consult her *Black Families in Therapy: A Multisystems Approach* (1989), which well describes the situation of African American families and suggests a flexible approach to psychotherapy, with interventions at many levels of systems that affect the family. Her approach is similar to the "bending the frame" approaches described in chapter 2. Another, related book is *Children, Families, and HIV/AIDS,* edited by Boyd-Franklin, Steiner, and Boland (1995). Two chapters are specifically relevant. One, on cultural sensitivity and competence (Boyd-Franklin, Aleman, Jean-Gilles, & Lewis, 1995), describes and illustrates application of a cultural competence model created by Sandra Lewis to work with African American, Latino, and Haitian families affected by HIV. Lewis's model, as described in the chapter, includes understanding family values regarding roles, child-rearing practices, and extended family involvement; understanding the role of spirituality; assessing the level of acculturation and empowering families to use their own strengths and resources. Another chapter, by Boyd-Franklin and Boland, describes application of the multisystems approach to HIV.

Those who work with Latinos should consult *Hispanics and Mental Health: A Framework for Research* (Rogler, Malgady, & Rodriguez, 1989), which also raises many important questions for clinicians. These authors and their colleagues at the Hispanic Research Center at Fordham University, Bronx, New York, continue to publish a variety of books and journal articles that can assist clinicians with Latino clients. See, for example, Malgady, Rogler, and Constantino (1987); Rogler (1993); and Rogler, Cortes, and Malgady (1991).

Clinicians with Asian or Asian-American clients should consult the work of Stanley Sue and his colleagues (for example, Sue, Nakamura, Chung, & Yee-Bradbury, 1994). The Asian AIDS Project in San Francisco can also serve as a resource. Chan (1989) has written about Asian-American lesbians and gay men and Gock (1992) has written about gay and lesbian Asian-Pacific Islanders.

A relatively new journal titled *Culture Diversity and Mental Health*, published by Wiley, should be regular reading for therapists who wish to develop cultural competence.

Finally, practitioners who want to understand the cultures of clients should look at publications and productions from the client's homeland, including movies, books, and magazines, with subtitles or in translation, and reports on the homeland. Discussions of these with the client could provide additional information and insight.

## *Clinician's Self-Appraisal*

One cannot begin to comprehend persons of different cultures, let alone work with them in mental health practices, if one does not value them and their cultures. If you have the heart—that is, you regard other cultures as valuable—then the learning of information comes easier. But few practitioners will admit they are not culturally sensitive.

It is often helpful to assess one's knowledge and interest in a topic, as a pretest, before becoming involved in an issue. Here is a two-part quiz. The first five questions measure knowledge of different cultures, and the rest ask about your values. Note your emotional responses to the pretest and to each question. Dig deeper into each emotional response, noting your feelings and trying to understand sources of these feelings. Please take the time to consider your answers before reading the rest of the chapter.

## *Cultural Quiz*

1. What is someone asking when he asks, "Are you a friend of Bill Wilson?"
2. A woman says she will be attending a pride parade. What is she saying to you?
3. Your client wants to cancel the next session because she is attending a Kwanzaa celebration. Kwanzaa refers to what?
4. Your client makes a reference to "the rapture." What is the meaning of this phrase?
5. The nurse making the referral tells you that your new client is taking INH p.o. What is INH (pronounced eye-en-aitch) and what does p.o. (pronounced pee-oh) mean?
6. You have two job offers as a mental health counselor and must

choose one. The first entails working with white, middle-class college students at a local university. The second is at another university campus, one that has a predominantly African American student body. Both jobs pay the same, have the same benefits and are equally accessible. Where would you prefer to work? Why?

7. Are the students at both campuses (a) equally prepared for college, (b) equally likely to succeed in careers, and (c) equally amenable to mental health care? Justify your answers.
8. Are you equally prepared to serve either campus? In what psychological ways are you not?

The first five questions test your knowledge regarding some of the major cultures that HIV providers are likely to deal with. The first question comes from the twelve-step culture of substance abuse treatment, the second from gay and lesbian cultures, the third from black culture, the fourth from a fundamentalist religious culture, and the fifth from the medical culture. The answers are available by asking people who know those cultures.

Questions 6–8 ask you to reflect on how you regard others of different cultures, and yourself. Since this is a private assessment, you need not tell yourself stories. Ask yourself if you really value minority individuals or, perhaps, overvalue majority-culture members — if you have prejudices. If you do have prejudices, welcome to the human race. The issue now is how you deal with them.

What was learned from this brief test? Some readers may realize that while they claim to be culturally sensitive, they actually have tunnel vision — they really haven't grasped some of the cultural issues around them. Perhaps the "regard" part of the test will help them discern their real feelings about racial minorities. Finally, I hope this test conveyed that there are many cultures around us, beyond those bound to ethnicity and skin color. In the medical center in which I work, for example, there is a plethora of disciplinary cultures: medicine, nursing, social work, psychology, to name a few, and each has its own belief system about causes of conditions and methods of treatment.

## *Tools for Clinical Practice*

As clinicians strive for cultural competence, these points may prove helpful:

- *It is a mistake to assume that because a person has certain cultural/ethnic characteristics, he or she strongly identifies with that culture.*

  The correct initial stance is to make no assumption and to conduct a detailed inquiry of the client's cultural and ethnic feelings. It may be that a person is ambivalent about his or her ethnicity and culture or has rejected it. Or it may be that a strong identification serves to defend against a majority culture seen as hostile. Many persons who are bicultural identify with one culture in some situations and with the other culture in different situations. These issues should be explored.
- *A time-worn clinical practice anecdote is: If there is an elephant in the room, the therapist and the client should acknowledge it. A difference in culture/ethnicity between therapist and client is an "elephant."*

  Too often, the client will not raise the issue, for a variety of reasons. The therapist must, and the client's feelings should be explored. The therapist should not be satisfied with a client's shrugging off the question. Feelings regarding ethnic/culture differences run deep in American society, and the client must be encouraged to express those feelings.
- *When working with a client from another culture, the mental health practitioner must make a commitment to learning about that culture.*

  Some major steps to take when working with a client from another culture:

  Ask yourself:

1. What are your experiences with people of that culture?
2. What feelings do people of that culture evoke in you? Are they positive or negative? What are the bases for those feelings?
3. What are your expectations of the client?
4. Are you able to enter into a relationship in which you consciously scrutinize the reenactment of power and control issues between the cultures/races?
5. Can you tell your supervisor about prejudices and feelings stirred up by the cross-cultural work?

Regarding the client:

1. Conduct a literature search in psychology, social work, and sociology to get a sense for the literature in and regarding that culture.

2. Find a supervisor who is of that culture or, at least, competent to work with that culture. If your institution cannot provide such a person, you need to look elsewhere. Ways to find that person include:

   — Contact professional organizations, such as those of Hispanic providers or African American psychologists.
   — Consult specialized lists on the Internet. Many professions have specialized bulletin boards and e-mail mailing lists.
   — From your literature search, determine if any authors of articles that may pertain to your client are in your geographic area, and then contact the author for supervision or to network for additional contacts.
   — Check with ethnically based organizations. Contact, for example, local, regional, or national groups such as those of Hispanic or African American advocates for their cultures and peoples.
   — Contact universities to find such programs as black studies or Asian studies and scholars in cultural areas.
   — Talk to members of gay and lesbian organizations and service groups and groups of persons with other sexual preferences or interests.

- *With a client from another culture, take a "Will you teach me?" stance.*

  Asking the client to describe and explain in detail his or her cultural background, including family background, is entirely consistent with quality psychotherapy. Ideally, we over time come to understand every client in a broad context. With clients from different cultures, we need always consciously to be curious about everything we do not know or only partially know. (Perhaps most dangerous is presuming that we do know, which results in not asking and not understanding). We need to listen and inquire with a culturally sensitive ear, using, in part, what we have learned about the client's culture from many sources.
- *In cross-cultural work with HIV, several themes emerge that are particularly problematic for majority-culture providers.*

  These themes include:

— *Power.* Power discrepancies in society that oppress and enrage are easily reenacted in mental health service delivery. Many providers and agencies that provide services are majority culture, and their styles reflect that culture. Many persons with HIV are of minority cultures, including gay and inner-city. Power differences are inherent in the helper (privileged) and client ("needy") relationship. Other dialectics may be: provider (healthy) and client (infected); psychiatrist (educated) and client (uneducated), case manager (resourceful) and client (resourceless). "[P]ower is a primary issue in racial dynamics and a focus on power assures attention to those aspects of race that can remain hidden even in the racial exploration" (Pinderhughes, 1989, xiii). Both the provider's and the client's interpretations of the relationship should be brought to the surface and scrutinized.

– *Sex.* American society's discomfort with sex has certainly facilitated the spread of HIV. Within the area of sexuality, consider white American society's extreme discomfort with black sexuality, which West (1993) calls "a taboo subject in America principally because it is a form of black power over which whites have little control – yet its visible manifestations evoke the most visceral of white responses, be it one of seductive obsession or downright disgust" (87). If, however, a majority-culture therapist is uncomfortable discussing sexuality with an African American man or woman, let alone exploring its meanings, how can HIV be comfortably discussed, and how can a psychotherapy occur? Again, the work of providing competent mental health services begins with the provider's analysis of self and working through these problematic areas.

- *The most difficult task of the majority-culture therapist is to allow oneself to be the target for the minority client's rage.*

If rage goes unexplored in any psychotherapy, the process's depth is questionable. If it goes unexplored between a majority-culture therapist and a minority-culture client, then, arguably, you may have only the illusion of psychotherapy.

It is difficult for a therapist to be the target of rage. Yet, a majority-culture therapist must encourage the expression of a minority client's rage, which may be a dominant theme in the therapy. It is no wonder that this occurs so seldom. Nevertheless, it must.

- *Some clients may use cultural explanations for irresponsible behavior. You need to be sufficiently knowledgeable so that you can challenge them.*

  Jacqueline Cherry, MSW, a former colleague and of Jamaican heritage, provided us this example: A Jamaican man in the United States, in talking with his therapist, justifies his significant marijuana abuse by saying that in his homeland marijuana use is common and well tolerated. Ms. Cherry notes that this is not at all the case — the client is telling a story that may be swallowed whole by the unknowing clinician.
- *Inquire regarding the possibilities of psychological trauma back in the homeland, and of relocation/immigration stress.*

  Many ethnic groups in their homelands have suffered unspeakable persecution. Others, such as Cambodians and some groups of Latin Americans, have been through horrific wars. Many immigrants, particularly those with few financial resources, find themselves in very difficult and stressful situations once in the United States. They often are relocated by refugee agencies to threatening neighborhoods, they have to contend with the English language, and without proper working papers they are either unhirable or exploited by employers who pay low wages and provide no benefits. Their living situations therefore can be very stressful and a source of psychological distress.
- *Acknowledge cultural expression of spirituality.*

  Many mental health providers underwent training in a secular environment, meaning that little mention of how to integrate religion or spirituality into mental health care occurred. The exception occurs in the training of pastoral counselors, a subset of mental health providers. While secular service provision may be a comfortable set for white providers, many clients and potential clients have deeply held spiritual views.
- *Watch for countertransferential "flags."*

  The following reactions to clients should be examined, with a supervisor, for cultural bias:

  — Immobilization. This may include failure to confront a client or failure to raise topics or issues. If you feel you are "walking on eggshells," it may be because you fear the client.
  — A significant emotional response, such as revulsion, to atti-

tudes and behaviors discussed by the client. These areas may include disciplining of children, sexual practices, and male and female roles. During the introspective process, you need to ask not only why the client reacts differently but why you are reacting differently from the client.
- Being pleased with a therapeutic relationship that is "polite" and emotionally shallow. It likely indicates that the therapist is failing to allow the client to express uncomfortable emotions, such as rage.
- Providing case management not just because it is needed but because the therapist decides the client is not an appropriate candidate for therapy. The therapist's part in the relationship requires scrutiny.

- *Institutions and agencies too often rely on hiring of minority providers to meet requirements for "cultural competence."*

  Minority staff members may work in settings where the majority culture dictates ways of viewing clients and their situations, as well as rules and procedures. Subtle and not-so-subtle majority culture mores — including value judgments, styles of dealing with emotion, and expressions of superiority — can communicate that minority staff members' cultural interpretations and contributions are not welcome or worthless. This undermines morale, increases staff tension, forces staff turnover, and negatively affects patient care. Institutions and agencies need to give real "voice" to their minority providers, not only by hearing their culturally based issues but by making these staff supervisors and teachers. If an agency or institution, such as an outpatient mental health clinic, does not have regular (monthly is not too often) cross-cultural training sessions, then it is deficient in its commitment to cultural competence. And if minority providers do not make the deficiency known, they have abdicated their responsibility to their colleagues.

## *Conclusion*

Despite practitioners' acknowledgement of our society's multiculturalism, training and practice in mental health remains predominantly reflective of a white, male, middle-class, and heterosexual society. Cultural competence is a process that begins with reflecting on one's prejudices and attitudes. With openness, one can begin learning cultural content. The majority-culture practitioner working with a minority-culture client has a difficult task — attempting to understand thoroughly the client's cultural aspects. But skillful practice demands that this hard work be done.

## REFERENCES

The author wishes to acknowledge the assistance of Maria Caban, M.A., in the writing of this chapter.

This chapter was made possible by grant number BRH 970165-02-0 from the Health Resources and Services Administration. Its contents are solely the responsibility of the author and do not necessarily represent the official views of HRSA.

Altman, N. (1993). Psychoanalysis and the urban poor. *Psychoanalytic Dialogues, 3,* 29–49.

American Psychological Association (1991). *Guidelines for providers of psychological services to ethnic, linguistic, and culturally diverse populations.* Washington, DC: Author.

Boyd-Franklin, N. (1989). *Black families in therapy: A multisystems approach.* New York: Guilford Press.

Boyd-Franklin, N., Aleman, J. del C., Jean-Gilles, M. M., & Lewis, S. Y. (1995). Cultural sensitivity and competence. In N. Boyd-Franklin, G. L. Steiner, & M. G. Boland (Eds.), *Children, families and HIV/AIDS* (53–77). New York: Guilford Press.

Boyd-Franklin, N., & Boland, M. G. (1995). A multisystems approach to service delivery for HIV/AIDS families. In N. Boyd-Franklin, G. L. Steiner, & M. G. Boland (Eds.), *Children, families and HIV/AIDS* (199–215). New York: Guilford Press.

Boyd-Franklin, N., Steiner, G. L., & Boland, M. G. (Eds.) (1995). *Children, families, and HIV/AIDS.* New York: Guilford Press.

Cancelmo, J. A., Millan, F., & Vazquez, C. I. (1990). Cultural and symptomatology — the role of personal meaning in diagnosis and treatment: A case study. *American Journal of Psychoanalysis, 50,* 137–149.

Chan, C. S. (1989). Issues of identity development among Asian-American lesbians and gay men. *Journal of Counseling and Development, 68,* 16–20.

Eaton, W. W. (1986). *The sociology of mental disorders.* New York: Praeger Special Studies.

Erikson, K. T. (1962). Notes on the sociology of deviance. *Social Problems, 9,* 307–314.

Flaskerud, J. H. (1986). Effects of culture-compatible intervention on the utilization of mental health services by minority clients. *Community Mental Health Journal, 22,* 127–141.

Flaskerud, J. H. (1990). Matching client and therapist ethnicity, language, and gender: A review of research. *Issues in Mental Health Nursing, 11,* 321–336.

Fromm, E. (1980). *Greatness and limitations of Freud's thought.* New York: Harper and Row.

Gates, H. L., Jr. (1995, October 23). Thirteen ways of looking at a black man. *New Yorker, 71(33),* 56–65.

Gock, T. (1992). Asian-Pacific Islanders: Identity integration and pride. In B. Berzon (Ed.), *Positively gay* (247–252). Berkeley, CA: Celestial Arts.

Gomez, J. R. R., & Caban, M. (1992). The problem of bilingualism in psychiatric diagnoses of Hispanic patients. *Cross-Cultural Psychology Bulletin, 26(2),* 2–5.

Grusky, O., & Pollner, M. (1981). *The sociology of mental illness.* New York: Holt, Rinehart & Winston.

Hegeman, E. (1995). Cross-cultural issues in interpersonal psychoanalysis. In M. Lionells, J. Fiscalini, C. H. Mann, & D. B. Stern (Eds.), *Handbook of interpersonal psychoanalysis* (823–846). Hillsdale, NJ: Analytic Press.

Horney, K. (1939). *New ways in psychoanalysis.* New York: W. W. Norton.

Lionells, M., Fiscalini, J., Mann, C. H., & Stern, D. B. (Eds.) (1995). *Handbook of interpersonal psychoanalysis.* Hillsdale, NJ: Analystic Press.

Malgady, R. G., Rogler, L. H., & Constantino, G. (1987). Ethnocultural and linguistic bias in mental health evaluation of Hispanics. *American Psychologist, 42,* 228–234.

McGoldrick, M., Giordano, & J. Pearce, J. (Eds.). (1996). *Ethnicity and family therapy (2nd ed.).* New York: Guilford Press.

Millan, F., & Elia, N. (In press). Model of multiple oppression in psychotherapy with HIV-infected injecting drug users. *Journal of Chemical Dependency.*

Navarro, V. (1980, November). Panel on culture and health. Symposium on cross-cultural and transcultural issues in family health care. University of California, San Francisco. Cited in Pinderhughes, 13.

Ortmeyer, D. H. (1995). History of the founders of intepersonal psychoanalysis. In M. Lionells, J. Fiscalini, C. H. Mann, & D. B. Stern (Eds.), *Handbook of interpersonal psychoanalysis* (11–27). Hillsdale, NJ: Analytic Press.

Pinderhughes, E. (1989). *Understanding race, ethnicity, and power.* New York: Free Press.

Rogler, L. H. (1993). Culturally sensitive psychiatric diagnosis: A framework for research. *Journal of Nervous and Mental Disease, 181,* 401–408.

Rogler, L. H., Cortes, D. E., & Malgady, R. G. (1991). Acculturation and mental health status among Hispanics. *American Psychologist, 46,* 585–597.

Rogler, L. H., Malgady, R. G., & Rodriguez, O. (1989). *Hispanics and mental health: A framework for research.* Malabar, FL: Robert E. Krieger.

Scheff, T. J. (1974). The labelling theory of mental illness. *American Sociological Review, 39,* 444–452.

Sue, S., Nakamura, C. Y., Chung, R. C-Y., & Yee-Bradbury, C. (1994). Mental health research on Asian Americans. Special Issue: Asian-American Mental Health. *Journal of Community Psychology, 22(2),* 61–67.

Sue, D., & Sue, S. (1987). Cultural factors in the clinical assessment of Asian Americans. *Journal of Consulting and Clinical Psychology, 55,* 479–487.

Tyler, F. B., Sussewell, D. R., & Williams-McCoy, J. (1985). Ethnic validity in psychotherapy. *Psychotherapy, 22,* 311–320.

West, C. (1993). *Race matters.* Boston: Beacon Press.

Winiarski. M. G. (1993). Integrating mental health services with HIV primary care: The Bronx experience. *AIDS Patient Care, 7,* 322–326.

# 7 | The Role of Psychiatry in HIV Care

*Karina K. Uldall*

Psychiatry plays a significant role in the treatment of the immense and complex mental health needs related to HIV/AIDS. Although psychiatrists have a unique place in overseeing psychopharmacological interventions, it would be a travesty if the role of psychiatry in HIV care were to be limited to prescription of psychiatric medications. As HIV disease develops into a chronic illness, psychiatry has the opportunity to span the gulf between biological and psychosocial/spiritual approaches.

Because the virus is prevalent in groups with multiple problems, such as homelessness, chronic mental illness, and substance use, diagnosis and treatment planning become increasingly complicated. One must identify symptoms as psychiatric or neurological; although accuracy in identifying symptoms improves with time and training, diagnoses are still missed and the patient is blamed for misbehavior. A psychiatrist is the best qualified person to answer such typical and complex questions as: Are psychiatric symptoms due to one's chronic mental illness, substance use, "physical" illness outside of HIV/AIDS, HIV/AIDS-related medical illness, medication toxicity, psychological reaction to distress, inadequate housing, nutrition, or some combination of these above?

Given the correct diagnoses, complex patient management can be handled by a diverse treatment team consisting of primary-care providers (physicians, physician assistants, nurse practitioners), psychiatrists, nurses, psychologists, social workers, and other mental health specialists.

I am a psychiatrist committed to caring for HIV-affected persons in Seattle, Washington, and work in a medical specialty clinic serving more than 850 persons with HIV disease. I currently direct a federally funded project that attempts to integrate psychiatry and primary care by training physicians to recognize acute neuropsychiatric problems arising from HIV/AIDS, such as delirium, as well as more chronic conditions, such as AIDS Dementia Complex.

I became interested in this work early in my medical training, while on a neurology rotation during my psychiatric residency. A young man named Dale entered the hospital with a headache, fever, and mental status changes. Before long, it became clear that he had cryptococcal meningitis. Therapy for this illness was inadequate then. I watched as Dale became increasingly ill from this infection. He had walked into his hospital room at the time of admission; now he was bed-bound. I relied heavily on the AIDS social worker to find a community placement where Dale could spend his final days. No nursing home would accept him because of his medical needs, because he had AIDS, and the hospital was not prepared to provide long-term care. Recreational therapy was grossly underfunded, but we had access to VCR equipment. One day I brought in a couple of musicals and watched them with Dale when things were quiet in the hospital. It was one of the greatest moments in my medical career. I learned a valuable distinction between curing and caring. Late one night on call, I telephoned Dale's parents to inform them that his condition appeared to be worsening. His elderly mother asked if they should come immediately. I explained that it was difficult to judge how long Dale would live but that she and her husband could probably wait until morning. Dale died in the middle of the night. Despite having known that his death was near, Dale's mother cried when I called back with the news. My experience with Dale and his family continues to influence my medical practice eight years later.

This chapter is about what I believe the roles of a psychiatrist are in HIV care — physician, consultant/liaison, educator, therapist, and visionary. I believe that comprehensive care of the HIV-affected person is multidisciplinary care. My clinical practice reflects that model.

## *Background Reading*

At the beginning of the HIV/AIDS epidemic, patients typically died quickly from acute infections, such as *pneumocystis carinii* pneumonia (PCP). The role of psychiatrists and other mental health providers was limited, if it existed at all. As more individuals became affected, experts in the field distinguished two groups of people with HIV/AIDS and mental illness: those with preexisting chronic and/or recurrent psychiatric illness who subsequently become HIV infected and HIV-infected persons who later develop neuropsychiatric or psychosocial problems related to their infection.

### *Persons with Preexisting Psychiatric Illness*

Studies addressing the number of acutely hospitalized psychiatric inpatients infected with HIV-1 found that between 5.2 percent and 7.1 percent of individuals studied were HIV-seropositive (Cournos, Empfield, & Horwath, 1991; Sacks, Dermatis, & Looser-Ott, 1992). Among longer-stay patients at a state hospital, HIV seroprevalence has been reported as 4 percent (Meyer, McKinnon, & Cournos, 1993). Injection drug use is a well-documented risk factor for HIV infection. Recent information shows that alcoholics and noninjection drug users also are at higher risk: Seroprevalence rates in these populations range from 4.5 percent to 11.4 percent (Lee, Travin, & Bluestone, 1992; Schleifer, Keller, & Franklin, 1990). One cohort of 300 alcoholic patients showed 10.3 percent of patients were HIV-infected, 77.4 percent of whom were undetected during inpatient alcohol treatment (Mahler, Yi, & Sacks, 1994).

Several investigators have identified higher-risk behaviors among persons with mental illness, including engaging in casual sex, trading sex for money or a place to stay, combining sex with substance use, having unprotected heterosexual intercourse with known HIV-positive partners, having unprotected anal intercourse with men, and sharing needles or drug paraphernalia (Kelly, 1992; Sacks, 1990). The understanding of AIDS risk behaviors appears to be compromised among psychiatric inpatients. But few programs developed to date address the special needs that chronic mentally ill patients have regarding AIDS education (Baer, 1988; Carmen & Brady, 1990).

In addition to prevention/education challenges, persons with mental illness who subsequently become HIV-infected also present providers with unique challenges around treatment compliance and diagnosis. What is the most effective method for keeping a homeless individual with schizophrenia and tuberculosis engaged for the several weeks to months of medications required both to ensure proper treatment of the lung infection and to minimize the risk of exposure to the general population? Are the current psychiatric symptoms seen in an immunocompromised patient an exacerbation of bipolar disorder or indicative of a central nervous system infection?

### *Persons Who Develop Neuropsychiatric or Psychosocial/Spiritual Problems as a Result of HIV/AIDS Infection*

The World Health Organization Neuropsychiatric AIDS Study, which attempted to study a population representative of the current epidemic, reported a higher prevalence of current mental disorders among symptomatic HIV-1 infected persons than among HIV-1 seronegative controls (Maj, Janssen, & Starace, 1994). AIDS dementia, characterized by cognitive impairment, motor dysfunction, and changes in mood/personality, typically occurs in significantly immunocompromised AIDS patients. Earlier reports suggested a prevalence at a single point in time from 8 percent to 16 percent, with prevalence over the life of the individual approaching 40 to 50 percent (McArthur, 1987; World Health Organization, 1989). More recent studies suggest that this illness occurs in 10 to 20 percent of AIDS patients.

Delirium, defined as an acute confusional state with a physiological cause, is characterized by disturbances of consciousness and attention, changes in cognition or perceptual disturbances, and acute onset with a fluctuating course (American Psychiatric Association, 1994). Many providers mistake delirium for dementia. Many take it for granted as a natural part of dying. Misconceptions result in underrecognition and inappropriate treatment of this condition. In one study of hospitalized AIDS patients, delirium accounted for 57 percent of the identifiable organic mental disorders seen in the study group (Fernandez & Levy, 1989).

The research literature also includes reports of other neurological diseases presenting with psychiatric symptoms: toxoplasmosis and psychosis; cryptococcal meningitis and mania; dementia and depression (Beresford, Blow, & Hall, 1986; Boccellari, Dilley, & Shore, 1988; Kermani, Borod, & Brown, 1985; Navia & Price, 1987; Perry & Jacobsen, 1986; Price & Forejt, 1988; Rundell, Wise, & Ursano, 1986; Schmidt & Miller, 1988). Adequate population-based descriptive studies that outline the frequency and the severity of psychiatric illness in HIV/AIDS patients, and the subsequent effect of such an illness on function and general health, remain missing from the literature.

In addition to neuropsychiatric illness, mental health providers working with HIV/AIDS patients commonly address spiritual or existential crises across the spectrum of HIV disease. Farmer and Kleinman (1989) describe AIDS as human suffering despite the rational-technical language of disease. Kuhn (1988) advocates viewing spirituality as a legitimate and purposeful area of medical investigation. The current literature certainly supports the need to comfort and to maintain hope in HIV/AIDS patients and their families as they deal with this devastating illness (Rabkin, Williams, Neugebauer, Remien, & Goetz, 1990). Mental health providers have entered the battle against HIV/AIDS around issues of suicide (McKegney & O'Dowd, 1992; Cote, Biggar, & Dannenberg, 1992), multiple losses/grief (Coates et al., 1987; Rabkin et al., 1990; Rait, 1991; Winiarski, 1991), and existential dilemmas (Farmer & Kleinman, 1989; Yarnell & Battin, 1988).

Psychiatrists working in the area of HIV/AIDS certainly possess a unique role in overseeing psychopharmacological interventions. Unfortunately, much of the literature in this area consists of anecdotal information and case reports. Only recently have controlled medication trials in HIV/AIDS patients for common psychiatric illnesses such as depression been published (Rabkin, Rabkin, Harrison, & Wagner, 1994). Many psychiatrists working with HIV/AIDS patients rely heavily on clinical experience, recognizing that medication usage in this population still remains an art as well as a science. General guidelines, such as "less is better" and "benzos (benzodiazepines) are bad," provide starting points in clinical decision making.

## *My Clinical Work*

The focus of the Seattle-King County Department of Public Health project, Integration of Psychiatry and Primary Care, directly met the challenge of providing comprehensive care for persons with HIV/AIDS. In 1991 we received a Ryan White C.A.R.E. Act Title II Special Projects of National Significance grant for psychiatric services in the Madison Clinic, an outpatient clinic serving more than 850 persons with HIV/AIDS. The project firmly established psychiatry as an integral part of the multidisciplinary treatment team of providers, allowing exploration of the unique role of psychiatry in the treatment of HIV disease. Primary care providers, nurses, social workers, mental health specialists and psychiatrists make up the team. Each team member brings his or her professional perspective, joining in a "horizontally integrated" team approach to patient care. No one member is the designated team leader. No group of members are delegated as perennial followers. The team member with a concern about a particular patient initiates discussion about that concern, bridging traditional boundaries of medical versus nonmedical, psychological versus social, and so on. For the team to work successfully, it is imperative that all providers involved in a patient's care meet and discuss their working relationship (Ferguson & Varnam, 1994).

## *The Roles of Psychiatry*

The unique role of psychiatry in the treatment of HIV/AIDS patients encompasses and balances each aspect of the biopsychosocial/spiritual model; the psychiatrist is at once physician, consultant/liaison, educator, therapist, and visionary.

### *Psychiatrist as Physician*

Charles sat in the office chair breathing heavily after his walk to the clinic. Diagnosed with alcohol dependence and bipolar disorder, he saw his psychiatrist more often than his medical provider. In fact, his recent problems around accepting his HIV status had led him to avoid seeing the internal medicine doctor. A bout of alcohol use two weeks ago resulted in a fall that fractured his upper arm; the pain made it difficult to move; his sleep was decreased. Depressed, tired, out of breath, and in pain, he waited for the psychiatrist.

Upon entering the room, the psychiatrist noticed that Charles looked different: He was short of breath; his color was pale; he had lost weight. Rather than focus only on the psychiatric medications, the doctor asked several questions about Charles' current symptoms. It rapidly became clear that Charles needed a physical examination followed by a chest x-ray to address his respiratory disease. The need for consultation with a primary-care provider was explained to Charles, and he agreed to an examination. The diagnosis was pneumonia.

In this clinical example, the psychiatrist was in the best position to appreciate the interaction between medical and psychiatric illness. Alcohol abuse led to a fracture of Charles's arm, which led to serious pain and decreased mobility, which facilitated the development of pneumonia, which ultimately resulted in depression and problems with sleep. If the psychiatric provider had merely addressed Charles's depression, sleep disturbance, alcohol abuse, and psychiatric medications, a serious infection would have gone untreated. As physicians, psychiatrists utilize a set of methods gleaned from basic science to understand the workings of the human body. These methods emphasize diagnosis, which determines appropriate treatment (Weissman, 1994). Identification and treatment of comorbid conditions can lead to increased level of function, decreased disability, and improved quality of life (Streim & Katz, 1995). Psychiatric facilitation of primary care for HIV patients may affect survival, given the association between survival and lack of medical care (Dorrell, Snow, & Ong, 1995), higher T-helper, also known as CD4, cell count at the initial visit (Hogg, Strathdee, Craib, O'Shaughnessy, Montaner, & Schecter, 1994), and *pneumocystis carinii* pneumonia prophylaxis and antiretroviral therapy (Osmond, Charlebois, Lang, Shiboski, & Moss, 1994).

### *Psychiatrist as Consultant/Liaison*

Peter approached the nursing station asking for juice. Despite his admission to the hospital only the previous evening, the staff were well aware of his presence on the unit. Throughout the night, he left his room to find the nurses and to make some request. He rapidly earned the reputation of being "high maintenance" and "intrusive." As the unit clerk was explaining who his nurse would be for that shift, Peter started to urinate in the hallway. Quickly, several staff members rushed to stop him. As they approached, he repeated his request for juice. He became agitated and hostile as staff returned him to his room. A psychiatric consult was requested to evaluate Peter's behavior, which the staff perceived to occur when his demands were not immediately met.

The consulting psychiatrist interviewed Peter and found him to be pleasant and cooperative; he demonstrated problems recalling information and moved very slowly; Peter denied having symptoms of mood, anxiety, or psychotic illness. Upon meeting with the staff, the psychiatrist discovered that Peter was repeatedly instructed in the use of his call button as the preferred way of calling for nursing assistance but that Peter "refused" to comply with these instructions. The consulting psychiatrist looked further into the medical record. Peter was clearly immunocompromised; the brain scan showed tissue wasting, and the lumbar puncture showed an elevated $\beta$-2-microglobulin level (a surrogate marker in spinal fluid for the presence of HIV dementia). After completing her evaluation, the psychiatrist diagnosed Peter as having dementia. Upon recognizing that Peter's behavior was due to frontal lobe disinhibition and memory impairment, the staff began a treatment plan to manage his behavior during hospitalization.

Consult/liaison psychiatry is a specialty area within the area of psychiatry. Peter's case illustrates how the role of psychiatric consultants in HIV/AIDS care goes beyond recommendation of psychiatric medications and facilitation of civil commitment. This function provides a remarkable opportunity to influence patient care without being directly responsible for the patient. This unique perspective often results in a more neutral evaluation than is given by primary-care providers, nursing staff, and social workers who have ongoing interactions with the patient and who may be emotionally involved.

One assumption in having psychiatrists serve as consultants is that direct-care providers recognize the need for psychiatric consultation. This is a documented problem throughout medicine and is not unique to HIV/AIDS (Koenig, Meador, Cohen, & Blazer, 1988; Mayou, Hawton, & Feldman, 1988; Ormel, Koeter, van der Bruik, & van de Willige, 1990; Regier, Goldberg, & Taube, 1978). Psychiatric liaison services tend to work toward better recognition of psychiatric illness in primary-care settings, as well as assist in the discussion of various legal and ethical issues confronted in the care of complicated patients. Liaisons take a more proactive role: affiliating with specific providers or clinics, providing continual reinforcement regarding the importance of psychiatric intervention, and bridging gaps between more medically oriented providers and psychosocial or spiritual healers.

The psychiatric consultant/liaison relies heavily on the relationships forged with direct-care providers. Without the information obtained from discussion with these providers or from review of their chart notes, the psychiatric consultant cannot complete her assessment. Without support from the staff caring directly for the patient, the best-formed treatment plan will surely fail.

### *Psychiatrist as Educator*

Petra's family adamantly refused to allow a psychiatric assessment. Over the last few weeks, her condition had deteriorated, and family members were bracing themselves for her death. In the family's community, good people, normal people, did not see psychiatrists. Petra had a fatal illness; her experiences of seeing visions and talking confusedly were merely a part of dying. With encouragement from Petra's home health nurse, who had seen Petra and her family through much of the illness, the family agreed to talk to the psychiatrist in the presence of the nurse.

The psychiatrist began by listening to the family. She acknowledged their fears and accepted their judgments about psychiatry as a discipline. The psychiatrist spoke to the family about her experience with HIV/AIDS patients, admitting that Petra might be dying but maintaining that death did not need to include "visions" and incoherent ramblings. The family ultimately agreed to allow the psychiatrist to see Petra and to review her medical records. The psychiatrist explained to the family that Petra was experiencing delirium, probably caused by recent, simultaneous increases in pain medication, sedatives, and antidiarrhea medications. After conferring with Petra's primary-care provider, medication changes were made. Petra died peacefully three weeks later, speaking coherently and sharing important moments with her family.

One key outcome of having psychiatrists serve as educators is the reduction of stigma associated with mental illness. This misunderstanding of psychiatric disease is not confined to the general public; medical professionals, despite their training, share many of these misperceptions. HIV/AIDS is a disease already characterized by shame, discrimination, and misunderstanding. When psychiatric illness is added to this tenuous situation, even the most empathic caregiver can succumb to stereotypes and frustration.

Psychiatrists, because of their unique biological perspective, can assist HIV/AIDS providers to recognize better psychiatric illness and understand better psychiatric pharmacological subtleties. Psychiatrists can educate other physicians, physician assistants, and nurse practitioners in prevention of iatrogenic disease due to medication toxicity. Psychiatrists, because of their appreciation for the psychosocial/spiritual characteristics of the patient, can listen carefully to providers' and family members' concerns, presenting their information in a manner that the recipient can relate directly to the patient or loved one. Optimal care for HIV/AIDS patients requires an educational component for patients, providers, and family members. Education, as a form of advocacy, empowers those who receive it.

### *Psychiatrist as Therapist*

Canda worked as a prostitute for fifteen years. She was already addicted to heroin on her sixteenth birthday. At thirty, she tested positive for HIV. As her dreams of becoming a wife, mother, student, and artist disappeared in the shadow of her HIV status, Canda sought help at the local HIV clinic. She expressed a desire to stop working as a prostitute and to decrease her heroin use. In the course of therapy, her low self-esteem became obvious. When Canda impulsively overdosed on heroin, her primary-care provider expressed frustration and hopelessness about her noncompliance with appointments and medical interventions.

Canda continued in psychotherapy, focusing on relationship and family issues that contributed to her current situation. At one point, she required medication for treatment of major depression. At other times, she needed reassurance that medications were not indicated; medicating her pain would have interfered with the process of psychotherapy and with her personal growth. Over time, Canda completely stopped using heroin and working as a prostitute; she ended a physically abusive relationship; she enrolled in school and obtained her G.E.D.; and her art was displayed by a local restaurant.

Psychiatry is not synonymous with psychotherapy. In fact, in recent years some psychiatrists have distanced themselves from the practice of psychotherapy and embraced the definition of psychiatry as strictly a medical discipline. Nevertheless, 50 percent of residents in psychiatric training are in therapy and believe that therapy is essential to becoming a psychiatrist (Weissman, 1994). The "art" of medicine resides in the understanding and expertise that addresses that which is human, such as relationships, conscious and unconscious thought, and the complexity of "volitional" behavior. Psychiatry, and medicine in general, would suffer tremendously if no medical discipline devoted its time and resources to the better understanding and practice of this art.

Concerns regarding cost of care and limited funding may preclude psychiatrists from only performing psychotherapy in the future. Psychiatric psychotherapy may one day be restricted to complicated patients with severe personality disorders or who require both medications and psychotherapy. Among injection drug-using individuals, there is evidence to suggest that the risk of drug overdose may exceed the progression of HIV disease; in one four-year study, drug overdose accounted for seventeen of twenty-five patients who died (Eskild et al., 1994). The role of a skilled psychotherapist with medical expertise needs to be better defined in working with such challenging patients. Because of their ability to integrate medical and psychosocial/spiritual perspectives, psychiatrists treating HIV/AIDS patients may be in a unique position to differentiate neurologic sequelae of the virus, psychiatric illness needing medications, psychological distress, and existential dilemmas. Research into the relationship between psychosocial factors and improved immunologic status and physical functioning needs to be a priority area for HIV psychiatric psychotherapy (Lutgendorf, Antoni, Schneiderman, & Fletcher, 1994).

### *Psychiatrist as Visionary*

The word *psychiatry* stems from the Greek for mind and soul; psychiatrists are healers of the mind and the soul. Advances in the late 20th century established a union among the mind, the soul, and the brain that should not end in divorce (Weissman, 1994). Psychiatrists must work diligently to strengthen this union if HIV/AIDS patients are to be served properly.

The changing demographics of the HIV/AIDS population suggest an increasing need for psychiatric services in the 21st century. As patients continue to live longer with the disease, there will be a greater opportunity for development of psychiatric illness, both as a result of HIV neurological disorders and as a reaction to living with a chronic illness. It is hoped that efforts to strengthen the collaborative partnerships among primary-care providers, nonphysician providers of mental health services, and psychiatrists will lead to increased recognition of psychiatric morbidity in HIV/AIDS patients, for diagnosis always precedes proper treatment. The epidemic's movement into populations with multiple problems increases the complexity of addressing psychiatric illness in HIV/AIDS patients.

Psychiatrists wishing to work with HIV/AIDS patients must prepare to leave the private practice and medical clinic settings in which they currently work. Creative treatment approaches, including housing programs for people with mental illness, substance use, and HIV disease, will need on-site psychiatric services in order to maintain these challenging patients in the community and to decrease the need for psychiatric or medical hospitalization. Mobile treatment units that meet patients where they live may be one option for the care of homeless, mentally ill, HIV-infected persons. Links among the public and the private sectors and university- and community-based agencies must be encouraged. Pooling academic and front-line resources will result in better understanding of the HIV population needing care, treatment ideas that work effectively, and archaic perspectives that must be abandoned.

Psychiatrists must fully engage in the effort to abolish the stigma associated with HIV/AIDS and mental illness. Working with other physicians, nonphysician providers of mental health care, patients, and families, psychiatrists can provide a unique perspective on the biopsychosocial/spiritual aspects of HIV disease and impact the highly political process that determines health policy. Until the economic stigma surrounding HIV disease and mental illness is decreased, HIV/AIDS patients needing psychiatric care will suffer.

The practice of psychiatry in the setting of HIV/AIDS must be determined by local circumstances and not merely by ideology (Ferguson & Varnam, 1994). The increasing complexity of mental illness in HIV-infected patients demands the best that all providers can offer. A collaborative model that empowers each care provider to address psychiatric illness in HIV from his or her unique perspective is the model of the future. In that model, psychiatrists clearly have a multifaceted role in the provision of services to HIV/AIDS patients, their families, and the other members of the treatment team.

General psychiatric practice of the future, as well as HIV-specific psychiatric practice, demands better definition of diagnostic subtypes in order to achieve improved treatment outcomes (Council on Long Range Planning and Development, 1990). Is the depression seen in an AIDS patient due to a "major depressive episode" or to depression associated with AIDS dementia? Do the two illnesses respond equally well to current modes of depression therapy, or does a different etiology require a different intervention? Improvement in diagnosis will also achieve more uniform application of diagnostic labels, resulting in better communication among care providers. Improvement in identification and communication will then allow a clearer definition of treatment outcomes, providing the opportunity for a clearer demonstration of benefit from psychiatric services. (Council on Long Range Planning and Development, 1990)

Future advances in the understanding of individual drug metabolism will facilitate more individualized dose-response targets for each patient (Michels & Markowitz, 1990). In other words, patients may one day benefit from truly individualized medication treatment plans, rather than population-based medication dosage recommendations. This is especially important in HIV/AIDS patients, who tend to be prescribed ten and twenty medications simultaneously (Greenblatt, Hollander, McMaster, & Henke, 1991), to be particularly susceptible to adverse medication effects (Harb, Alldredge, Coleman, & Jacobson, 1993), and to exhibit altered patterns of drug metabolism (Lee, Wong, Benowitz, & Sullam, 1993).

## *Tools for Clinical Practice: Utilizing a Psychiatrist*

Psychiatrists can serve many roles in the provision of care to HIV/AIDS patients, even when those patients receive the bulk of their care from other providers.

### *Psychopharmacology*

Many patients seek mental health care from a nonphysician provider because medication is not their treatment of choice. Patients deserve to have clear explanations of the risks and benefits of medication for a given psychiatric illness in making this choice.

*It is important for nonphysician providers of mental health care to HIV/AIDS patients to form a relationship with a psychiatrist for purposes of medication consultation and referral, by taking these steps:*

1. If possible, find a consultant with HIV/AIDS experience and interest. Medication management in HIV/AIDS patients is complex. Differentiating medication side effects from underlying illness or other possible causes requires special understanding of the biopsychosocial/spiritual aspects of HIV/AIDS.
2. Develop a relationship with the consultant before it is needed. It is always easier to call and ask a question of someone you know than it is to call someone "out of the blue." Be clear about your agenda in establishing a relationship with a consultant, and determine what the consultant sees as limitations to that relationship.
3. Remain neutral in your discussion with the client about the "best" treatment options. As in any other area of the therapeutic relationship, neutrality is vital. Allow exploration of issues such as whether to use medications or which particular medication is most appropriate. Help the individual to clarify his or her own biases without introducing your own.
4. If a referral for a medication evaluation is made, obtain releases of information, and provide the consultant with as much information about

the individual's illness and potential need for medication as possible. Important information to include in your referral includes:

- Demographics, such as age, ethnicity, and relationship status.
- HIV disease status, including category (A,B,C), T-helper (CD4) count/CD4%/viral load (if known). If you do not know or feel comfortable about gathering this information, give the psychiatrist the name and the phone number of the patient's physician.
- Past psychiatric diagnoses, including substance use.
- Current psychiatric diagnoses, including substance use.
- Current symptoms that suggest a need for medication (i.e., why you are making a referral).
- Past medication trials, if any, including the patient's experience with the medicine.
- Concerns the patient has expressed about seeing a psychiatrist or using medication.

In making a referral for a medication evaluation, it is important to be clear with the client and the consultant about the working relationships between each of you and how information will be shared after the consultation occurs.

### *Diagnostic Dilemmas*

In addition to helping to resolve psychopharmacology questions, psychiatrists can assist with diagnostic conundrums. As discussed previously, HIV/AIDS patients may have several things going on simultaneously: mental illness, substance use, HIV-related illness, and other physical illness. Obtaining a second opinion on a patient's condition can help clarify your treatment approach as well as reassure the patient, who may be concerned that symptoms represent the first stages of some frightening illness, such as dementia.

A unique aspect of HIV/AIDS is the psychiatric presentation of many serious, and in some cases life-threatening, neurological diseases. In cases where a client presents with psychiatric symptoms in the setting of severe immunocompromise (T-helper or CD4 count less than 200; CD4% less than 14), a psychiatric referral is indicated to ensure that a medical explanation for the symptoms cannot be found. In cases where the client is mildly to moderately immunocompromised (CD4 count between 200 and 500), a phone consultation is warranted to determine if further evaluation is necessary. It is important to remember that any change in mental status, even a relatively subtle one that develops over a period of weeks, may reflect an underlying physical problem. It is best to err on the side of referral. The nonphysician provider may be the first to encounter this change in the client and therefore has the responsibility of informing the patient's other providers if the patient cannot do this her- or himself.

## *Conclusion*

With HIV disease, the borders between the biological, psychological, social, and spiritual disappear. Individual practitioners, regardless of their disciplines, need to acknowledge this and practice accordingly. Institutions and agencies can no longer retain divisive care systems when dealing with a condition that demands new, integrated models of care. I believe that psychiatry has the opportunity to improve patients' lives significantly — to heal mind, soul, and brain. We now need dedication to that task.

## REFERENCES

This chapter was supported in part by grant BRH970127-02-0 provided by the Health Resources and Services Administration, Special Projects of National Significance. The views expressed are those of the author and do not represent those of HRSA.

American Psychiatric Association (1994). *Diagnostic and statistical manual of mental disorders* (4th Ed.) (DSM-IV). Washington, DC: Author.

Baer, J. W. (1988). Knowledge about AIDS among psychiatric inpatients. *Hospital and Community Psychiatry, 39,* 986–988.

Beresford, T. P., Blow, F. C., & Hall, R. C. W. (1986). AIDS encephalitis mimicking alcohol dementia and depression. *Biological Psychiatry, 21,* 394–397.

Boccellari, A., Dilley, J. W., & Shore, M. D. (1988). Neuropsychiatric aspects of AIDS dementia complex: a report on a clinical series. *Neurotoxicology, 9,* 381–389.

Carmen, E., & Brady, S. M. (1990). AIDS risk and prevention for the chronic mentally ill. *Hospital and Community Psychiatry, 41,* 652–657.

Coates, T. J., Stall, R., Mandel, J. S., Boccellari, A., Sorensen, J. L., Morales, E. F., Morin, S. F., Wiley, J. A., & McKusick, L. (1987). AIDS: a psychosocial research agenda. *Annals of Behavioral Medicine, 9,* 21–28.

Cote, T. R., Biggar, R. J., & Dannenberg, A. L. (1992). Risk of suicide among persons with AIDS. *Journal of the American Medical Association, 268,* 2066–2068.

Council on Long Range Planning and Development (1990). The future of psychiatry. *Journal of the American Medical Association, 264,* 2542–2548.

Cournos, F., Empfield, M., & Horwath, E. (1991). HIV seroprevalence among patients admitted to two psychiatric hospitals. *American Journal of Psychiatry, 148,* 1225–1230.

Dorrell, L., Snow, M. H., & Ong, E. L. (1995). Mortality and survival trends in patients with AIDS in north east England from 1984–1992. *Journal of Infection, 30,* 23–27.

Eskild, A., Magnus, P., Sohlberg, C., Kittelsen, P., Olving, J. H., Teige, B., & Skullerud, K. (1994). Slow progression to AIDS in intravenous drug users infected with HIV in Norway. *Journal of Epidemiology and Community Health, 48,* 383–387.

Farmer, P., & Kleinman, A. (1989). AIDS as human suffering. *Proceedings of the American Academy of Arts and Sciences, 118,* 135–160.

Ferguson, B. G., & Varnam, M. A. (1994). The relationship between primary care and psychiatry: an opportunity for change. *British Journal of General Practice, 44,* 527–530.

Fernandez, F., & Levy, J. K. (1989). Management of delirium in terminally ill AIDS patients. *International Journal of Psychiatry and Medicine, 19,* 165–172.

Greenblatt, R. M., Hollander, H., McMaster, J. R., & Henke C. J. (1991). Polypharmacy among patients attending an AIDS clinic: utilization of prescribed, unorthodox, and investigational treatments. *Journal of Acquired Immune Deficiency Syndromes, 4,* 136–143.

Harb, G. E., Alldredge, B. K., Coleman, R., & Jacobson, M. A. (1993). Pharmacoepidemiology of adverse drug reactions in hospitalized patients with human immunodeficiency virus disease. *Journal of Acquired Immune Deficiency Syndromes, 6,* 919–926.

Hogg, R. S., Strathdee, S. A., Craib, K. J., O'Shaughnessy, M. V., Montaner, J. S., & Schecter, M. T. (1994). Lower socioeconomic status and shorter survival following HIV infection. *Lancet, 344,* 1120–1124.

Kelly, J. A. (1992). AIDS/HIV risk behavior among the chronically mentally ill. *American Journal of Psychiatry, 149,* 886–889.

Kermani, E. J., Borod, J. C., & Brown, P. H. (1985). New psychopathologic findings in AIDS: case report. *Journal of Clinical Psychiatry, 46,* 240–241.

Koenig, H. G., Meador, K. G., Cohen, H. J., & Blazer, D. G. (1988). Detection and treatment of major depression in older medically ill hospitalized patients. *International Journal of Psychiatry and Medicine, 18,* 17–31.

Kuhn, C. C. (1988). A spiritual inventory of the medically ill patient. *Psychiatric Medicine, 6,* 87–99.

Lee, B. L., Wong, D., Benowitz, N. L., & Sullam, P. M. (1993). Altered patterns of drug metabolism in patients with acquired immunodeficiency syndrome. *Clinical Pharmacology and Therapeutics, 53,* 529–535.

Lee, H. K., Travin, S., & Bluestone, H. (1992). Relationship between HIV-1 antibody seropositivity and alcohol/nonintravenous drug abuse among psychiatric inpatients. *American Journal of Addiction, 1,* 85–88.

Lutgendorf, S., Antoni, M. H., Schneiderman, N., & Fletcher, M. A. (1994). Psychosocial counseling to improve quality of life in HIV infection. *Patient Education and Counseling, 24,* 217–235.

Mahler, J., Yi, D., & Sacks, M. (1994). Undetected HIV infection among patients admitted to an alcohol rehabilitation unit. *American Journal of Psychiatry, 151,* 439–440.

Maj, M., Janssen, R., & Starace, F. (1994). WHO neuropsychiatric AIDS study, cross-sectional phase I. *Archives of General Psychiatry, 51,* 39–49.

Mayou, R., Hawton, K., & Feldman, E. (1988). What happens to medical patients with psychiatric disorder? *Journal of Psychosomatic Research, 32,* 541–549.

McArthur, J. C. (1987). Neurological manifestations of AIDS. *Medicine, 66,* 407–437.

McKegney, F. P., & O'Dowd, M. A. (1992). Suicidality and HIV status. *American Journal of Psychiatry, 149,* 396–398.

Meyer, I., McKinnon, K., & Cournos, F. (1993). HIV seroprevalence among long-stay patients in a state hospital. *Hospital and Community Psychiatry, 44,* 282–284.

Michels, R., & Markowitz, J. C. (1990). The future of psychiatry. *Journal of Medicine and Philosophy, 15,* 5–19.

Navia, B. A., & Price, R. W. (1987). The acquired immunodeficiency syndrome dementia complex as the presenting or sole manifestation of human immunodeficiency virus infection. *Archives of Neurology, 44,* 65–69.

Ormel, J., Koeter, M., van der Bruik, W., & van de Willige, G. (1990). Recognition, management and course of anxiety and depression in general practice. *Archives of General Psychiatry, 48,* 700–706.

Osmond, D., Charlebois, E., Lang, W., Shiboski, S., & Moss, A. (1994). Changes in AIDS survival time in two San Francisco cohorts of homosexual men, 1983 to 1993. *Journal of the American Medical Association, 271,* 1083–1087.

Perry, S. W., & Jacobsen, P. (1986). Neuropsychiatric manifestations of AIDS-spectrum disorders. *Hospital and Community Psychiatry, 37,* 135–142.

Price, W. A., & Forejt, J. (1988). Neuropsychiatric aspects of AIDS: a case report. *General Hospital Psychiatry, 8,* 7–10.

Rabkin, J. G., Rabkin, R., Harrison, W., & Wagner, G. (1994). Effect of imipramine on mood and enumerative measures of immune status in depressed patients with HIV illness. *American Journal of Psychiatry, 151,* 516–523.

Rabkin, J. G., Williams, J. B. W., Neugebauer, R., Remien, R. H., & Goetz, R. (1990). Maintenance of hope in HIV-spectrum homosexual men. *American Journal of Psychiatry, 147,* 1322–1326.

Rait, D. S. (1991). The family context of AIDS. *Psychiatric Medicine, 9,* 423–439.

Regier, D., Goldberg, I. D., & Taube, C. A. (1978). The de facto mental health services system. *Archives of General Psychiatry, 35,* 685–693.

Rundell, J. R., Wise, M. G., & Ursano, R. J. (1986). Three cases of AIDS-related psychiatric disorders. *American Journal of Psychiatry, 143,* 777–778.

Sacks, M. (1990). Self-reported HIV-related risk behaviors in acute psychiatric inpatients: a pilot study. *Hospital and Community Psychiatry, 41,* 1253–1255.

Sacks, M., Dermatis, H., & Looser-Ott, S. (1992). Seroprevalence of HIV and risk factors for AIDS in psychiatric inpatients. *Hospital and Community Psychiatry, 43,* 736–737.

Schleifer, S. J., Keller, S. E., & Franklin, J. E. (1990). HIV seropositivity in inner-city alcoholics. *Hospital and Community Psychiatry, 41,* 248–254.

Schmidt, U., & Miller, D. (1988). Two cases of hypomania in AIDS. *British Journal of Psychiatry, 152,* 839–842.

Streim, J. E., & Katz, I. R. (1995). The psychiatrist in the nursing home. *Psychiatric Services, 46,* 339–341.

Weissman, S. (1994). American psychiatry in the 21st century: the discipline, its practice, and its work force. *Bulletin of the Menninger Clinic, 58,* 502–518.

Winiarski, M. G. (1991). *AIDS-related psychotherapy.* New York: Pergamon Press (now distributed by Allyn & Bacon, Needham Heights, MA).

World Health Organization (1989). Report of the consultation on the neuropsychiatric aspects of HIV infection. *AIDS: Profile of an Epidemic,* Scientific Publication No. 514, Washington, D.C.

Yarnell, S. K., & Battin, M. P. (1988). AIDS, psychiatry and euthanasia. *Psychiatric Annals, 18,* 594–603.

# 8 | Secondary Prevention: Working with People with HIV to Prevent Transmission to Others

*Kathy Parish*

When John and Susan married eighteen years ago, they thought his hemophilia would be their greatest health challenge. Having learned to live with its unpredictability and treatment needs, they went on to have two children, at which point they decided that their family was complete. John had a vasectomy, and they threw away Susan's diaphragm. About twelve years ago, though, they started hearing concerns about AIDS being transmitted through the blood supply. John was told that he might be at risk for contracting the AIDS virus but that the blood supply was thought to be pretty safe by then and that, anyway, not treating his hemophilia with the blood product factor concentrate would most certainly have negative consequences, as compared to the small possibility that he would get AIDS.

In 1986 John was tested and learned he was infected with HIV. Susan was tested as well, and she was not infected. Thus, they learned they were a "serodiscordant couple," and they were advised to practice safer sex by using condoms. They had many reactions: shock, disbelief, and fear about his diagnosis; different coping styles that sometimes clashed; fear of John's dying; fear of giving or getting the virus; anger at the doctors and the government; confusion, distrust, resentment, and discomfort about having to use condoms, when they had no experience using them and had no need for birth control. This was not a simple safer-sex crisis. A multitude of emotional, psychological, and social reactions to the infection and the threat of disease all combined with the need to change their sexual behavior, draining them of their coping abilities.

John heard from other men with hemophilia that HIV was rarely transmitted in heterosexual couples. Susan was told by her physician that if they avoided anal intercourse, they would have nothing to worry about. They tried to use condoms occasionally but felt that it interrupted the spontaneity of lovemaking and served as a reminder of his illness, robbing them of romance. They didn't always have condoms when they needed them and would usually just skip them entirely if they had had anything to drink. After a while, they found they were having sex less often and feeling less emotional intimacy, as well. Neither one could talk about his or her fears, out of concern of upsetting the other. Their families and friends did not know about John's HIV infection, so there was no one else with whom to talk. Susan became depressed; John became angry and estranged. The children had no idea what was happening but knew that there was a great deal of tension and unhappiness in the home. They worried that their parents might divorce.

I first met John and Susan at the hemophilia treatment center where I had been hired as a psychologist focusing on risk-reduction counseling. They arrived for their first appointment, a part of John's annual evaluation for his hemophilia, with many questions, much anxiety, and considerable embarrassment about addressing such a personal area. My role was to provide a secondary prevention intervention, but clearly this would be a complex task.

As a risk-reduction counselor and psychologist, I need to be concerned with all aspects of the patient's and the partner's functioning — physical, emotional, and social — and acutely aware of the interplay of each of these with relationship dynamics and sexual behavior. This vignette portrays some of the array of issues that may be present in people who are facing the potential for transmitting HIV from one partner to the other and the demands placed upon the counseling task.

## *Background Reading*

If public health efforts for reducing the risk of transmission of HIV were to be concentrated where they would have the most potential for positive effect, it would make sense to start with those people currently in a position to directly affect transmission: the people with HIV themselves and their sexual partners (Wenger, Kusseling, Beck, & Shapiro, 1994). HIV infection does not preclude sexuality and sexual behavior. Many HIV-positive people continue to have sex, and those uninvolved may seek romantic relationships, although their attitudes about relationships and condoms may vary (Norman, Parish, & Kennedy, 1995). It is not known how often HIV-infected people put someone else at risk, although studies have indicated that up to 40 percent might have unprotected sex after notification of their positive HIV serostatus (Parish, Mandel, Thomas, & Gomperts, 1989; Wenger et al., 1994; Wiley, Hannan, Barrett, & Evatt, 1994). In men with hemophilia, a heterosexual population with a high rate of HIV infection, approximately 10.6 percent of the female sexual partners are known to be HIV-infected as well (Wiley, Hannan, Barrett, & Evatt, 1994).

Surprisingly, though, most of the literature on HIV risk reduction deals with primary prevention, defined as working with uninfected persons, and sometimes with populations that face only minimal risk, such as college students, but which are more accessible for study. In an extensive review of HIV prevention literature, Choi and Coates (1994) identified very few studies dealing with secondary prevention, defined as working with infected persons, and those studies involved primarily discordant heterosexual couples. By a large margin, primary prevention is emphasized in intervention planning and evaluation, focusing on self-interest as a motivator.

Furthermore, even those writings that deal with the health needs and the medical treatment of people who are infected with HIV pay minimal or no attention to prevention of HIV transmission. If anything about transmission is noted, the focus is on transmission rates and predisposing factors for unsafe sex, rather than on interventions (Sherr, 1993). Risk-reduction programs for secondary prevention belong directly in primary-care clinics caring for HIV-positive patients (Wenger et al., 1994), combining state of the art treatment and behavioral approaches (Francis et al., 1989).

Perhaps there is an assumption that without a self-protective motive it would be difficult to persuade people to change their sexual behavior. Indeed, the motivation in the case of people who already have HIV infection needs to be altruistic: to protect someone else by giving up something valuable (unprotected sex). Probably there exists some doubt that people would be that altruistic, that they would care about their partners' safety more than their own basic gratification. Sometimes, the partners themselves might not be cooperative, believing that it is their fate to take the risk and perhaps to die along with their mates, in a Romeo-and-Juliet scenario. Unfortunately, the timing rarely works out that way when a partner becomes infected, and regrets, remorse, guilt, and anger are more likely outcomes.

Some believe that the sex drive is so strong, the sense of altruism so remote, and the behavior change to abstinence or safer sex so complex and difficult that there is no way to stop transmission once one partner in a couple has HIV, and thus there is little point in trying. At least some of the time, perhaps much of the time, people with HIV do care to keep their partners from getting the virus that infects them. It is true that it is difficult to change sexual behavior, because the activity of unsafe sex is highly reinforcing, strongly motivated, and often well established (Kelly, 1991). As with any other behavior change goal, however, people are more likely to practice safer sex when they believe the recommended means to be efficacious (that condoms really do work to prevent HIV transmission) (Centers for Disease Control, 1993; Feldblum, 1991); when they believe that they are self-efficacious and possess the necessary skills (that they are capable of negotiating and using condoms consistently) (Kelly, 1991); and when they believe that there are strong advantages to using condoms (such as making sex safe and removing fear). Couple counseling with serodiscordant couples has been shown to be effective in changing sexual behavior (Kamenga et al., 1990; Padian, O'Brien, Chang, Glass, & Francis, 1993). Simply notifying people of their HIV status, however, is not adequate intervention. After a group of blood donors were notified of their positive serostatus, more than one third still engaged in unsafe sex (Cleary et al., 1991).

In dealing with the epidemic of this disease, secondary prevention is critical. Sexual partners of people with HIV are the most at risk, and they should be the primary targets of risk-reduction efforts, since such interventions are likely to have the most directed impact. Furthermore, secondary prevention with women with HIV or female partners of men with HIV involves intervening to reduce the risk of HIV transmission perinatally to offspring, by means of informed decision making about getting pregnant, carrying a baby to term, accepting medical treatment, and declining to breast-feed (Benson & Shannon, 1995; Kurth, 1995).

Efforts at secondary prevention that are reported in the literature include several populations and approaches. In studying HIV-positive women and childbearing decisions, Kline and VanLandingham (1994) noted that partner-related factors, such as whether a partner is seronegative, whether the woman has a sense of power in the relationship, and whether there are conflicts between the woman and her partner, were important for HIV-positive women in determining their approach to safer sex and childbearing decision making. Another study found that after HIV testing, those women who were HIV-positive demonstrated a considerable decline in their desire for pregnancy and an increase in their use of condoms, but only to 54 percent (Lai, 1994). The author cited the need for adequate counseling, beyond disclosure of serostatus, to help bring about critical behavior changes.

The sexual practices of persons with hemophilia and HIV were described and the potential for heterosexual transmission was raised as a concern by Lawrence and colleagues (1989), but their recommendation that female partners should be sure to abstain or change their sexual behavior suggests a lack of appreciation for the role played by gender power differences within relationships.

There appears to be an important link between safer sex and communication, which has important bearing on secondary prevention. HIV-positive persons having unprotected sex with partners at risk for HIV transmission often relate discomfort in discussing HIV with others (Wenger et al., 1994). Sexual partners are often unaware of the other person's HIV infection (Marks, Richardson, & Maldonado, 1991; Wenger et al., 1994). Marks and colleagues (1991) state that people who are HIV-positive and who have sex have a social and legal responsibility to disclose their infection to their partners, or else there is increased potential for transmission and infecting others. In one study, HIV-infected women stated that ethical responsibility and concern for partners' health led to disclosure to partners and that a desire for support was the reason for disclosing to family and friends (Simoni et al., 1995). Cultural factors also influence rates of disclosure; the same study found lower rates of disclosure among Spanish-speaking Latinas than among English-speaking Latinas, African Americans, and Anglo Americans. Catania et al. (1992), in a study of 1,229 San Francisco households, found a correlation between sexual communication and condom use across gender and sexual orientation and concluded that condom promotion programs should build sexual communication skills. Discussion of safer sex by an HIV-infected person with a partner was the strongest predictor of consistent condom use in a study of 351 adults with hemophilia, supporting the conclusion that sexual communication is a key factor in risk reduction (Parish, Mandel, Thomas, & Gomperts, 1989). In one study, repeated counseling was shown to lead to increased disclosure of serostatus to partners of HIV-positive adults, and perceived social support further predicted self-disclosure (Perry et al., 1994). However, one third of the sexually active subjects still did not disclose their HIV infection to any current sex partner after counseling, although very few reported unsafe sex. Thus, self-disclosure and safer sex may be related in some cases, but not necessarily in all.

## *My Clinical Work*

At Huntington Hospital Hemophilia Center in Pasadena, California, my work as a psychologist has involved clinical practice and clinical intervention research in secondary prevention of HIV transmission. The patient population comprises people with hemophilia and related bleeding disorders, most of whom are followed on a lifelong regular basis for comprehensive medical and psychosocial care by hemophilia treatment centers. Hemophilia is a genetic blood-clotting disorder affecting all racial, cultural, and socioeconomic groups and thus creating a community otherwise representative of the general population.

By the mid-1980s it became clear that the agent causing AIDS was linked to blood and that people with hemophilia were infected in large numbers. Approximately 70 percent of people with hemophilia, including 90 percent of severe factor VIII deficiency, the most common type of hemophilia, were infected before the pooled blood product used in their treatment could be produced safely (Gomperts, 1990). In 1986 the U.S. Maternal and Child Health Bureau and the Centers for Disease Control stepped in with programming and funding to provide psychosocial support and risk reduction, spurred on by the potential for a second wave of the epidemic that would involve sexual partners and their newborns. Even before this point, however, hemophilia treatment centers had begun to encourage safer sex practices among their patients (Mason, Olson, & Parish, 1988).

At Huntington Hospital Hemophilia Center, a risk-reduction clinical model was developed that would provide a separate risk-reduction session for patients during their annual comprehensive evaluations, in addition to social work, nursing, and physician meetings, to which partners are invited as well. As part of the risk-reduction services, we offer free confidential or anonymous testing for partners; free condoms and safer sex literature; counseling for adolescents as a frank and routine part of their medical care; and separate counseling for partners or for parents of adolescents, as requested. The risk-reduction sessions for children are designed to make it comfortable to address any questions about HIV, hemophilia, or sexuality and to promote communication skills and self-esteem as a foundation for later dealing with safer sex.

Our center is also participating as a site for the adult Hemophilia Behavioral Intervention Evaluation Project, in collaboration with the Centers for Disease Control and Prevention and five other national sites. This project involves developing and piloting an individualized intervention to reduce HIV transmission between men with HIV and hemophilia and their female partners. The intervention makes use of a stage-based behavioral approach, developed from the Transtheoretical Model of Behavior Change (Prochaska, DiClemente, & Norcross, 1992), in which sexual behavior change is conceptualized as a process through stages, each approached with different strategies. The intervention that was developed for this project is designed to enhance communication skills and was offered to participants either individually or in group retreat settings. The interventions were very well received by participants, and components of this stage-based, communication skills approach may be valuable in secondary prevention with other populations, as well.

Several tenets emerge as important in HIV transmission prevention counseling for people who are HIV-infected and their sexual partners. First is the belief that people with HIV, like anyone else, need and deserve to have closeness, caring, and connectedness in their lives. It is normal and healthy to seek sexual expression and intimacy. Becoming sexually involved when an individual has HIV does, however, raise some unique issues. These issues include disclosing HIV status to a partner, communicating feelings and concerns about sexuality, and negotiating and making decisions about having safe and healthy sex. Effective HIV safer-sex counseling, then, is best delivered in a trusting relationship, in which information about reducing the risk of transmission is offered thoroughly and sensitively and with respect for the needs, problems, and cultural context of the individual or couple being counseled. Safer-sex counseling is best offered in the context of supporting people in dealing with HIV, and with life in general, in a broad, whole-person perspective. It deals with both sexuality and loss. It requires that the counselor be self-aware of values, beliefs, and feelings elicited by the work, especially about sexuality, illness, and death, and be willing to deal with these honestly and to get help when needed.

## *Barriers to Effective Secondary Prevention*

The barriers to effective secondary prevention of HIV transmission are many but fall into categories: those arising from the HIV-infected persons, from the partners, from the culture/social system, and from the counselor or agency. The case study about John and Susan at the beginning of the chapter demonstrates a few of the barriers.

- One barrier is a sense of unfairness. John and Susan had already been faced with one illness and had managed that one, and they had taken other measures to avoid pregnancy — a vasectomy — and figured that they wouldn't have to deal with birth control (i.e., condoms) again. For others, the problem is that they still wish to have children, and their goals for safety and pregnancy conflict; actually, in the first years of safer-sex recommendations, the birth rate among people with hemophilia increased. These issues involve losses and resentments that, unresolved, stand in the way of making healthy behavioral choices and changes.
- John and Susan had never used condoms before, having relied on birth control pills and the diaphragm, as did most of their contemporaries, so condom use presented a further barrier, the need to learn a new behavior. Their negative feelings about condoms and their failure to keep them always available stood in the way of using them all the time. It is often the case that use of alcohol or drugs reduces the likelihood of condom use, too.
- At first, John's doctor was reluctant to have him tested for HIV, because he felt that it would upset him beyond his coping abilities and because there was no treatment to offer. Years later, this reluctance is less common, but many HIV-infected people say that they began to practice safer sex consistently only after receiving their test results. Thus, any barrier to testing — attitudes, fears, stigma, or practical matters of cost, access, or confidentiality — has the potential to impede safer sex.
- Lack of accurate information, or misinformation, represents another barrier to secondary prevention. John and Susan had both been given inaccurate information from lay and professional peo-

ple, giving them a false sense of security about having unprotected sex.

- John and Susan's decision not to disclose John's HIV infection to family and friends left them isolated and growing apart from each other. Many people make the decision to keep HIV a secret because they fear rejection and discrimination, having heard of people forced out of school or work or burned out of their house. Not only does secrecy cut people off from receiving the support of others; it impedes a self-acceptance that is a critical part of the process of behavior change and the decision to protect a partner or oneself.
- Sometimes, partners know little or nothing about the risk they face, and not being able to talk with a partner directly is a barrier for the counselor. When the partner is not informed, he or she cannot share the responsibility for safer sex. Other times, a partner knows of the HIV infection but takes the position that "if he goes, I might as well go, too," something of a Romeo and Juliet theme. Such situations suggest an overuse of denial. At the same time, it is important to note that denial is often encouraged and reinforced among people dealing with chronic disease: Such behavior is seen as brave or stoic. It shouldn't be surprising that denial is so widely employed, especially by people with lifelong chronic illness, such as hemophilia.
- Some messages about safer sex conflict with some religions, social behavior in some groups, and values held by people of various ages, races, or political beliefs. The relative lack of power held by women in many relationships stands in the way of their asserting their right to refuse unsafe sex or to insist on condoms.
- Sex is considered a highly private, sensitive area of most people's lives, and reactions to discussions of safer sex may range from being uncomfortable to being insulted to being completely unwilling to discuss the subject with a counselor or any health care provider. Professionals themselves may feel embarrassed, unskilled, or intrusive about opening up sexual issues and may avoid the topic or communicate their wish to end the conversation quickly.
- Illness symptoms can get in the way of secondary prevention. Dementia, fatigue, distorted thinking, reduced capacity to reason or problem-solve, and suspicion can manifest with HIV/AIDS,

and each of these problems makes it difficult for a person to understand, decide, make changes, and trust. People with HIV infection and their partners experience behavioral and physical barriers to using condoms: discomfort, loss of sensation, outright dislike, loss of spontaneity, and allergic sensitivity to latex or lubricants. On a more subtle plane, clients tell us that talking about and practicing safer sex can serve as painful reminders of the disease, thereby taking away a sense of pleasure and intimacy in sex, or lead to negative emotional reactions in one's partner, creating powerful emotional barriers (Parish, Cotton, Huszti, & Parsons, 1993).

## *Tools for Clinical Practice*

The following are important points to consider in risk-reduction counseling:

- *Risk-reduction sessions must be tailored to the client and carefully planned from a menu of topics, and they should include a risk-reduction plan.*

  The following topics are typically covered during a risk-reduction session. Not all topics are relevant for each person, and not all are covered each time. Also, the order of presentation will vary. The counselor can make an attempt to assess which of these are important for the patient and the situation and focus on these topics first.

  — Sexual history. The meaning of sexuality in the person's life is explored, as well as sexual activity in the past year and before. Changes in sexual behavior, interest, and attitudes are assessed. Beyond these basics, it is also important to ask about how illness and disability affect sexuality and sexual self-image for the patient and the partner, keeping in mind that sexual development continues through the lifespan, not only in adolescence.

  — Update of current information about reducing the risk of sexual transmission. Use and efficacy of condoms is reviewed. Condom breakage or other problems are assessed, and suggestions are discussed to address these. Choice of condom type/brands, other contraceptives, female condoms, and allergies or sensitivities are discussed. Information about other STDs and protection from and treatment for these is presented.

— Deciding on a risk-reduction plan. In this area, the health care provider covers various sexual practices and how to evaluate risks and protect against transmission. The discussion also includes an exploration of communication and negotiation with the sexual partner and elicits issues and concerns or problems in talking about and practicing safer sex with that partner. The counselor can suggest strategies to support behavior change and to avoid "relapse" to unsafe sexual behavior.

— Building and enhancing a safer-sex repertoire. Sexual practices other than penetrative intercourse can be explored, evaluating risk in each case. The idea is to promote thinking about and experiencing sex and intimacy creatively. For those clients who no longer have sex, or who have it less often than they wish, discussion may be opened about any desire to restore sexual activity and to increase intimacy and sexual satisfaction while still protecting one's partner from transmission.

— Casual transmission. Equal in importance to discussion about how HIV is transmitted is discussion about how it is not transmitted. It is important to explore for myths and unsubstantiated concerns that are hampering an individual's behavior towards others, participation in routine activities, or positive self-image. At the same time, routine household blood safety precautions and feelings and behaviors about these practices are reviewed.

— Relationships with partners. This area includes a broader discussion about needs for intimacy and how to meet them. Single patients may want to talk about their concerns regarding dating, getting involved, and coping with loneliness, and patients with partners may have concerns about relationship satisfaction and maintaining intimacy in a healthy relationship.

— Partner testing. The importance and purpose of repeated HIV testing for partners is presented. It is also important to cover the meaning of test results and any difficulties or barriers to testing, ranging from access to attitudes. Former partners may need to be notified about their possible risk, and patients may need assistance in getting word to them and encouraging them to be tested.

— Communicating with the partner. Here, the patient's experience in talking with a partner about safer sex and his or her ability to do so is assessed. This kind of communication involves an open sharing of needs, feelings, and problems. Communication skills, including problem-solving and assertiveness skills, can be taught and encouraged. For those people without partners, the most essential communication task is the disclosure of one's HIV status to a new partner. This disclosure can be discussed, planned, and practiced with a supportive provider.

— Communicating with others. Closely tied to communication with partners are issues about disclosing HIV status to family members and to support systems, along with concerns about discrimination, stigma, and rejection. For those patients with children, there is a unique need to determine if, when, and how to talk with them about a parent's HIV disease.

— Having children. The desire to have children, the decisions that are facing couples, and the feelings involved are discussed. Risks of transmission to mother and offspring are presented, and options (including donor insemination, adoption, involvement with the children of others, and methods to reduce risk in conceiving) and the pros and cons of each are explored. For those who have put aside plans to have children, support is offered for dealing with feelings about not having one's own children.

— Coping. The patient's overall well-being, ability to function emotionally and socially, and ability to cope with hemophilia and HIV within his or her life circumstances are assessed. Coping strategies and mechanisms that work or backfire are explored, and together the patient and health care provider problem-solve for responses to some of the challenges. This area is closely tied to safer sex, as a person's ability to cope in general with life demands highly influences his or her ability to maintain relationships and safer-sex practices.

— Loss and grieving. The patient with HIV faces multiple losses in functioning, opportunities, dreams, and intentions, as well as in physical health and anticipated life span, and the counselor needs to become aware of and to acknowledge these losses. Assistance is offered in understanding and addressing the needs of other family members. Support is offered for grieving what is lost in relationships and sexuality, in particular, as an essential step before a person can move on to live fully within the limits imposed by HIV infection.

- *To be effective in secondary prevention, the counselor is advised to begin with the client's agenda.*

  Although you may want to move into talking about safer sex right away, this may not be where the client's attention is directed. Since the focus of these interventions is on relationships, it is important to establish one with the client that communicates respect and interest in the client's needs and issues.
- *Keep a broad perspective.*

  Sex, and safer sex, are integral parts of a person's life, connected to needs and relationships in more general terms — intimacy and loneliness, physical and emotional well-being, self-image and self-esteem, personal strength, child-bearing, and hope for the future.
- *Deal with coping with HIV as well.*

  HIV and safer sex are fairly inseparable. Each serves as a reminder to the person of the other. Learning to live with HIV helps make safer sex possible. It's about multiple losses: As more and more aspects, capabilities, and dreams are lost, the sense of loss can be overwhelming, and having to give up freedom in expressing sexuality can feel like the last, impossible straw.
- *Deal with grief.*

  All the multiple losses add up to having one's usual life die off, one or a few pieces at a time. In sexuality, there is grief over what is no longer safely or physically possible: sex without condoms, sex with health and vigor, sex without fatigue and pain, sex to conceive a child. To resolve these losses, it is necessary to mourn, to feel sorrow and other grieving feelings, before a person can move on and look to live life and experience sexuality or intimacy differently. (See chapter 5.)
- *Address fears.*

  It is important to discuss fears, founded or not. Some people are so afraid of transmitting the virus that they avoid even casual contact with others. Clearly, they need a different message from those who don't appear to care about unprotected sex. Single people with HIV infection may fear getting involved and being rejected. Once in a relationship, some individuals fear becoming dependent on a partner or caring so much that dying is made more painful. Fears about getting sick and dying get involved in sexual behavior, along with fear that those events will adversely affect the people for whom they care. In working through a person's fears, listening with empathy and concern is much more helpful than advice and halfhearted solutions. Counseling can provide a precious opportunity to talk, to be acknowledged, to be listened to, about the most taboo issues in our culture—sex and death.

- *Talk about disclosure of HIV serostatus to partners and others.*

  Disclosure of one's HIV infection can mark the beginning of working together on risk reduction, but it is fraught with risk of rejection. As a relationship grows, disclosure becomes ever more difficult, especially if sex, even protected, has occurred without the partner's being aware that he or she faces HIV risk. Exploring the options, working on different ways of presenting the information, and practicing with a counselor and feeling supported in taking on a difficult task can help a client sort out the pros and cons of disclosing.
- *Consider facilitating networking or group support.*

  It is believed that people who have social support are more likely to maintain safer sex behavior, perhaps mediated by increased self-esteem. HIV is a tremendously isolating disease, and even after committing to practice safer sex, HIV-infected people may need social support to help maintain the new behavior. Support groups and retreats for people with HIV and even newsletters and Internet chats can provide an important sense of connection.
- *Encourage empathy, sexual assertiveness, and communication skills.*

  For people with HIV infection, the motive for HIV-transmission prevention has to be altruistic, rather than self-protective or overtly self-beneficial. Exploring questions such as, "How would you feel if someone were carrying an infection that could be devastating to you and didn't tell you?" and role-playing the role of a partner are possible means of facilitating an altruistic response. For HIV-infected individuals as well as their partners, the ability to say no to unsafe sex and to communicate what they can feel comfortable with are important communication skills that a counselor can help develop.

- *Individualize the intervention, taking into consideration the person's readiness to change.*

  For people who are not yet ready to make a change to safer sex, raising their consciousness about the importance of protection and exploring with them the pros and cons of safer sex will likely prove helpful. For people who have been using condoms faithfully for months or years but who don't want to risk relapsing, however, these approaches will likely hold little value, compared to evaluating interpersonal and intrapersonal mechanisms to make maintenance of the behavior easier.

- *Welcome further questions; admit what you don't know; develop resources to get answers for clients.*

  It is of no help to clients to give information about which you're unsure, especially when the consequences of misinformation can be so serious. It is a better idea to work hard to learn and keep up with developments and to be honest about what you don't know and then offer to get answers and get back to the client. There are many resources for up-to-date information, including AIDS projects, the National AIDS Clearinghouse, the Centers for Disease Control, newsletters, and researchers, and every counselor can develop the resources needed to get information (see appendix B).

  Many times as a counselor doing secondary prevention work, you can be left feeling that there is much more to cover, more that needs to be imparted, more that needs to be changed. It's far better to create or build on a good working relationship with a client who will be willing to return, however, than to overwhelm or fail to establish adequate rapport with the client and never have another chance to talk. Sometimes, it is possible only to plant a seed, to lay a groundwork for the next step.

To follow these recommendations for secondary prevention, the counselor must work at self-awareness and the processing of feelings, reactions, and values that are regularly churned up in this work. She or he must work to enhance and expand communication, relating, and counseling skills, to reach out creatively to varied people with many needs, and to be nonjudgmental and empathic. Finally, the counselor should consider the impact she or he can have not only on an individual but on a partner, a couple, a family, a network, a community, as well as on society and on institutional and governmental entities, in facilitating understanding, sensitivity, and changes that create a supportive climate for the prevention of further HIV transmission.

## REFERENCES

Benson, M., & Shannon, M. (1995). Nevirapine: Ethical dilemmas and care for HIV-infected mothers. *Focus: A Guide to AIDS Research and Counseling, 10*(7), 5–6.

Catania, J. A., Coates, T. J., Kegeles, S., Thompson-Fullilove, M., Peterson, J., Marin, B., Siegel, D., & Hulley, S. (1992). Condom use in multi-ethnic neighborhoods of San Francisco: The population-based AMEN (AIDS in Multi-Ethnic Neighborhoods) study. *American Journal of Public Health, 82,* 284–287.

Centers for Disease Control (1993, August 6). Update: Barrier protection against HIV infection and other sexually transmitted diseases. *Morbidity and Mortality Weekly Report, 42,* 589–591, 597.

Choi, K., & Coates, T. J. (1994). Prevention of HIV infection. *AIDS, 8,* 1371–1389.

Cleary, P. D., Van Devanter, N., Rogers, T. F., Singer, E., Shipton-Levy, R., Steilen, M., Stuart, A., Avorn, J., & Pindyck, J. (1991). Behavior changes after notification of HIV infection. *American Journal of Public Health, 81,* 1586–1590.

Feldblum, P. (1991). Results from prospective studies of HIV discordant couples. *AIDS, 5,* 1265–1266.

Francis, D. P., Anderson, R. E., Gorman, M. E., Fenstersheib, M., Padian, N. S., Kizer, K. W., & Conant, M. A. (1989). Targeting AIDS prevention and treatment toward HIV-1-infected persons. *Journal of the American Medical Association, 262,* 2572–2576.

Gomperts, E. (1990). HIV infection in hemophiliac children: Clinical manifestations and therapy. *American Journal of Pediatric Hematology and Oncology, 12,* 497–504.

Kamenga, M., Ryder, R. W., Jingu, M., Mbuyi, N., Mbu, L., Behets, F., Brown, C., & Heyward, W. L. (1990). Evidence of marked sexual behavior change associated with low HIV-1 seroconversion in 149 married couples with discordant HIV-1 serostatus: experience at an HIV counselling center in Zaire. *AIDS, 5,* 61–67.

Kelly, J. A. (1991). Changing the behavior of an HIV-seropositive man who practices unsafe sex. *Hospital and Community Psychiatry, 42,* 239–240, 264.

Kline, A., & VanLandingham, M. (1994). HIV-infected women and sexual risk reduction: the relevance of existing models of behavior change. *AIDS Education and Prevention, 6,* 390–402.

Kurth, A. (1995). HIV disease and reproductive counseling. *Focus: A Guide to AIDS Research and Counseling, 10(7),* 1–4.

Lai, K. K. (1994). Attitudes toward childbearing and changes in sexual and contraceptive practices among HIV-infected women. *Cleveland Clinic Journal of Medicine, 61,* 132–136.

Lawrence, D. N., Jason, J. M., Holman, R. C., Heine, P., Evatt, B. L., & the Hemophilia Study Group (1989). Sex practice correlates of human immunodeficiency virus transmission and acquired immunodeficiency syndrome incidence in heterosexual partners and offspring of U.S. hemophilic men. *American Journal of Hematology, 30,* 68–76.

Marks, G., Richardson, J. L., & Maldonado, N. (1991). Self-disclosure of HIV infection to sexual partners. *American Journal of Public Health, 81,* 1321–1323.

Mason, P. J., Olson, R. A., & Parish, K. L. (1988). AIDS, hemophilia, and prevention efforts within a comprehensive care program. *American Psychologist, 43,* 971–976.

Norman, L. R., Parish, K. L., & Kennedy, M. (1996). Close relationships and safer sex among HIV infected men with hemophilia. Manuscript submitted for publication.

Padian, N. S., O'Brien, T. R., Chang, Y., Glass, S., & Francis, D. P. (1993). Prevention of heterosexual transmission of human immunodeficiency virus through couple counseling. *Journal of Acquired Immune Deficiency Syndromes, 6,* 1043–1048.

Parish, K. L., Cotton, D. A., Huszti, H. C., Parsons, J., & the Hemophilia Behavioral Intervention Evaluation Project Group (1993, June). Qualitative analysis of behavioral determinants: HIV risk reduction and adults with hemophilia. Poster session presented at the Ninth International Conference on AIDS, Berlin, Germany.

Parish, K. L., Mandel, J., Thomas, J., & Gomperts, E. (1989, June) Prediction of safer sex practice and psychosocial distress in adults with hemophilia at risk for AIDS. Poster session presented at the Fifth International Conference on AIDS, Montreal, Canada.

Perry, S. W., Card, C. A. L., Moffatt, M., Jr., Ashman, T., Fishman, B., & Jacobsberg, L. B. (1994). Self-disclosure of HIV infection to sexual partners after repeated counseling. *AIDS Education and Prevention, 6,* 403–411.

Prochaska, J. O., DiClemente, C. C., & Norcross, J. C. (1992) In search of how people change: Applications to addictive behaviors. *American Psychologist, 47,* 1102–1114.

Sherr, L. (1993). Discordant couples. In L. Sherr (Ed.), *AIDS and the Heterosexual Population,* (83–102). Chur, Switzerland: Harwood Academic Publishers.

Simoni, J. M., Mason, H. R. C., Marks, G., Ruiz, M. S., Reed, D., & Richardson, J. L. (1995). Women's self-disclosure of HIV infection: rates, reasons, and reactions. *Journal of Consulting and Clinical Psychology, 63,* 474–478.

Wenger, N. S., Kusseling, F. S., Beck, K., & Shapiro, M. F. (1994). Sexual behavior of individuals infected with the human immunodeficiency virus. *Archives of Internal Medicine, 154,* 1849–1854.

Wiley, S., Hannan, J., Barrett, S., & Evatt, B. (1994, October). Surveillance of hemophilia, HIV, and HIV risk reduction at federally funded hemophilia treatment centers, 1990–1993. Poster session presented at National Hemophilia Foundation Annual Meeting, Dallas, Texas.

# II Specialized Aspects of HIV/AIDS Clinical Care

# 9 | Psychoeducational Group Work for Persons with AIDS Dementia Complex

*Michele Killough Nelson*

In the early 1980s, a number of neurological manifestations of HIV were noted, most commonly a decline in cognitive and behavioral functioning. It is now widely recognized that most HIV-infected individuals have at least mild neurobehavioral changes that are related to the virus (Koralnik et al., 1990), but the prevalence rates of AIDS Dementia Complex (ADC) vary from 6 to 30 percent (Day et al., 1992; Janssen, Nwanyanwu, Selik, & Stehr-Green, 1992; Maj et al., 1994; McArthur et al., 1993).

ADC is characterized by a gradual decline in cognitive functioning with specific deficits in the integration of motor functioning, information-processing speed, attention and concentration, memory, and affective and social functioning (Heaton et al., 1995). ADC causes significant declines in social and occupational functioning and is similar to other subcortical dementias (e.g., Huntington's disease) that affect the white matter of the brain, which lies below the grey matter.

Clients may not always be aware of their decline, and it may co-occur with other psychiatric disorders, making diagnosis more difficult. When a client is aware of some cognitive difficulties, he or she may typically say, "I forget things that used to be easy for me to remember, like what I wanted to get at the store, and I get lost when I try to follow conversations." Later in the decline, a person with ADC may have slowed speech and thought processes, difficulty concentrating on and finishing tasks, trouble making good decisions, confusion, and decreased insight regarding the deficits.

ADC is an AIDS-defining illness and generally occurs in the late stages of the disease. Before combination therapies and viral load testing, median survival time after the diagnosis of ADC has been approximately 6 months (Day et al., 1992; McArthur et al., 1993; Navia, Cho, Petito, & Price, 1986).

Clinically, the diagnosis of ADC is often more emotionally difficult for clients to accept than is the diagnosis of other AIDS-related illnesses. Many HIV-infected people expect a decline in their physical health but not in their cognitive functioning. Dementia is also unexpected because most clients are relatively young. There are profound implications for self-esteem, self-care, and legal issues (e.g., competency to execute a will, ability to operate motor vehicles). Finally, there are few treatment options for clients with ADC, and clinical improvement is not usually maintained for long periods of time since ADC is progressive (Reinvang, Froland, & Skripeland, 1991; Sidtis, Gatsonis, Price, & Singer, 1993).

## *My Clinical Work*

In my practice as a clinical psychologist at the Medical College of Virginia, I was struck by the broad psychological and social ramifications of ADC. Clients had strong, negative reactions to the diagnosis of ADC or, in some cases, did not recognize the decline in their function and refused to accept that there had been any changes. Most were referred after they or their health care workers noticed changes in the clients' cognitive function. For those clients who were still trying to function independently or with minimal assistance and who recognized their decline, I became aware of the profound helplessness they felt. They did not know how to compensate for their deficits and often felt depressed, isolated, alone, and defective. I also received frequent phone calls from members of these clients' support systems, who were concerned over their loved ones' continued decline. They were eager to know what could be done to stabilize or improve the clients' functioning. Initially, I worked with clients with ADC in individual psychotherapy and tried to help them process their feelings about their situation and generate new coping strategies, but this approach was not helpful for most people.

After I spoke with a number of clients with ADC about what they wanted, it became clear that a group format was preferable to individual psychotherapy to help clients feel supported and less alone (Yalom, 1995). It was also clear, however, that clients wanted to learn compensatory skills to minimize the deficits they had secondary to ADC.

As a first step, I reviewed the literature on cognitive retraining and rehabilitation. I found that most of the literature pertained to people with traumatic brain injuries and strokes; there was no body of literature on cognitive retraining for HIV-infected persons, largely because ADC is a relatively new diagnosis and little research has been conducted beyond defining the pathogenesis of the infection and clinical manifestations of the disorder. In addition, most of the literature focused on helping people regain employment, which is generally not possible or desirable for people in the late stages of AIDS. It became clear that a new approach was needed, one that borrowed from other fields but incorporated the unique challenges posed by ADC and AIDS.

A second step involved neuropsychological testing of persons who wished to participate in the group. They were administered a series of tests that included subtests from the Wechsler Adult Intelligence Scale-Revised (WAIS-R; Wechsler, 1981), Logical and Figural Memory with delayed recall from the Wechsler Memory Scale (WMS; Wechsler, 1945), Trail Making Tests A and B (Reitan, 1979), California Verbal Learning Test (Delis, Kramer, Kaplan, & Ober, 1987), Incidental Recall for Digit Symbol from the WAIS-R, the Purdue Pegboard Test (Tiffin, 1968), and the Benton Controlled Oral Word Association Test (Benton & Hamsher, 1983). Most of the tests we give have age, education, and gender-corrected norms, making it possible to come up with meaningful results that help us decide whether or not the client has had a decline. Results from these tests gave us a picture of our clients' specific areas of difficulty, including problems with short-term memory, learning new information, completing tasks quickly and efficiently, concentrating, and functioning independently. The tests are often emotionally difficult for clients because they are made aware of their deficits by their inability accurately and quickly to answer questions or complete tasks that would have been easy for them in the past. Obviously, although the information gained from these tests is important, clinicians must be sensitive to their clients' feelings during the assessment and must help their clients maintain their dignity.

## *Designing the Group*

The therapy group was designed with three goals in mind:

1. *Issues specific to ADC and AIDS needed to be considered.*

Unlike most groups designed to help people improve their cognitive and emotional functioning, this group comprises people with a terminal illness and a median life expectancy of six months. This basic fact makes it clear that the group needs to be brief and focused. It is also likely that at least one group member will become seriously ill or die during the course of the group, so this needs to be anticipated.

Assurances of confidentiality will be necessary to recruit clients and help them to risk exposing their areas of deficits to others. Many people do not want others to know about their HIV status but are even more anxious about the discovery of cognitive decline. Talking about confidentiality with each client before he or she enters the group and restating the policy at the beginning of each session will help clients feel more comfortable. Also, it may be beneficial to talk openly about clients' strengths and weaknesses as revealed by their neuropsychological test data. Some people, for example, may have average verbal memory but impaired visual memory. If visual memory techniques are discussed, then those who could benefit most should be encouraged to pay close attention. It will therefore be helpful to let clients know that some of their test results may be shared with the group as appropriate.

ADC is progressive, so maintenance of cognitive functioning may be a more realistic goal than improvement, which is the traditional goal of cognitive retraining. It is important to help clients set appropriate expectations and not believe that the group will fix their problems. It may also be difficult to convince others that this is a reasonable form of treatment because much of the focus is on improving quality of life rather than making significant, permanent changes. In fact, Auerbach and Jann (1989) discuss the current financial pressures associated with health care and suggest that the cost-effectiveness of rehabilitation for clients with HIV may be questioned.

Unfortunately, not all clients with ADC who want to attend will be appropriate for the group. Appropriate clients will have to be cognitively, psychologically, and physically strong enough to participate in a psychoeducational group. We normally exclude persons with a major mental illness, such as schizophrenia, or a problematic personality disorder. There may also be problems if clients have remarkably different levels of cognitive functioning, although some variations may be helpful to stimulate discussion. Obviously, clients with severe ADC will not be able to participate in or gain much from the group, even if they want to come, and those with mild ADC may be saddened and scared by seeing others with more advanced ADC.

Finally, for group leaders, many feelings of frustration, helplessness, and sadness may be evoked by this population. Clients with ADC represent a subset of the AIDS population, and some of the problems posed by this group may seem amplified. Some clients with ADC, for example, may continue to engage in activities such as drug use or prostitution, which is frustrating enough for health care professionals and therapists to contend with when the client is healthy, let alone cognitively impaired. Others may have family members or significant others who refuse to admit that the client has declined. There may be external pressures on clients to continue driving, caring for children, or managing finances, even when these activities are clearly beyond their abilities. In contrast, some families and friends may infantilize them and inappropriately try to take away responsibilities. Finally, many persons with AIDS and ADC are homeless or live in suboptimal situations. It may be clear that these clients could do better if they were in other situations, but they may have to or choose to stay in their current ones. It can be sad to work with these clients, only to watch their continued physical and cognitive decline, regardless of what the therapist does. These feelings need to be processed with other professionals to reduce the possibility of burnout. Using two group leaders is also strongly recommended.

2. *Cognitive retraining principles needed to be understood and applied to meet the needs of persons with ADC.*

Cognitive retraining has been defined as "those activities that improve a brain-injured patient's higher cerebral functioning or help the patient to better understand the nature of those difficulties while teaching him or her methods of compensation" (Klonoff, O'Brien, Prigatano, & Chiapello, 1989, 37). In retraining, a series of interventions is used to focus on either improving the area of deficit or developing new or compensatory strategies. The literature suggests three general methods of remediation: direct remediation, indirect remediation or strategy learning, and compensatory remediation or external aids (Glisky & Schacter, 1986; Tankle, 1988). Domain-specific training has also been proposed by some authors (Parente & Anderson-Parente, 1989).

Direct remediation requires first clearly defining the specific deficit area and understanding the contributory factors. After the problem is defined, a strategy (e.g., rehearsal) is used to correct the core deficit. Direct remediation is not generally considered successful because it assumes that a damaged area can be fixed or improved by practice, and this has not been supported in the research (Glisky & Schacter, 1986).

Indirect remediation involves using unimpaired cognitive skills in place of impaired ones to reduce the negative consequences associated with the deficit. As with direct remediation, it is imperative to understand the client's specific strengths and weaknesses in order to identify relatively intact areas. Unfortunately, indirect strategies have been difficult to teach to brain-injured patients because they require elaborate cognitive processing and are, therefore, not practical in most situations. Verbal and visual mnemonic strategies in particular have received significant attention in the literature, but their benefits are greatest for clients with only mild deficits (Glisky & Schacter, 1986).

Compensatory remediation or external aids have been widely used with brain-injured and stroke patients. This strategy relies on creating external aids to reduce the consequences of the deficits (Glisky & Schacter, 1986; Milton, 1985). Checklists, alarm watches, structured environments, and daily schedules are examples of frequently used external aids. There has been limited research on their effectiveness, but they are generally thought to be the most helpful strategy (Tankle, 1988; Glisky & Schacter, 1986).

In addition to the strategies already mentioned, some therapists use domain-specific training, which attempts to "match the task demands in therapy to those of the real world" (Parente & Anderson-Parente, 1989, 61). In this method, people are taught information that is directly pertinent to their lives. Simulations of situations that the client will likely face are developed so that the client can become competent in those specific areas (e.g., taking medications) or pieces of knowledge (e.g., one's phone number or address). Factors that predict a good response include client motivation, ability to control one's behavior and impulses, premorbid functioning, and ability to interact with the therapist and other clients (Klonoff, O'Brien, Prigatano, & Chiapello, 1989; Milton, 1985).

Orr and Pinto (1993) described their strategies for dealing with problems faced by clients with ADC who were also in a residential drug treatment program. These included using external aids, encouraging clients to take whatever time they needed to express themselves and to complete tasks, making travel plans in advance and with supervision, encouraging participation in social activities, limiting distractors, breaking down large tasks into smaller ones, structuring the environment, and educating others about ADC.

For purposes of this group, I combined both the remediation and the support strategies discussed earlier to accomplish a well-rounded group for clients. I felt that offering multiple strategies would increase a client's chances of finding one that was helpful, especially given the wide variety of functional deficits associated with ADC.

3. *We had to create a forum for clients to discuss their feelings about ADC and the impact it has on their lives.*

As previously mentioned, persons with ADC frequently report feeling alone, anxious, and saddened by their declines. They discuss feeling embarrassed in social situations, being afraid of getting lost or forgetting friends' names, and having a new, poignant understanding of their prognosis. Given the significant cognitive decline and intense emotions experienced by people with ADC, it was decided to have a guided discussion of clients' feelings that taught them to recognize their own patterns of distorted thinking, which increased their anxiety and depression.

## *The Group*

Based on the three issues discussed in the previous section, it was decided to have an eight-session psychoeducational group for patients with ADC. Each session would last fifty minutes and would occur once a week. This format was decided on because it allowed time to cover all of the necessary topics in a thorough way but did not appear too taxing for most clients. Most people who participated were capable of maintaining reasonable levels of attention for fifty minutes, but each person was evaluated on the basis of his or her performance during the initial ADC assessment and in a screening interview for the group. Those who were not capable of participating in fifty-minute sessions were invited to do individual remediation work that was much more focused.

Anyone who had the diagnosis of ADC was invited to be screened for the group, and most referrals were made by physicians, social workers, and nurses. All clients who were referred were screened for appropriateness, including motivation, ability to attend regularly (e.g., transportation, child care, and physical problems were addressed), current substance abuse or other high-risk behaviors, and ability to participate appropriately (e.g., no patients with severe ADC). Collaboration with clients' case managers and health care workers was pursued when possible to facilitate clients' attendance and participation. All clients were asked for permission to share their test data in group as appropriate, and all were asked what they wanted the group leaders to tell other group members in the event of their absence due to illness. The issue of group confidentiality was discussed in advance and clients had to agree to the policy prior to being accepted in the group. The screening interview was used as a chance to build rapport between the leaders and each group member.

Following is a description of the content of each of the sessions.

### *Session 1: Introduction and Checklists*

Clients and group leaders introduced themselves and gave brief descriptions of the effects of ADC on their daily lives. Clients were encouraged to raise issues that had been especially difficult for them so that others could share strategies that had worked, find commonalities, and get support. Issues raised most frequently included going shopping but forgetting what was supposed to be purchased, forgetting people's names, difficulty following conversations, and being embarrassed by slowed speech. Virtually all clients reported that they were avoiding some situations because of their anxiety. Most had also begun making long checklists in an effort to organize themselves and reduce their stress.

After working to establish rapport among group members, the leaders began discussing how to make better checklists. Those clients who had checklists with them were encouraged to share them with the group. Commonly identified problems were the length of the checklists and the lack of order and priority among the items. A sample checklist was generated using items from the clients' lists. The coleaders suggested that the checklist be put on lined paper and broken into two categories: things that need to be done today and things that the client would like to get done soon. The "today" column was then broken into three sections: morning, afternoon, and evening. This structure appeared to help clients prioritize the items, and most were able to make reasonable decisions about which items should go in each category. All important things (e.g., taking medications, paying bills, going to appointments) were to be listed and checked off as soon as the activity was completed. Apparently some clients had problems remembering whether they had completed an activity, even when it was on their list, so checking off items became an important new skill for some people. The coleaders then distributed copies of a blank checklist with the categories mentioned for clients to use. Clients were instructed to bring in a completed checklist the following week for review. Group goals were also presented.

*Session 2: Memory, Part I*

Given that there has been little work on cognitive retraining for clients with ADC, all of the memory remediation strategies discussed earlier were included, primarily to provide clients with a range of choices that might be helpful to them. Handouts were given to all clients with the following strategies listed and discussed:

- Rehearsal. This is the method most children are taught to use to encode information, so adults frequently revert to it. It can facilitate overlearning and is helpful when a person is under stress. We encouraged group members to rehearse no more than five items at a time.
- Chunking. This involves breaking information into smaller "chunks" to make it manageable. For example, a grocery list of twelve items may be broken into three lists of four items (e.g., four dairy products, four cleaning supplies, and four canned foods). We spent several minutes teaching chunking, because some people were too overwhelmed to generate ideas on their own.
- Association. This involves joining two items to form a connection. Mnemonics is a form of association. Several examples were given, especially for remembering people's names.
- Rhythm and rhyming. Clients were encouraged to make up rhymes or sayings to remember things that needed to be done. One example generated by a group member who frequently forgot to lock his doors at night was "Check the door before I leave the floor." Another group member volunteered, "Take my meds before I go to bed." This exercise added humor to the group, although it was unclear if clients actually used these sayings in daily life.
- Remembering written information. Clients were encouraged to read printed material for the big picture instead of getting lost in the details, as many were beginning to do. We encouraged them

first to scan the document for the general idea, then read it thoroughly, and finally read it again to ensure comprehension. Although cumbersome, this method provided structure for clients who were overwhelmed by printed material and encouraged them to focus on understanding the main idea. Highlighting of important information was also encouraged.

- Note taking. Note taking often makes people more active listeners and provides them with something to refer to after leaving the situation. Clients were encouraged to take notes at their doctors' appointments, case management meetings, and other important events and to have someone check their notes for accuracy and completeness. Most of the physicians, nurses, and social workers who were asked to check clients' notes were happy to do so and felt it was a useful strategy. When possible, the coleaders approached health care staff first to let them know that clients would be requesting this.
- Eliminating distractors. Clients were encouraged to learn information in quiet situations when they were not feeling stressed.

All clients were encouraged to keep track of the techniques they used during the week and decide which ones were most helpful for them.

### *Session 3: Memory, Part II*

Compensatory strategies were discussed in this session with a focus on addressing the specific problems clients had raised in earlier sessions. The following strategies were discussed and demonstrated: checklists, calendars, flashcards, audiotaping, alarm clocks, alarm watches, posted signs, color coding, and pill boxes.

### *Session 4: Coping with Feelings of Anxiety, Frustration, and Depression, Part I*

The first part of this session was spent with clients talking about the feelings they had been experiencing. They were then asked to talk about feelings that interfered with their ability to do things well. Most clients reported increased self-doubt and self-criticism, with many clients reporting that they felt "stupid" or as if they were "losing" their minds. With some guidance, they were able to see how their thoughts about themselves fed into a cycle of avoidant behavior and increased self-doubt and anxiety. These were termed "unhelpful thoughts," largely on the basis

Figure 9.1.
*Sample Unhelpful Thoughts*

| Type of unhelpful thoughts | Examples generated by clients |
|---|---|
| All or nothing thinking | If I can't do it right, I won't do it at all. |
| Overgeneralization | I can't do anything right. |
| Disqualifying the positive | I know my family cares for me, but it doesn't matter. They don't understand. |
| Jumping to conclusions | I know my friend thinks I'm an idiot—you should have seen the look he gave me. |
| Catastrophizing | I've screwed up everything because I forgot my appointment with my social worker. |
| Emotional reasoning | I've had bad nerves all day—I know something will go wrong. |
| Mislabeling | I'm a loser. |

of writings by Beck, Rush, Shaw, and Emery (1979) and Burns (1980). Examples are given in Figure 9.1.

### *Session 5: Coping with Feelings of Frustration, Anxiety, and Depression, Part II*

This session focused on helping clients respond to and modify their unhelpful thoughts. Basic cognitive interventions were used. Clients were encouraged, for example, to identify the unhelpful thought, label it, and come up with a more rational response to refute it. Statements that clients had made during the group sessions were used in a practice exercise. Figure 9.2 contains examples taken from the group.

Clients were also encouraged to keep track of their unhelpful thoughts to see if they happened more frequently in some situations than in others (e.g., when the client felt anxious or tired). They were also taught thought-stopping (Beck, Rush, Shaw, & Emery, 1979) as a method of controlling negative, ruminative thoughts and encouraged to keep journals as a way to express themselves. Other suggestions for managing stress included taking time to have fun, distraction, relaxation techniques, light exercise, spending time with friends or family, planning ahead, and asking others for help when needed.

### *Session 6: Reaction Time and Attention and Concentration*

One of the most frequent complaints of clients with ADC is feeling cognitively slowed. Many are able to articulate specific problems with slowed information processing and psychomotor speed and have concerns

Figure 9.2.
*Refuting Unhelpful Thoughts*

| Unhelpful Thought | Type | Rational Response |
|---|---|---|
| I can't do anything right. | Overgeneralization | I make some mistakes, but I do a lot of things right—like taking my medicines and keeping my house clean. |
| My friends must think I'm stupid. | Jumping to conclusions | I need to explain my problem to my friends so that they know why I have trouble remembering things. |
| My mom calls me sometimes, but if she really cared she'd be here. | Disqualifying the positive | I wish my mom would come stay with me, but I'm glad that she calls. Maybe I could ask her to come. |

about their ability to continue driving, living independently, and making important decisions. Clients were encouraged to think through situations that were difficult for them or that might become difficult in the future. Most agreed that feeling pressured to do something quickly caused them to become more anxious and to make more mistakes. Many felt unable to get out of these situations gracefully. We spent approximately twenty minutes role-playing these situations and encouraged clients to experiment with different ways of excusing themselves from having to do things they were uncomfortable with. Many patients had not considered saying no as an option and needed permission to do this. Others wanted face-saving excuses they could use in multiple situations, such as "I'm a little tired, so could you (drive, get dinner, etc.) today?"

The rest of the session was spent talking about ways clients could maximize their attention and concentration. The following ideas were suggested:

- Take regularly scheduled breaks before getting tired.
- Ask someone else to help you with projects.
- Eliminate internal and external distractors.
- Take notes.
- Use active listening skills, and ask questions when confused.
- Break tasks down into smaller parts.
- Get adequate rest.
- Focus on staying calm and not letting anxiety interfere with concentration.

*Session 7: Decision Making*

Many clients reported new difficulties with decision making. In this session, they frequently voiced complaints about feeling pressured by others to make quick decisions, making "snap" decisions and later feeling frustrated by them, having trouble generating options, obsessing over details, focusing on impossible or impractical solutions, feeling that there is a "right" choice, letting others make decisions for them, vacillating, and making decisions on the basis of emotions rather than facts.

General decision-making strategies were reviewed, and clients were encouraged to share decisions they needed to make with the group for discussion. The following steps in decision making were discussed:

- List all options.
- Eliminate impossible or impractical options.
- Identify the options you like best.
- List the pros and cons of these options, including your feelings about them.
- Pick the best of the options based on the information generated in the earlier steps.
- Realize that no decision is perfect and few are permanent.
- Ask someone you trust to review your decision with you if you are still unsure.
- Stick with your decision to give it a chance before changing your mind.

*Session 8: Review and Goodbye*

In the final session, a handout summarizing all the major points from the other sessions was distributed. Clients were encouraged to discuss whatever issues or concerns they had, and these were addressed. Clients were asked to provide feedback about the helpfulness of the group in written and verbal form. Part of the time was also spent praising group members for coming and sharing their struggles and successes. Finally, group members and leaders talked openly about saying goodbye to each other.

Clients reported feeling most positively about the memory, the coping, and the decision-making sessions. The compensatory remediation strategies, especially checklists and alarm watches, were rated as most helpful.

They reported appreciating having a forum in which to discuss their feelings with others who understood their frustrations, and they all believed that they benefited from learning to recognize and change unhelpful thoughts that deepened their negative feelings about themselves. The decision-making group was rated highly because members felt that it was pertinent to their lives and offered practical, concrete ways to make decisions. Some members suggested that more role playing would have been helpful as a technique to help them reduce their anxiety about stressful situations.

## *Barriers to Successful Group Therapy for ADC Clients*

Many potential obstacles were encountered or anticipated while developing this group, including these:

1. There is limited research on the effectiveness of cognitive retraining and no body of literature on cognitive retraining for clients with ADC. This made it difficult to select appropriate topics and interventions. Given that our group was based on clinical need rather than on empirical information, it was less focused and probably less effective than one based on sound data would have been.
2. The continuing decline of group members' health over the eight weeks affected the group process and cohesion. Some clients also experienced symptoms consistent with organic mania associated with advanced AIDS and ADC, leading others to worry about whether this would happen to them as well. Much reassurance was needed and given. Collaboration with multidisciplinary team members was important for facilitating client attendance, maximizing client participation and gain, and reinforcing skills that were learned.
3. Clients had markedly different levels of premorbid and ADC functioning, so it was challenging to present information in a way that was easily understood by all and interesting to those who were higher functioning. Clients also came from dissimilar economic and social backgrounds (e.g., long-term drug users and high-functioning professionals), so rapport and trust between group members was slower to develop than anticipated.
4. Given the current health care climate and the need to justify services, there may be questions about the cost-effectiveness and utility of this group. Is it cost-effective or desirable to provide psychoeducational

services to people whose median life expectancy is just six months? Do improved social support, self-esteem, and coping justify the time and the cost of the group, especially given that most of the gains will be time-limited, since clients will continue declining? These are reasonable questions to consider and address when contemplating such a group.

## *Recommendations for Future Practice*

The sessions described in this chapter constitute a reasonable beginning, but the focus now needs to be on gathering data about the most helpful cognitive and psychological strategies for coping with the numerous effects of ADC. It may also be helpful to include specialists from different disciplines when designing the group curriculum. Traditional cognitive retraining programs, for example, include speech, occupational, and mental health therapists, physicians, nurses, social workers, and rehabilitation psychologists.

The group format appears to be an effective way to deliver these services, and I believe it should be continued. It is more cost- and time-effective than delivering the services to individuals, and it provides a forum for clients to solicit help and strategies from others who have similar problems. A shorter group may be more practical, but this will need to be explored through clinical experience and research.

## *Tools for Clinical Practice*

Other concerns should be considered by mental health practitioners concerned with ADC in clients, including the following:

- *Individuals with symptoms that may be ADC are likely to have a complicated presentation of neuropsychological functioning based on current HIV status, history and effects of substance use that includes alcohol, baseline IQ and learning disabilities, and current levels of anxiety and depression.*

  The diagnostic picture for these clients is complex. In making diagnoses, you should consider:

  - Is the decline significant enough to cause impairment in the person's social and occupational functioning?
  - Can the decline be explained by other factors, such as poor nutrition, depression, or delirium?

- Is the nature of the decline consistent with ADC (e.g., decline in psychomotor speed and memory followed by general cognitive decline)?
- What roles do substance abuse, learning disabilities, previous head injuries, premorbid functioning, and other illnesses play in the decline?

- *It can sometimes be difficult to distinguish dementia from delirium or depression.*

  Delirium, as described in the *Diagnostic and Statistical Manual of Mental Disorders* (4th ed.) (*DSM-IV*, American Psychiatric Association, 1994) includes the following diagnostic criteria: disturbance of consciousness, change in cognition or the development of a perceptual disturbance that is not accounted for by a dementia, rapid onset of the disturbance, and a medical condition as the causative agent.

  Depression, as described in *DSM-IV* (American Psychiatric Association, 1994) includes at least five of the following diagnostic criteria occurring during at least a two-week period and representing a change from previous functioning: depressed mood, consistently diminished interest or pleasure in most daily activities, significant weight loss or gain, consistent insomnia or hypersomnia, psychomotor agitation or retardation, fatigue or loss of energy, feelings of worthlessness or excessive guilt, diminished ability to think or concentrate, and recurrent thoughts of death.

  Obviously, some of the symptoms of depression and delirium are similar to those of ADC, but the neuropsychological test data, thorough clinical interview, and data from other sources will be invaluable in making the final diagnosis.
- *Clients with ADC often feel alone and may develop avoidant patterns in an attempt to mask their decline. This avoidance decreases their self-esteem and increases their sense of helplessness and impotence.*

  This pattern needs to be identified and changed to help clients function at the highest possible level. Ways to do this include:

  - Helping clients recognize the pattern and discussing their feelings about it
  - Teaching clients new strategies to cope with difficult or frightening situations
  - Providing supportive counseling

- Helping clients learn that it is okay to ask for help from others and then teaching them how to ask appropriately for help
- Pointing out areas in which the client is still functioning well

- *Group coleaders need to have names of responsible friends or family members who can act decisively when necessary in case of an emergency.*

  The need for the involvement of family members became apparent at several points in our group, but one situation was especially memorable. One group member had moderate ADC and limited insight into his decline. Unfortunately, he insisted on continuing to drive, even though his license had been revoked because of several traffic violations that had occurred after the onset of ADC, and on gambling large sums of money that were to be used for his health care. He discussed these activities freely in the group and made it clear that he would not change his behaviors. Fortunately, we had obtained his permission prior to the beginning of the group to speak with his wife if concerns arose during the group and, after informing him of our concerns and our intent to contact her, did so at once. She was unaware that he was continuing to drive and very upset to discover how low their bank balance was. She was able to take steps to ensure that he was no longer able to drive his car (she took away his keys and disabled the battery), told his friends that he was not to drive their cars, and eliminated his ability to withdraw money from their bank account. These steps averted other possible catastrophes. We spent significant time helping him process his feelings about his new restrictions. He was angry with us but had become attached to the group and continued to participate.
- *When a client becomes debilitated with ADC, the mental health professional needs to consider many issues to maximize the client's functioning and quality of life.*

  Some of the issues that need to be addressed are long-term placement options, such as nursing homes or supervised adult homes; education and support for the client's caregivers to prevent burnout; supportive counseling for the client; and close contact with the client's health care providers to coordinate treatment appropriately.

## *Conclusion*

After doing this work for three years with more than fifty clients, I am acutely aware of the necessity for mental health providers to attend to the neuropsychological issues of their clients, whatever the provider's discipline. The clients, for their part, have responded to the sessions by saying that their self-confidence had improved significantly and that they felt better able to cope with the new pressures in their lives. One client said, "I don't feel like such a dummy anymore. I understand what's happening, and so does my family. That means a lot." Another said, "Now I can talk to my doctor and remember what she said." Finally, one client stated, "I remembered all the names of my care team members. I surprised them all at our second weekly dinner by calling them all by name. They knew this had been hard for me to do and that I was going to practice it, and when I did it, they clapped for me." Providing clients with new skills is a goal that many mental health providers have, and these strategies can help clients learn to cope with their new psychological and neuropsychological needs.

## REFERENCES

The author wishes to acknowledge Rochelle Klinger, M.D., Maria Devens, M.A., and Robert Higginson, PA-C, for their contributions and facilitation of these groups. This chapter was written with the support of Grant 601-45416-491-03 from Ryan White Title II funds, Michele Killough Nelson, principal investigator.

American Psychiatric Association (1994). *Diagnostic and statistical manual of mental disorders* (4th ed.). Washington, DC: Author.

Auerbach, V., & Jann, B. (1989). Neurorehabilitation and HIV infection: Clinical and ethical dilemmas. *Journal of Head Trauma Rehabilitation, 4(1),* 23–31.

Beck, A. T., Rush, A. J., Shaw, B. F., & Emery, G. (1979). *Cognitive therapy of depression.* New York: Guilford Press.

Benton, A. L., & Hamsher, K. (1983). *Multilingual Aphasia Examination.* Iowa City, IA: AJA Associates.

Burns, D. D. (1980). *Feeling good.* New York: Morrow.

Day, J. J., Grant, I., Atkinson, J. H., Brysk, L. T., McCutchan, J. A., Hesselink, J. R., Heaton, R. K., Weinrich, J. D., Spector, S. A., & Richman, D. D. (1992). Incidence of AIDS dementia in a two year follow-up of AIDS and ARC patients on an initial Phase II AZT placebo-controlled study: San Diego cohort. *Journal of Neuropsychiatry and Clinical Neurosciences, 4(1),* 15–20.

Delis, D. L., Kramer, J. H., Kaplan, E., & Ober, B. A. (1987). *California Verbal Learning Test, Adult Version.* San Antonio, TX: Psychological Corp.

Glisky, E. L., & Schacter, D. L. (1986). Remediation of organic memory disorders: Current status and future prospects. *Journal of Head Trauma Rehabilitation, 1(3),* 54–63.

Heaton, R. K., Grant, I., Butters, N., White, D. A., Kirson, D., Atkinson, J. H., McCutchan, J. A., Taylor, M. J., Kelly, M. D., Ellis, R. J., Wolfson, T., Velin, R., Marcotte, T. D., Hesselink, J. R., Jernigan, T. L., Chandler, J., Wallace, M., Abramson, I., and the HNRC Group (1995). The HNRC 500—Neuropsychology of HIV infection at different disease stages. *Journal of the International Neuropsychological Society, 1,* 231–251.

Janssen, R. S., Nwanyanwu, O. C., Selik, R. M., & Stehr-Green, J. K. (1992). Epidemiology of human immunodeficiency virus encephalopathy in the United States. *Neurology, 42,* 1472–1476.

Klonoff, P. S., O'Brien, K. P., Prigatano, G. P., & Chiapello, D. A. (1989). Cognitive retraining after traumatic brain injury and its role in facilitating awareness. *Journal of Head Trauma Rehabilitation, 4(3),* 37–45.

Koralnik, I. J., Beaumanoir, A., Hausler, R., Kohler, A., Safran, A. B., Delacoux, R., Vibert, D., Mayer, E., Burkhard, P., & Nahory, A. (1990). A controlled study of early neurologic abnormalities in men with asymptomatic human immunodeficiency virus infection. *New England Journal of Medicine, 323,* 864–870.

Maj, M., Satz, P., Janssen, R., Zaudig, M., Starace, F., D'Elia, L., Sughondhabirom, B., Mussa, M., Naber, D., Ndetei, D., Schulte, G., & Sartorius, N. (1994). WHO Neuropsychiatric AIDS study, cross-sectional Phase II: Neuropsychological and neurological findings. *Archives of General Psychiatry, 51,* 51–61.

McArthur, J. C., Hoover, D. R., Bacellar, H., Miller, E. N., Cohen, B. A., Becker, J. T., Graham, N. M. H., McArthur, J. H., Selnes, O. A., Jacobson, L. P., Visscher, B. R., Concha, M., & Saah, A. (1993). Dementia in AIDS patients: Incidence and risk factors. *Neurology, 43,* 2245–2253.

Milton, S. B. (1985). Compensatory memory strategy training: A practical approach for managing persisting memory problems. *Cognitive Rehabilitation, 3(6),* 8–16.

Navia, B. A., Cho, E. S., Petito, C. K., & Price, R. W. (1986). The AIDS dementia complex: II. Neuropathology. *Annals of Neurology, 19,* 525–535.

Orr, D. A., & Pinto, P. F. (1993). The clinical management of HIV-related dementia and other memory disorders in the residential drug treatment environment. *Journal of Substance Abuse Treatment, 10,* 505–511.

Parente, R., & Anderson-Parente, J. K. (1989). Retraining memory: Theory and application. *Journal of Head Trauma Rehabilitation, 4(3),* 55–65.

Reinvang, I., Froland, S. S., & Skripeland, V. (1991). Prevalence of neuropsychological deficit in HIV infection. Incipient signs of AIDS dementia complex in patients with AIDS. *Acta Neurologica Scandinavica, 83,* 289–293.

Reitan, R. M. (1979). *Trail Making Test.* Tucson, AZ: Reitan Neuropsychology Lab.

Sidtis, J. J., Gatsonis, C., Price, R. W., & Singer, E. J. (1993). Zidovudine treatment of the AIDS dementia complex: Results of a placebo-controlled trial. *Annals of Neurology, 33(4),* 343–349.

Tankle, R. S. (1988). Application of neuropsychological test results to interdisciplinary cognitive rehabilitation with head-injured adults. *Journal of Head Trauma Rehabilitation, 3(1),* 24–32.

Tiffin, J. (1968). *Examiner's Manual.* Chicago: Purdue Pegboard Science Research Associates. Available from Lafayette Instruments Co., Lafayette, IN.

Wechsler, D. (1945). A standardized memory scale for clinical use. *Journal of Psychology, 19,* 87–95. Available from Psychological Corp., San Antonio, TX.

Wechsler, D. (1981). *Wechsler Adult Intelligence Scale—Revised.* San Antonio, TX: Psychological Corp.

Yalom, I. D. (1995). *Theory and practice of group psychotherapy* (4th ed.). New York: Basic Books.

# 10 | Rural Practice

## *I. Michael Shuff*

HIV disease has come to small-town and rural America. It may be less visible because of the relatively thin spread of cases over larger geographic areas and because those affected by the disease in less populated areas feel that they must keep it secret.

Thought to be a problem of the big city, AIDS doesn't fit in with the heartland's conventional self-perception. But HIV/AIDS is here, now, and the longer the epidemic drags on the more undeniable that fact becomes. In the Midwestern state in which I live, Indiana, one half of all the reported AIDS cases live in towns with populations under 30,000 or in rural areas (Rural Prevention Center, 1994).

Some issues encountered in the delivery of mental health services to those living in smaller communities are unique. Others represent variations on themes encountered in urban areas. But the issues encountered in rural areas are no less complex than those encountered in the largest cities. While the absolute numbers of cases may be fewer, other circumstances make HIV/AIDS-related mental health care in less populated areas complex and challenging.

When considering mental health service delivery in non-urban America, keep in mind that small towns and rural communities suffer as much from stereotyping as do any other segments of our society. Remarkable diversity resides within these communities, making generalizations misleading and even dangerous.

## *Background Reading*

Research and professional writing concerning the impact of HIV/AIDS on small town and rural areas has been scarce. This can partially be explained by the delayed expansion of the epidemic into rural areas, the secrecy surrounding the occurrence of cases, and the overwhelming spread of the disease and its impact on urban areas. The relatively higher concentration of research and professional resources found in urban centers has also led to greater research interest in HIV disease in those areas.

To have a literature to review, it was necessary to include material relating to health service delivery in general as well as mental health care specifically. Many of the issues encountered in rural mental health care are also common to other areas of health service delivery, for example, the availability of hospice care and home health care. Material specific to mental health care delivery in rural areas is scant. The majority of the health service literature devoted to HIV/AIDS in nonurban America makes only indirect reference to mental health services. The situation mirrors the inattention to health and mental health services for those with HIV/AIDS in small towns and rural areas.

For ease of presentation, the literature will be divided into four general areas: general policy and public health, service provider preparation, rural practice, and homophobia.

### *General Policy and Public Health*

Articles in newsletters targeting health care audiences have pointed to the dramatic increase in the number of AIDS cases in small towns and rural areas (American Health Consultants, 1995; Hearn, 1994; Rural Prevention Center, 1994). Quoting findings from the National Commission on AIDS, the *Rural Prevention Report* (1994) noted that in 1989 the number of AIDS cases in rural areas increased 37 percent while the case increase in urban areas was 5 percent for the same year. American Health Consultants (1995) reported that data from studies on opportunistic infections, controlling for the 1993 change in the definition of AIDS, revealed that between 1989 and 1994 the percentage increase in AIDS cases among rural men infected through sexual contact with other men increased by 69 percent, while the percentage increase for those in the same risk category in urban areas was 19 percent. (See also Graham, Forrester, Wysong, Rosenthal, & James, 1995.)

These articles also point out that HIV disease is highly stigmatized in rural areas and note the relative inadequacy of health care resources in those areas. With health care resources already strained and rural areas underserved, health care providers are anxious about taking on new challenges. Stigma by association with HIV disease only adds another barrier to an already overburdened and uncertain future.

One of the most potent and revealing contributions to the literature is Vergheses' (1994) *My Own Country.* Written by a physician practicing in East Tennessee, this memoir vividly conveys the human suffering occasioned by the shame, guilt, and isolation produced by community reaction to the disease.

Articles tracing the epidemiology and the geography of AIDS have provided interesting insights into the spread of the disease. In an *Atlantic Monthly* article, Gould and Kabel (1993) described computer-assisted math modeling that traced the diffusion of AIDS across Ohio. Their research documented that in terms of geography, AIDS spreads in exactly the same manner as other sexually transmitted diseases, from urban areas outward and along the interstate highway system.

Research in the demography and the epidemiology of AIDS in rural areas has focused on documenting trends in the progression of the epidemic and tracking the effects of migration of individuals living with HIV disease from urban to rural areas in the Southeastern states (Davis & Stapelton, 1991; Rumley, Shappley, Waiver, & Esinhart, 1991; Whyte & Wilber, 1992). Researchers have been particularly concerned about an underestimate of AIDS cases in rural areas. This underestimate occurred because national prevalence statistics for AIDS do not take into account the mobile nature of our society and the underreporting of AIDS cases.

Researchers are concerned about whether the limited health care resources available in rural areas will be equal to the task of caring for an influx of AIDS patients, first diagnosed in urban areas, who return home to nonurban areas to be cared for through the final stages of their illness. Since federal funding for HIV/AIDS care has been tied to prevalence reports, urban areas have received the lion's share of funding, with medium and low impact states receiving little assistance.

One study (Wasser, Gwinn, & Fleming, 1993) focused on urban and nonurban women of childbearing age. Rates of HIV infection for these women ranged from 0 to 12.2 per 1,000 population. Rates were highest in East Coast urban areas, but high rates were also found in nonurban areas, especially in the South. Incidents of HIV infection were three to thirty-five times higher for black women than for white women in nine states, regardless of urbanicity. Research such as this indicates that the complexion of HIV/AIDS in nonurban areas is multifaceted, adding to the service delivery challenge posed there.

Two policy papers have been generated by the Health Resources and Services Administration (HRSA) (Berry, McKinney, McClain, & Valero-Figueira, 1995; Health Resource and Services Administration, 1991). The first reports on four case studies, commissioned by HRSA, of rural areas in the South Atlantic and the Mountain census divisions. The study identifies issues important to the development of HIV services in nonurban areas. These issues are identified as the perception among rural residents that HIV is an urban problem; efforts at professional education that do not reach rural health care providers; the fact that HIV disease in rural areas is only one component of a more complex set of problems related to poverty, alcohol and drug abuse, and sexually transmitted diseases; and the need for government-supported research and development concerning health services for persons with HIV/AIDS in nonurban areas.

The second paper focuses on a series of five broad recommendations for public policy initiatives in the area of HIV education and service delivery: information needs; planning, coordination, and resource allocation; training and skill development; dissemination; and financing. The paper calls attention to the diversity of nonurban areas and to differences among special populations within those areas. While attention is paid to differences between urban and rural populations, significantly less interest is shown in the diversity found in nonurban areas.

### *Service Provider Preparation*

Three studies relevant to mental health service provider training and preparation are worth mention. Two studies (D'Augelli, 1989; Pollard & D'Augelli, 1989) focused on knowledge, attitudes toward AIDS, and attitudes toward gays and lesbians. The first of these studied rural nurses and the second, rural volunteers in an AIDS prevention program. Results indicated that nurses had a great deal of knowledge about AIDS but unrealistic fears regarding transmission. One third of the nurses held strongly negative attitudes toward homosexuality. This attitude decreased when they reported knowing a gay man. The incidence of AIDS phobia and that of homophobia were correlated.

The volunteers in the second study (Pollard & D'Augelli, 1989) demonstrated a relatively high level of knowledge about AIDS, but a large majority rated their knowledge as inadequate. Participants were not particularly worried about contracting AIDS. Attitudes toward homosexuals were either mixed or negative. Once again, fear of AIDS was correlated with homophobia. The authors concluded that quality of care may be compromised if caregivers' negative attitudes toward gay individuals are not remedied. Specifically, they called for the inclusion of information regarding psychosocial and attitudes toward homosexuals as part of HIV/ AIDS training.

Aruffo, Thompson, Gottlieb, and Dobbins (1995) reported on the effects of training on a group of mental health service providers in rural Arkansas. Results of pre- and posttests showed that training effects were positive, and the authors concluded that training is important for developing a knowledgeable and accessible base of mental health service providers in rural areas.

### *Rural Practice*

The rural practice literature relating to HIV/AIDS, though limited, is dominated by the work of Kathleen Rounds. Her article (Rounds, 1988a) reports a qualitative study of care providers working in rural areas and contains an excellent overview of issues encountered by health and human service providers as they attempt to care for those with HIV/AIDS. Findings of the study were categorized under the headings: structural (including geographical distance), concerns for client confidentiality, fear of AIDS contagion, and homophobia. She concludes with a number of suggestions specific to the development of HIV services that should serve to enhance service delivery.

The guidance offered in this study and in a companion article (Rounds, 1988b) concerning community development work in rural areas is especially worth a serious reading. The author notes, among other things, that community development work in nonurban areas follows informal networks of personal and professional relationships. She advocates the use of these networks in building HIV/AIDS service delivery systems.

Rounds, Galinsky, and Stevens (1991) reported on a unique approach to HIV support groups tailored to rural areas. They established a telephone support group for HIV-infected individuals. The article reports on the protocol for the development of the group and the results of a pilot group. The group offered a unique and interesting approach to outreach to individuals who might never attend a conventional support group, either because of distance or because of fears concerning confidentiality.

Fuszard, Sowell, Hoff, and Waters (1991) reported results of a national study of rural American hospitals and their readiness to care for HIV/AIDS patients. While the vast majority of hospitals had acute-care services in place and had educated employees about universal precautions, the study found that other services were lacking. Community services were basically unavailable in rural areas, as were many other patient care services. Unavailable services specific to HIV care included adequate discharge planning, chronic care, and patient and family education services.

Seeley, Wagner, Mulemwa, Kengeya-Kayondo, and Mulder (1991) reported on the development of community-based HIV/AIDS counseling services in rural Uganda. While the focus of the present chapter is on nonurban America, the Ugandan experience is instructive and noteworthy if for no other reason than that it is one of the few articles in the professional literature that deals primarily with mental health services and HIV/AIDS in rural areas. The authors relate their experience in making entry into two separate rural communities. Lessons learned regarding community development in Uganda only serve to reinforce those reported by Rounds (1988a, 1988b). These authors also look at counseling models developed primarily in Europe and America and conclude that these models must be adapted to African culture by placing greater emphasis on family support.

### *Homophobia*

Various authors have researched and written about the interrelationship of AIDS phobia and homophobia. Others have written about the pervasive nature of homophobia, especially in small-town and rural areas (D'Augelli, 1989; Pollard & D'Augelli, 1989). It is beyond the scope of this chapter to review that extensive literature. Suffice it to say, however, that the homophobia associated with HIV/AIDS has a powerful and multifaceted impact on the availability of health and human services in nonurban areas, the quality of care given when these services are available, and the patterns of help-seeking behavior in which those living with HIV disease engage.

## *My Clinical Work*

I write after more than a decade of labor in HIV service delivery, in settings that varied from large urban centers to medium-size cities to small-town and rural areas.

In 1991 and 1992 I received funding for two independent but interrelated projects that serve as the experiential basis for this chapter: the Indiana Integration of Care Project and the Heartland Care Center. Both projects have provided a wealth of experience in mental health service delivery across an essentially nonurban Midwestern state.

The purpose of the integration project was to demonstrate the integration of community-based mental health services into the primary health care of the HIV-infected across the state of Indiana. The project consisted of four components: referral network building, integration into existing health and human service systems, training and support for mental health service providers, and research and project evaluation. Although the project was not conceived to target rural areas specifically, in point of fact, half the AIDS cases reported in Indiana are in nonurban areas. The past five years of training, consultation, and network building across the state have provided a considerable fund of experience regarding HIV mental health service delivery and community development.

Coincidental with the development of the integration project, the Heartland Care Center came into being. It is one of twelve state-supported HIV-dedicated care coordination centers in Indiana and serves an essentially rural area composed of seven counties in west-central Indiana. It is housed on the campus of Indiana State University and offers care coordination, counseling and testing, support groups, and individual and couples counseling to the HIV-affected in the Wabash Valley.

Heartland Care Center is unique in Indiana in that it is located on the campus of a state university and graduate students in the Department of Counseling, working under faculty supervision, provide services to clients. Thus it has a training function, for both students and faculty supervisors, in addition to that of service delivery.

The observations and lessons in this chapter have been the outgrowth of these two projects.

## *Barriers to HIV/AIDS Service Delivery in Rural Areas*

Two barriers to care for HIV/AIDS are the most salient in nonurban and rural areas:

1. *Geography.* This is the most obvious barrier, both for those with HIV disease and for those who attempt to respond to their needs in nonurban areas. The essential problem is the broad spread of HIV cases over a large geographic area. The relatively thin spread probably does not justify the development of HIV-dedicated services within specific communities, so the task becomes one of integrating HIV services into existing community-based health and human service agencies.

   Existing agencies are typically already stretched beyond their capacities. The addition of services targeting those living with HIV disease, along with the attendant stigma, is not a welcome development to service providers.

   Nonurban geography insulates service providers, who consequently tend to view AIDS as not something that affects their communities. Little importance is attached to development of HIV services. Given the best of motives, nonurban service providers are not likely to have encountered many HIV-affected individuals requesting care. Thus, considering other problems that press for attention, they are unlikely to see as a priority the development of HIV services or training that would increase their competence in this area. In fact, they often see planning and training efforts as punishment because they detract from more pressing issues.
2. *Homophobia.* From the beginning of the epidemic in America, AIDS has been labeled the "gay plague." A minister who was one of the first transfusion-related AIDS cases and who lived in Indiana said toward the end of his life, "The issue is homophobia pure and simple." He continued, "I never had any conception of what it was like before I became infected. Once infected, I was tarred with the same brush of homophobia that tars the gay man who is HIV infected."

## *Recommendations for Future Practice*

While geography forms a barrier to providing care to those with HIV disease in nonurban areas, it can be overcome.

Emphasis should be placed on regional centers for the development of HIV services. Most small-town and rural areas have a larger town or small city as their geographic focus for retail trade, entertainment, and medical care. These regional centers may serve as focal points for the development of HIV services that can serve larger geographic areas. (Note that these regional areas do not necessarily follow state boundaries.) Since a proportionately larger number of HIV cases can be expected in these regional trading and medical centers, the development of HIV services there would make greater economic sense. These regional centers frequently also have institutions of higher education and medical residency programs associated with hospitals. Medical educators and faculty in regional colleges and universities are often more approachable regarding development of HIV services in their geographic area and may even be counted on to provide leadership for service delivery planning and development.

In most instances, leadership for HIV community-based resource development and maintenance will have to come from outside the specific small town or rural area. The regional centers are ideally positioned to bridge the gap between federal and state-level resources and the needs and realities of the local nonurban area. A focal point for sustained leadership, such as a regional care center, is critical to the establishment and integration of HIV service delivery in nonurban settings.

Development of telephone and computer-based "warm lines" for case consultation can assist mental health and other health and human service providers by providing needed information, guidance, and support. But such technology-assisted resources will be used only to the extent that they emerge out of trusting relationships between professionals. This is especially true in the area of mental health care. Those staffing "warm lines" must have a great deal of credibility and demonstrated skill in the area of HIV service delivery and mental health. They must also possess excellent training, supervision, and consultation skills. Periodic field visits are necessary to reinforce relationships with mental health professionals who utilize these support services.

## *Tools for Clinical Practice*

I have found these points to be critical in developing a system for HIV/AIDS services delivery in nonurban areas:

- *The importance of the community-level sanctioning process cannot be overstated in the development of HIV services in small towns and rural areas.*

  Rounds (1988a) and Seeley et al. (1991) have pointed out the importance of informal social networks for providing support and care in nonurban areas. Experience bears this out. People in small towns and in rural areas typically have different expectations regarding caregiving, founded in an ethic of self-reliance and a deep-seated distrust of government. People are expected to take care of themselves and their own, and reliance on outside organizations can be construed as a failure of self-reliance, the family, and community.

Different approaches are required, therefore, in making entry into nonurban communities and developing HIV-related services (Rounds, 1988b). Formal organization and public meetings with accompanying media coverage should be eschewed in the beginning because they provide opportunity for the venting of reactionary opposition. More efficient entrance can be made by using naturally existing informal support networks and working through one supportive individual at a time. These individuals who live within the local community can then provide leads to others who might be supportive or have resources. This "snowball" approach to community resource development is slow but has the advantage of allowing for the development of a network of service providers and resources in a nurtured and relatively safe environment. Once a sufficient number of people has become involved to give a certain amount of community sanction to HIV service delivery, a more public approach can be taken.

With service providers afraid for their reputations and their practices should it become known that they are the "AIDS Doc" or the "AIDS mental health service provider," it is essential that they know that there is a segment of the community who will support them. It takes an unusually strong individual to buck public sentiment in a rural area, where the economic and personal consequences for running counter to public opinion can be grievous. Those individuals who do run this risk are often motivated by deeply held moral and religious beliefs. Religious sentiment, however, in a local community is more likely to be dominated by fundamentalistic Protestantism and may be strong enough to inhibit such individuals from action on the HIV front.

- *When networks of service providers are established in small towns and rural areas, they are likely to be thinly staffed and very fragile.*

A whole service delivery network in a rural area may depend on one concerned professional or lay person. If that person leaves or becomes ill, the network falls into crisis. Maintenance becomes a constant issue and can be difficult, given the far-flung geographic spread of the service delivery system.

Similarly, a disruptive client can damage a fragile delivery system. Too often, once a client has been diagnosed with HIV disease, everything else about the client recedes into the background; service providers focus on the HIV to the exclusion of everything that has gone before. But many individuals who become HIV-infected have had multiple problems before infection. The HIV diagnosis is simply another overwhelming stress, and they may not have particularly good coping skills.

Service providers' immediate reaction to such disruptive clients is often a decision, based on one experience, that all HIV clients are impossible to treat, and they terminate their participation in the service delivery network.

A great deal of effort and leadership is required to support the network and to ensure its viability. The mind-set of those developing HIV services in small towns and rural areas can only be one of long-term effort working toward long-term goals.

- *Many people in rural areas have negative attitudes regarding mental health services.*

  Mental illness still carries a great stigma of its own, and this stigma is readily apparent in many rural areas. An attitude exists within much of the population that leads people to believe that mental health care is for "crazy people." Similarly, a person with HIV/AIDS may view his or her situation as strictly one of physical illness and reject mental health care as inappropriate. Physicians frequently make mental health referrals only as "referrals of last resort" and may present such referrals to difficult patients as the alternative unless they become more compliant.

- *HIV/AIDS mental health care and health service delivery in nonurban areas is an exercise in multiculturalism.*

  While much of multicultural education encountered in the graduate training of mental health care providers focuses on issues of gender and race, experience in small-town and rural areas leads us to believe that such a definition of multiculturalism in not nearly broad enough. Certainly multiculturalism in rural America can be illustrated by, for example, the presence of large numbers of racial-ethnic minorities such as African Americans and Hispanics in given localities. But another example of cultural diversity is the presence of migrant farm workers, which represents a very mobile population. Some nonurban areas are populated by religious sects such as the Amish. The mental health provider needs to take these cultural and community differences into account in planning and delivering services.

- *Confidentiality, difficult to maintain in small towns and rural areas, creates paradoxes of service seeking.*

  It is practically impossible not to know people through multiple contacts and in multiple roles. It is not uncommon for the receptionist at the doctor's office to be someone with whom the client went to high school. News travels quickly, since there are fewer people to engage in the process of dissemination.

  HIV clients have reason to be concerned about confidentiality. Jobs are still lost, families still disintegrate, homes are still given up, insurance can still be lost because of breaches in confidentiality. Some of those living with HIV disease still have their homes burned when their HIV status is revealed.

  Conversely, for those living with HIV disease in small-town and rural areas, geographical distance may spell assurance of confidentiality, and herein lies a paradox: While the client is asymptomatic and service delivery needs are the least complex, services are typically sought at a distance. When the client becomes more symptomatic, gets too sick to travel, and needs the most experienced care, services are sought locally. Yet, services available locally may not be adequate to the need. HIV service delivery planning for nonurban areas needs to take this pattern of service seeking into account.

- *The development of integrated health service delivery for those living with HIV/AIDS depends on the cultivation of relationships not only within individual systems, e.g., mental health centers, hospitals, and HIV/AIDS dedicated social service agencies, but also between agencies, care providers, and informal support networks.*

  The provider in a nonurban setting cannot afford to sit comfortably in an office and only provide services. That person must be a networker. That means the devotion of constant attention to the informal network of personal relationships in terms of case finding, service delivery, and referral resource development.

- *Distance and lack of transportation are barriers to accessing care.*

  Although fairly obvious, this is often lost on discharge planners in large, urban, tertiary-care hospitals. Hospital staff need to work closely with community-based care providers to determine if plans for follow-up care are possible, much less probable. The realities of nonurban life and the distance between available sources of needed care may impose severe limits on such plans.

- *The darker side to the often laudable and proud tradition of "taking care of our own" in small towns and rural areas is the relatively narrow definition regarding who is deserving of care.*

  By and large, gay men and injection drug users do not fit into this category. Issues of social class and race may also bear on this question. Typically, small towns and rural areas export nonconventional individuals to urban areas, and, of course, many are uncomfortable with the conformity espoused by local communities. Given this, small-town or rural communities can pretend that these kinds of differences do not exist. And, of course, if there are no gay individuals, for example, living within the community for the local population to know, there is no reason for their stereotypes to be dispelled. The mental health provider can respond by advocating tolerance if not acceptance of these individuals. Mental health service providers already enjoy some degree of social sanction for advocating unpopular causes. This social sanction can be capitalized on to broaden the boundaries of community acceptance.

- *Infected gay men coming home to die is a scene repeated daily across the small towns and rural communities of America.*

  Such homecomings are fraught with difficulties. In many cases the offspring's homosexuality was never openly acknowledged in the family or community. The family must thus cope with the conscious knowledge that a member is gay and that he is dying. Often the original leave-taking was not accomplished under the best of circumstances, and much unfinished business has been left incomplete. The return home tends to reactivate these old and perhaps festering issues. Fractures often appear in the marriage of the parents as they attempt to cope with this situation.

  Such homecomings may have a very high cost attached. Experience indicates that sometimes families agree to take their offspring back and provide care through the final illness only if he or she agrees not to have contact with any gay or lesbian friends. In more extreme cases, the HIV-infected person is asked to renounce his or her sexual orientation. Religious rites of reconversion may also be a part of the bargain.

The mental health provider involved in this situation is faced with ameliorating the crisis that such a homecoming produces. At the same time, opportunity may exist within the destabilized family system to make significant impact on long-standing and maladaptive patterns of interrelating.

- *Homophobia is more likely to be internalized within gay and bisexual individuals who remain in small towns.*

Certainly, the manifestations of internalized homophobia are easier to spot in the lives of gay and bisexual men who are HIV-infected and who have lived most of their lives in rural areas. Internalized homophobia can be found in the number of gay and bisexual men in heterosexual marriages, the understanding of their own sexual orientation in terms limited to sexual activity, reluctance to seek HIV testing and treatment even when they know they are infected, and the amount and pervasiveness of religious guilt present, especially during the final stages of the disease.

One outcome of this internalized homophobia is the number of multiple infections found in single families. Wives and newborn infants thus end up paying the price for this endemic homophobia. Internalized homophobia also affects men of color who have sex with other men. It is not uncommon to find these men claiming infection through injection drug use, when in fact they have never engaged in needle sharing and simply find admitting to injecting preferable to homophobic stigmatization.

Internalized homophobia makes for difficulty in accessing those who are in need of services, slow going in counseling and psychotherapy, and complicated ethical problems. Closeted clients may not be willing to come for services to a service center that is identified with caring for the HIV-infected. In some cases, it may be necessary to meet them on their own turf, at least initially. Complicated ethical issues present themselves when individuals fail to warn partners that they are HIV-positive, potentially putting them at risk.

- *Institutional manifestations of homophobia in nonurban areas run the gamut from denial of hospital visiting privileges to lovers to denial of access to services altogether.*

A particularly interesting twist on institutionalized homophobia is the referral of gay and lesbian clients to openly gay and lesbian service providers in mental health centers. This phenomenon also exists in private practice but is not as prevalent in nonurban areas.

On the one hand, this practice can ensure that gay clients are matched with professionals who may have a vital interest in HIV service delivery. On the other hand, as long as HIV clients can be referred to specific professionals on the basis of sexual orientation, other professionals do not have to become knowledgeable or explore their own negative attitudes that may form barriers to accessing care.

- *Because nonurban areas are generally underserved, mental health care providers working with HIV/AIDS clients often have to play multiple roles and serve multiple functions for the client.*

It may be necessary for the mental health service provider, lacking other resources, to act as informal monitor of the quality of medical care that the client receives or as client advocate for access to housing or other social services necessary for the maintenance of well-being. This role overlap can be confusing for the client as well as for the mental health service provider. It also assumes that the service provider has a knowledge base sufficient to know when to question the quality of care an HIV/AIDS client may be receiving from another professional. Interpersonal tact is also necessary in large measures to perform this role while still maintaining relationships with other professionals who are providing care to the client.

## REFERENCES

American Health Consultants. (1995, October). AIDS care now straining rural health systems. *AIDS Alert, 10,* 124–127.

Aruffo, J. F., Thompson, R. G., Gottlieb, A. A., & Dobbins, W. N. (1995). An AIDS training program for rural mental health providers. *Psychiatric Services, 46(1),* 79–81.

Berry, D. E., McKinney, M. M., McClain, M., & Valero-Figueira, E. (1995). *Rural HIV service networks: Patterns of care and policy issues.* Rockville, MD: Office of Science and Epidemiology, Bureau of Health Resources Development, Health Resources and Services Administration.

D'Augelli, A. R. (1989). AIDS fears and homophobia among rural nursing personnel. *AIDS Education and Prevention, 1,* 277–284.

Davis, K., & Stapelton, J. (1991). Migration to rural areas by HIV patients: Impact on HIV-related healthcare use. *Infection Control and Hospital Epidemiology, 12,* 540–543.

Fuszard, B., Sowell, R. L., Hoff, P. S., & Waters, M. (1991). Rural nurses join forces for AIDS care. *Nursing Connections, 4(3),* 51–61.

Gould, P., & Kabel, J. (1993, January). The last count: The geography of AIDS. *Atlantic Monthly,* 90–91.

Graham, R. P., Forrester, M. L., Wysong, J. A., Rosenthal, T. C., & James, P. A. (1995). HIV/AIDS in the rural United States: Epidemiology and health services delivery. *Medical Care Research and Review, 52,* 435–452.

Health Resources and Services Administration. (1991). *HIV infection in rural areas: Issues in prevention and services.* Rockville, MD: Author.

Hearn, W. (1994, July 25). AIDS in the country. *American Medical News,* 17–20.

Pollard, J. D., & D'Augelli, A. R. (1989). AIDS fears and homophobia among volunteers in an AIDS prevention program. *Journal of Rural Community Psychology, 10(1),* 29–39.

Rounds, K. A. (1988a). AIDS in rural areas: Challenges to providing care. *Social Work, 33,* 257–261.

Rounds, K. A. (1988b). Responding to AIDS: Rural community strategies. *Journal of Contemporary Social Work, 69,* 360–364.

Rounds, K. A., Galinsky, M. J., & Stevens, L. S. (1991). Linking people with AIDS in rural communities: The telephone group. *Social Work, 36,* 13–18.

Rumley, R. L., Shappley, N. C., Waiver, L. E., & Esinhart, J. D. (1991). AIDS in rural eastern North Carolina — patient migration: A rural AIDS burden. *AIDS, 5,* 1373–1378.

Rural Prevention Center (1994). HIV infection and AIDS in rural America. *Rural Prevention Report, 1(1),* 1–3.

Seeley, J., Wagner, U., Mulemwa, J., Kengeya-Kayondo, J., & Mulder, D. (1991). The development of a community-based HIV/AIDS counselling service in a rural area of Uganda. *AIDS Care, 3,* 207–217.

Verghese, A. (1994). *My own country.* New York: Vintage Books.

Wasser, S. C., Gwinn, M., & Fleming, P. (1993). Urban-nonurban distribution of HIV infection in childbearing women in the United States. *Journal of Acquired Immune Deficiency Syndromes, 6,* 1035–1041.

Whyte, B. M., & Wilber, J. A. (1992). HIV infection and AIDS — Georgia, 1991. *Morbidity and Mortality Weekly Report, 41,* 876–878.

# 11 | Mental Health Issues of HIV-Negative Gay Men

*Ariel Shidlo*

I wish I just became HIV-positive and got it over with.

These words were spoken in a therapy session by a high-functioning, intelligent, and successful gay man. This patient was suffering from the physical pain of a shingles episode and he was anxious about whether this meant he was HIV-positive. He was obsessively reviewing his sexual past to make sure that he had not done anything "risky," questioning whether the shingles inflammation was a sign from God to stop having sex with other men, and revisiting internalized homophobia that associated being gay with disease and punishment.

This HIV-negative gay man was angry. His recent experience of dating a man, falling in love and becoming sexual had been spoiled by the fear that he had become infected with HIV and that he had done something wrong. He complained of feeling that intimacy and love were contaminated for him by the fear of HIV and the wait to become infected.

This seronegative gay patient had never engaged in unprotected sex. He felt confident that he was not about to engage in risky sex. And yet he still had a nagging feeling that it was only a matter of time before he seroconverted. Being a gay man meant for him that eventually he too would get AIDS, no matter how careful he was (see Frederick & Glassman, 1996).

I myself am an HIV-negative gay man who came out in 1980, just one year before AIDS was identified. When I first tested for HIV antibodies in 1987, I expected to test seropositive. Even though I had practiced safer sex since the mid-1980s, I assumed that I had become infected with HIV before that. When I got my seronegative results, instead of feeling relieved and happy, I found myself depressed and mournful. It seemed inconceivable to me that I could be HIV-negative.

I frequently asked myself, "Why me?" How could it be that I hadn't been infected? I would envision a plane crash, the people next to me lying dead while I walked away unhurt. In light of the suffering of my peers, I felt guilty about being HIV-negative. I went through years of disbelief, suspicious that one day my real HIV results — positive — would finally emerge. My feelings of guilt and disbelief were compounded when, in the late 1980s, I learned that a man whom I had dated in 1980 had seroconverted and another man with whom I had been involved had died.

When they were published, I read Johnston's (1995) and Odets's (1995) writings on HIV-negative gay men. They described feelings that I had not been able to articulate previously — that HIV-negative gay men suffer considerably from the shadow of HIV, that we should allow ourselves to contemplate a personal future without illness, that we can survive this epidemic.

It has taken me nine years since I first tested seronegative to develop a stable belief that I am and will remain HIV-negative.

## *HIV-Negative Men in the Gay Community*

About the middle of the 1990s, we witnessed a new movement in the gay community. We started to acknowledge and articulate the stresses that many *HIV-negative* gay men are experiencing. Community forums in major U.S. cities, support and therapy groups, books, newspaper articles, videos, and counseling programs are addressing the concerns of HIV-negative gay men.

This activity has been spurred in part by our admitting aloud our worry at the resurgence of HIV seroconversion rates in gay men since the early 1990s (Gay Men's Health Crisis, 1995a). From one third to half of gay men in certain major U.S. urban centers are estimated to be infected with HIV (Morris & Dean, 1994). At the current rate of seroconversion, a twenty-year-old gay man has less than a 50 percent probability of remaining HIV-negative during his lifetime (Hoover et al., 1991).

Already many gay men in cities such as Los Angeles, San Francisco, and New York, where the gay community is dense and enmeshed, have experienced a multitude of deaths and ill friends. As many as 274,192 gay and bisexual men have been diagnosed with AIDS in the United States; tens of thousands have died (Centers for Disease Control and Prevention, 1996).

Odets (1995) has described many urban gay HIV-negative men as living in a world of shadows, survivors, and ghosts. As a result of so many losses, some HIV-negative gay men may experience significant survivor guilt. This guilt may be especially powerful when a partner or close friends are HIV-positive.

Many HIV-negative gay men find it difficult to discuss their feelings about how the specter of AIDS has affected their relationships, love, sex, their identities and their futures. Many HIV-negative gay men feel secretive and shameful about their serostatuses. They are afraid to tell their HIV-positive friends for fear of hurting them, making them envious, or burdening them with perceived trivialities. Some HIV-negative men even lie to others, pretending to be HIV-positive. They do not talk about their serostatuses with HIV-negative friends because it is supposed to be a nonissue, a lab result that one should accept quietly and gratefully. In a climate where the meanings of HIV serostatus are not openly explored and discussed, HIV-negative gay men's identities can become fragmented and confused (Ball, 1995).

Many gay men find it exceedingly difficult to discuss their feelings about protected and unprotected anal intercourse with prospective sexual partners or even with established life-partners. This lack of open communication about unprotected anal intercourse occurs in a climate where 20 to 43 percent of gay men aged 18 to 25 in large urban centers report having engaged in it over the previous year or two (see Dean & Meyer, 1995; Hays, Kegeles, & Coates, 1990). Similarly, more than 50 percent of a sample of gay and bisexual African American men in the San Francisco Bay Area reported having unprotected anal intercourse in the previous six months (Peterson et al., 1992), and 41 percent of a predominantly white Seattle community sample reported unprotected anal intercourse over the previous year (GayMap survey results, 1994). Recent figures from Project ACHIEVE in New York City reveal that 31 percent of men under age 30 and 25 percent of men age 30 and above in a cohort of 600 HIV-negative gay men reported insertive unprotected anal intercourse in the previous three months with an HIV-positive or unknown serostatus partner (*Achievements,* 1995). Figures for receptive unprotected anal intercourse in this sample were 25 percent for men under age 30 and 17 percent for men age 30 and above.

My clinical practice suggests that many HIV-negative gay men are mistrustful and fearful of being lied to about serostatus by their sexual partners. Intimacy and trust have paid a high price in this climate of suspicion and fear (Odets, 1995; Rofes, 1996). Prevention material exhortations to "use a condom with every partner" have been interpreted by many men to mean "trust no one, not even your lover" and "every man for himself." A young man in his twenties who seroconverted recently told me that his boyfriend had known for several years that he was HIV-positive and had withheld that information, yet had had unprotected anal intercourse with him. Only after my patient seroconverted and confronted his boyfriend, the only sexual partner with whom he ever had unprotected anal intercourse, did the boyfriend admit that he had been too afraid to tell him.

The majority of HIV-positive gay men may never have unprotected anal intercourse with an HIV-negative partner. Still, it is our responsibility to disillusion those HIV-negative men who *assume* that their sexual partners' or lovers' willingness to engage in unprotected anal intercourse signifies that their partners are seronegative (Gold, 1995). We have to help our HIV-negative clients learn to *ask* partners about their serostatus *before* deciding to engage in unprotected anal intercourse. Couples may view unprotected anal intercourse as a sign of commitment and trust in each other (Schoofs, 1995). They need to be supported in sharing the responsibility of staying uninfected through an open dialogue that values maintaining seronegativity as an expression of love and caring for each other.

Gold (1995) has written that asserting that the gay community is a safer-sex culture may make it very difficult for gay men who practice unprotected anal intercourse to discuss their behavior with friends. This conspiracy of silence has facilitated development of shame and secretiveness in those struggling with the riskiness of this behavior when partners are seropositive or of unknown status. Those who practice unprotected anal intercourse with a monogamous seronegative partner also do not feel readily able to talk about it because it is contrary to the "use a condom every time with every partner" exhortation of prevention campaigns. This scarcity of dialogue about risky sex has deprived gay men of the chance to provide emotional support and guidance to each other on these issues. Grass-roots groups such as the New York-based Community AIDS Prevention Activists are creating new and exciting forums for such dialogues.

Rofes (1996) has asked whether a gay culture filled with warnings about the hazards of anal sex has had the paradoxical effect of channeling gay men's erotic desires more strongly toward anal intercourse. As many gay men have staked out a terrain as "sexual outlaws" who are viewed as deviant or sinful by homophobes, Rofes poses the challenging question of whether unsafe sex has become the defining act of a renegade status. In my clinical work, one patient reported finding and enjoying comradeship with his partners in unprotected anal intercourse. He enjoyed the thrill of discovering whether a prospective sexual partner would (silently) consent to or signal interest in having intercourse without a condom. On a related note, Ostrow, DiFranceisco, & Kalichman (1996) investigated whether some men have a "risk-taking" personality trait that leads them to enjoy the dangers of unprotected anal intercourse with partners of unknown HIV status.

## *Odets's Conceptual Groundwork*

Odets (1994, 1995) has created a conceptual groundwork for understanding the lives of HIV-negative gay men.

First, he writes that there has been an obfuscation of an essential difference between the lives and the fates of HIV-negative and HIV-positive gay men. It is painful to acknowledge a qualitative difference between those who are uninfected and can look forward to longevity and those who face a chronic and often terminal illness. Uninfected gay men, HIV-positive men, and persons with AIDS are *not on a continuum,* as some prevention campaigns have claimed. The promotion of the continuum idea, while having positive connotations of unity between HIV-negative and -positive gay men, also contains the damaging implication that a progression along the continuum is inevitable. (One slogan of 1980s gay AIDS activism was "We are all people with AIDS.") As a community under siege from the right wing and from religious homophobes, gay men have not felt the luxury of articulating this potentially divisive fissure in the gay community. Instead, HIV-negative men have felt protective of their HIV-positive friends and lovers and fearful of any public articulation of the painful difference between negatives and positives.

Second, according to Odets, many HIV primary prevention efforts have confused outcome and target groups. Stating the obvious, only HIV-negative men can be helped to stay uninfected: They are therefore the only outcome group of primary prevention. HIV-negative and

-positive men should be viewed as distinct target groups for prevention activities, each with its own concerns and motivations. Educational material and counseling should acknowledge these realities rather than obfuscate them.

Third, the meaning and the importance of anal intercourse and the exchange of semen (orally or anally) for many gay men have been ignored. Anal intercourse has been trivialized as dispensable, and the desire for and the practice of unprotected anal intercourse have been pathologized. Odets attributes this trivialization and devaluing of the importance of anal intercourse between men to homophobia; it is expressed in the prevention message that this is an expendable activity that is interchangeable with other sexual behaviors. He has observed that, in contrast, married heterosexual couples who test seronegative for HIV are generally not told to use a condom every time they have vaginal intercourse or asked to view intercourse as a dispensable aspect of their sexual lives.

Another contribution of Odets's (1995) analysis is the recognition that HIV-related survivor guilt may activate earlier developmental guilt. In addition to whatever historical guilt issues both gay and nongay individuals may deal with, Odets points out that many gay men have a unique developmental history of guilt based on their experience of taking from their parents the "normal" heterosexual son that they expected. Many families experience their sons' homosexuality as an abandonment and their sons may thus emotionally equate survival as gay men with the abandonment of others.

An important generalization in understanding the interaction between preexisting characterological and developmental issues and being HIV-negative is that any developmental conflict may interact with the psychological experience of HIV-negative gay men living in the AIDS epidemic (Odets, 1995). A history of difficult conflict about homosexuality, serious depression, long-standing personal isolation and similar difficulties may interact destructively with AIDS.

## *HIV-Negative Identity*

The idea that being HIV-negative should be or even can be viewed as an identity or as a component of identity is being debated in the gay community (Johnston, 1995; Odets, 1995; Rofes, 1996). Arguments against its being viewed as an identity have included fears that it would promote what has been called "viral apartheid" and facilitate a dangerous demarcation between HIV-positive and -negative gay men. Others believe that promoting an HIV-negative identity is an important means to help keep gay men from seroconverting (Dalit, 1996; Odets, 1995).

An HIV-negative identity has several important characteristics:

- It is defined by the absence of a viral infection rather than by the presence of a defining feature.
- It is associated with a precarious sense of grace from which one can fall anytime. Seroconversion frequently appears as an omnipresent threat.
- It is a status that is seldom talked about with others.
- It is frequently unintegrated with other aspects of gay men's identity.

HIV-negative men who have not had the opportunity to talk openly about their serostatuses frequently describe their experience of being in an HIV-negative group as a "coming out" process that is reminiscent of having coming out as gay men. Odets (1995) posits that not coming out as HIV-negative compromises gay men's commitment to that identity and to their actual physical condition. HIV-negative gay men require social structures within the gay community that support their feelings and their identities and that are invested in maintaining their seronegative statuses. The preservation of an HIV-negative serostatus has to continue shifting from a solely individual responsibility to a communal effort. In this process, an open dialogue between HIV-negative and HIV-positive gay men is an essential component. Groups such as Community AIDS Prevention Activists and Gay Men's Health Crisis in New York have done important work in this direction by sponsoring CrossTalk community forums that bring together seronegative, seropositive, and untested men for the purpose of *talking* to each other.

## *My Clinical Work*

The program I direct, TalkSafe, is a peer counseling program for gay and bisexual men who self-identify as HIV-negative. The program provides time-limited individual, couple, and group peer counseling. TalkSafe is founded on the following principles:

- HIV-negative men need a safe space to talk openly about their feelings without fear of neglecting, offending, or hurting HIV-positive men or incurring their resentment or anger (Odets, 1995).

- Staying HIV-negative is an ongoing process that is impacted by psychological, interpersonal, and community factors.
- Gay men need help in the process of staying HIV-negative.
- Gay men who view HIV-negative serostatus solely as a lab result need to be supported in developing an identity as HIV-negative men and in integrating this identity into their multiple identities.
- No one factor explains why an individual would engage in unprotected anal intercourse, but a unique constellation of factors affects each individual.
- Gay men need help to talk about how they determine the situational riskiness of unprotected anal intercourse (see Lowy & Ross, 1994).
- HIV-negative couples need help to examine their decision-making around unprotected anal intercourse.
- Couples with mixed HIV statuses need help to examine each partner's feeling toward the other's serostatus.
- Clients who are candidates for peer counseling need a mental health assessment by a professional provider to link those with a significant psychological or substance abuse disorder with appropriate mental health services.
- Counseling for relatively intact clients can be successfully provided by peers who are trained and supervised by a professional mental health provider.
- Peer counselors can use disciplined self-disclosure and model for clients their own coping with the anxieties of an HIV-negative status.
- Gay men sometimes need help in developing nonsexual intimacy; they may need help to learn how to talk with each other.
- Since it is not clear what interventions are useful in helping HIV-negative gay men remain seronegative, we need ongoing program evaluation to determine what works (Choi & Coates, 1994).

## *Barriers to Services*

When I was asked in 1995 to design a peer counseling program for HIV-negative gay men at St. Vincent's Hospital and Medical Center in New

York, I was initially fearful of negative reactions from the gay community. Would we be vilified for creating a program that excluded HIV-positive men or accused of diverting limited resources from services for HIV-positive people? Providers considering HIV-negative services may be faced with hostility from within the AIDS health care community (Johnston, 1995; Odets, 1995; Rofes, 1996). Within our AIDS Center I overheard a (joking) remark about my project staff: "They're only the prevention program people. They're not important."

Both providers and clients may need consciousness raising to recognize that many HIV-negative gay men experience significant psychological distress associated with their serostatuses. Clients and providers may collude in avoiding difficult feelings or therapeutic issues by focusing instead on AIDS information and safer-sex guidelines. Many HIV-negative gay men are habituated to focusing on worries about the health concerns of HIV-positive partners and friends. Dalit (1996) reports on a member of an HIV-negative gay men's group who brought to a meeting copies of the latest research on protease inhibitors. The members were easily drawn into a discussion on these new anti-HIV medicines; they were startled that the group leader interpreted this group behavior as symptomatic of the difficulty many HIV-negative gay men have in focusing on issues related to their own serostatuses. The tendency to focus on HIV health issues should be similarly attended to when treating a couple with a mixed HIV serostatus.

## *Tools for Clinical Practice*

Clinicians working with HIV-negative men should consider these points:

- *Assess your clients' attitudes regarding their HIV-negative serostatus.*

  Gay men who are HIV-negative may experience a multitude of conflicting feelings about their serostatus. The following dimensions bear assessment: level of guilt, shame, and secrecy about being seronegative; level of precariousness about HIV-negative serostatus; and level of sense of legitimacy at viewing HIV-negativity as a problem compared to the concerns of friends and lovers who are HIV-positive. Clients who have not discussed their HIV-negative statuses with other HIV-negative gay men may benefit from viewing a short video that presents the isolation that some gay men feel about their seronegative statuses (Gay Men's Health Crisis, 1995b).

- *HIV-negative gay men need to be helped to develop an identity that integrates being uninfected into other aspects of their lives.*

  They need to be given permission to feel that being HIV-negative is something that they can feel good about and tell others about. Encourage your clients to articulate negative and positive feelings about being seronegative and to tolerate the confusion of contradictory sentiments. Adaptive identity integration of seronegative status can be accomplished only after exploring negative feelings.

  Facilitate the process of grieving the intrusiveness and contamination of AIDS on love, dating, relationships, sex, and sense of self as gay men. Help your clients examine to what extent they have constructed their identities and plans for the future around AIDS (Dalit, 1996). Some HIV-negative gay men may experience a tremendous burden at finding out they are seronegative. These are men who did not expect to grow old and therefore avoided dealing with issues of planning for a future, professionally and financially. One of Dalit's clients (Personal Communication, March 1996) who had recently tested negative reported never having paid taxes because he did not expect to have a long life.
- *Educate your clients regarding errors in assumptions.*

  Many HIV-negative gay men interpret the willingness of a sexual partner to have unprotected anal intercourse with them as evidence that their partner is also seronegative (Gold, 1995). Some men may not readily believe that a seropositive man would offer to have anal intercourse without a condom. They assume that their sexual partners are the same as they are – seronegative. Your clients need to be educated that their seropositive partners may themselves make an assumption of *sameness of serostatus,* thinking, "You're willing to have unprotected anal intercourse? This must mean *you are the same as me;* we are both HIV-positive so it's okay to do it without a condom." Help your clients to feel comfortable discussing serostatus issues with men they are dating, their lovers or life-partners and their sexual partners.
- *Help your clients articulate the meanings of specific sexual behavior.*

  Your clients may appear comfortable talking about sex but have difficulty exploring the meanings that sexual acts hold for them. Each gay man may have a unique constellation of meanings attached to sex and AIDS. Help your clients articulate aloud what anal intercourse with and without a condom means to them, what oral sex with and without a condom means to them, what having a man ejaculate inside them means to them, what ejaculating inside another man means to them, what kissing another man means to them, and what being sexually desired by another man means to them. Ask them what it means to them to have sex or make love with an HIV-negative partner, an HIV-positive partner, and a partner of unknown serostatus (see Elovich, 1995).

- *Examine the specific psychological impact that your clients experience as a result of the ambiguity over oral sex transmission data and prevention guidelines.*

  Many gay men have considerable anxiety about unprotected oral sex because the evidence about transmission is ambiguous. The most recent findings suggest that unprotected oral sex is classifiable as safer sex or as safe compared to safest (Nimmons & Meyer, 1996). The de facto standard of safer sex among many gay men includes unprotected oral sex. Examine whether anxiety and anger about the ambiguity of the riskiness of oral sex leads your clients to engage in unprotected anal intercourse ("No one knows what's really safe anyway; I might as well have anal intercourse without a condom.")

  I believe that providers should consider that there may be a danger of overfocusing or labeling oral sex as "high risk." This may lead clients to view the risk of unprotected oral sex as equivalent to that posed by unprotected anal intercourse. Remember: Only a handful of transmissions due to oral sex between gay men have been documented (Nimmons & Meyer, 1996). All other sexual transmission between men has occurred through unprotected anal intercourse. Recognize that a majority of gay men who engage in oral sex do so without a condom. Use of a condom in oral sex may not be a realistic goal for many clients. Do not collude with your clients in having them state that they intend to use condoms with oral sex unless they have a strong commitment to doing so. Instead, review the ways of reducing the risk of unprotected oral sex (Nimmons & Meyer, 1996): Keep the mouth, teeth, and gums healthy; do not floss before receptive oral sex; avoid using stimulant drugs that dull sensation, which may be associated with permitting trauma to the mouth and throat, thereby increasing susceptibility to infection;

do not have a large numbers of partners within a short period of time, since doing so can also cause trauma to protective tissue; avoid ejaculation in the mouth, which can lower the risk of transmission of HIV and other STDs.

- *Help your clients assess the unique factors that might lead them to engage in unprotected anal intercourse with partners of unknown status or with seropositive partners.*

  Each individual differs in the relative importance of the following factors that in my clinical experience may be associated with unprotected anal intercourse:

  — Internalized homonegativity (Shidlo, 1994) — negative attitudes toward one's homosexual feelings, behavior, relationships, and identity.
  — Shame about sex with other men.
  — Hopelessness and indifference about the future and one's personal well-being; fatigue of living in an epidemic without an apparent end: "We'll all get it sooner or later; it's just a question of time"; and "All my friends are sick or dead; I don't have much to look forward to."
  — Identity issues as a seronegative gay man: shame, secrecy, guilt, isolation, alienation, lack of visible role models.
  — Difficulty saying no to an attractive or sexually desirable partner who requests unprotected anal intercourse.
  — Experience of rejection by other gay men and associated negative mood states (Gold, 1995; Odets, 1995).
  — Impact of body image; poor self-esteem around body image may increase vulnerability to risky unprotected anal intercourse.
  — Risk-seeking trait; pleasure at placing oneself at risk (Ostrow, DiFranceisco, & Kalichman, 1996).
  — Poor communication and assertiveness skills; difficulty asking partner's serostatus, telling partner one's status, initiating condom use, insisting on condom use.
  — Informational fallacies, erroneous beliefs that insertive partners ("tops") can't get infected in unprotected anal intercourse, unprotected anal intercourse without ejaculation is safe, unprotected anal intercourse limited to insertion of tip of penis is okay.

– Distrust of safer sex credo; the role of the ambiguous data on oral sex as leading to unprotected anal intercourse.
– Sense of invulnerability; a feeling of personal immunity sometimes confirmed by a history of repeated HIV-negative test results in spite of history of risky unprotected anal intercourse.
– Untreated affective disorder.
– Untreated substance and alcohol abuse or dependence (Ostrow, DiFranceisco, & Kalichman, 1996; Ostrow et al., 1993).
– Need for intimacy; closeness and feeling of trust provided by unprotected anal intercourse may take on paramount significance over longevity and health (Odets, 1995). For some men, exchange of semen may be deeply valued and meaningful.
– Unacceptable negative meanings associated with condom use. Some men may view condoms as signifying "promiscuity," lack of trust, betrayal, and evidence of unacknowledged seropositivity in partner (see Schoofs, 1995).
– Condom-associated sexual dysfunction; erectile difficulties in insertive partner.
– Interethnic negative attitudes; differential perception of seroprevalence in particular ethnic groups; sadistic or masochistic impulses toward partner of different ethnicity.

- *Monogamous couples where both partners have tested HIV-negative sometimes opt to have unprotected anal intercourse. To minimize the risks of this decision, they need to be encouraged to think through and talk openly about their choice.*

  The Victorian AIDS Council/Gay Men's Health Centre in Australia (1994) has helpful education for couples considering unprotected anal intercourse. It recognizes that issues of trust and communication are crucial in the decisions. I have adapted their guidelines as follows:

1. The couple discusses the importance and meanings of unprotected anal intercourse for each partner.
2. If they both strongly want to engage in unprotected anal intercourse, both partners have an HIV test (preferably together) and commit to be completely honest with each other about the results.
3. The couple continues to use condoms every time they have anal intercourse for six months.

4. The couple then has another HIV test together.
5. If both test seronegative, the couple agrees that neither partner will engage in unprotected anal intercourse outside the relationship. *The couple commits and promises to tell each other immediately if this agreement is broken.* If the agreement is broken, they restart condoms for anal sex and go through all the preceding steps again.

If both partners test HIV-positive, they should consider the effects of reinfection when deciding whether to have unprotected anal intercourse with each other. If one of the partners is HIV-seropositive, they should continue to use condoms every time they have anal intercourse. Couples of mixed HIV status need help in talking to each other about the complex feelings each partner may have about the meanings of the difference between them in serostatus.

- *Conceptualize how characterological and developmental issues may be exacerbated by AIDS-related issues.*

  Help clients identify which aspects of their psychological distress or maladaptive behavior are in direct response to the stresses of the AIDS epidemic versus those aspects that are reactivations of earlier wounds and vulnerabilities. Assess whether earlier developmental issues related to internalized homophobia and gay identity formation need to be revisited by the clients. For some clients, AIDS may serve as a repository of toxic material. Ball (1995) reports having seen clients whose previous therapists interpreted anxiety, panic, and depression as solely characterological in origin, failing to contextualize them as normal reactions to the ongoing traumatization of the AIDS epidemic.
- *Actively support your clients when they report dating, falling in love, being in relationships, and having sex.*

  Gay men need to hear that loving other men is a good thing and that sex with other men is a healthy and desirable thing. In the context of the "AIDSification of gay identity" and the "homosexualization of AIDS" (Odets, 1995), it is an essential function for the provider to act as a counterforce that helps clients celebrate being gay. Challenge the tendency of clients to pathologize inappropriately their relationships and their sexual behavior. Help them examine what they actually mean when they report that they are "addicted" to sex. Is this an accurate description of dyscontrol and compulsion, or is it an AIDS-phobic and gay-phobic misinterpretation of high levels of sexual desire?

- *Clients may have different needs for individual, couple, and group modalities.*

  Clients who are early in the process of examining issues about being seronegative may require individual intervention. If appropriate, offer couple counseling for seronegative and negative/positive couples. The obvious but sometimes forgotten clinical wisdom is that not all HIV-negative gay men are appropriate for a group intervention. Screening for membership in group should be conducted according to established principles (Yalom, 1995).

- *Primary prevention programs and counseling materials need to recognize explicitly HIV-negative gay men and HIV-positive gay men and target each population distinctly* (Odets, 1995).

  When creating educational material, avoid obfuscating the differences between the concerns and the feelings of HIV-negative and HIV-positive gay men. HIV-negative men need to be helped to value self-preservation in addition to supporting their HIV-positive peers. HIV-positive men need to be helped to value avoiding reinfection in addition to maintaining the health of their HIV-negative peers. Both groups need help in valuing the continuity of the gay community and in keeping the next generation of gay men alive and healthy.

## REFERENCES

I would like to thank my partner, Jim Jasper, for his editorial help, patience, and love during the writing of this chapter. My colleague, Boaz Jacob Dalit, Psy.D., program coordinator at TalkSafe, has been instrumental in helping me think through issues of HIV-negative gay men and generous with sharing his clinical material.

*Achievements: A Newsletter for the Men of Project ACHIEVE* (1995, July). New York: Project ACHIEVE.

Ball, S. (1995, October). Positively negative. *In the Family,* 14–17.

Centers for Disease Control and Prevention (1996). *HIV/AIDS Surveillance Report, 8(1).*

Choi, K. H., & Coates, T. J. (1994). Prevention of HIV infection. *AIDS, 8,* 1371–1389.

Dalit, B. J. (1996, July). *Identity issues in HIV-negative gay men.* Paper presented at the Eighteenth National Lesbian and Gay Health Conference and the Fourteenth National AIDS/HIV Forum, Seattle, WA.

Dean, L., & Meyer, I. (1995). HIV prevalence and sexual behavior in a cohort of New York City gay men (Aged 18–24). *Journal of Acquired Immune Deficiency Syndrome and Human Retrovirology, 8,* 208–211.

Elovich, R. (1995, May 16). Harm's way. *Advocate,* 43.

Frederick, R. J., & Glassman, N. S. (1996). HIV in the lives of uninfected gay men. *HIV/AIDS & Mental Hygiene, 5(3),* 1, 5.

GayMap survey results (1994, October 21). *Seattle Gay News,* 7.

Gay Men's Health Crisis (1995a). *Swimming against the second wave. HIV prevention among gay men: A white paper.* New York: Author.

Gay Men's Health Crisis (1995b). *Talk about it* [Videotape]. (Available from Substance Use Counseling and Education [SUCE], GMHC, 129 West 20th St., New York, NY 10011)

Gold, R. (1995). Why we need to rethink AIDS education for gay men. *AIDS Care, 7, Supplement 1,* S11-S19.

Hays, R. B., Kegeles, S. M., & Coates, T. J. (1990). High HIV risk-taking among young gay men. *AIDS, 4,* 901–907.

Hoover, D. R., Munoz, A., Carey, V., Chmiel, J. S., Taylor, J. M. G., Margolick, J. B., Kingsley, L., & Vermund, S. H. (1991). Estimating the 1978–1990 and future spread of Human Immunodeficiency Virus Type 1 in subgroups of homosexual men. *American Journal of Epidemiology, 134,* 1190–1199.

Johnston, W. I. (1995). *HIV-negative: How the uninfected are affected by AIDS.* New York: Plenum Press.

Lowy, E., & Ross, M. W. (1994). "It'll never happen to me": Gay men's beliefs, perceptions and folk constructions of sexual risk. *AIDS Education and Prevention, 6,* 467–482.

Morris, M., & Dean, L. (1994). Effect of sexual behavior change on long-term Human Immunodeficiency Virus prevalence among homosexual men. *American Journal of Epidemiology, 140,* 217–232.

Nimmons, D., & Meyer, I. (1996). *Oral sex and HIV risk among gay men: Research summary.* New York: Gay Men's Health Crisis.

Odets, W. (1994). AIDS education and harm reduction for gay men: Psychological approaches for the 21st century. *AIDS & Public Policy Journal, 9(1),* 1–15.

Odets, W. (1995). *In the shadow of the epidemic: Being HIV negative in the age of AIDS.* Durham, NC: Duke University Press.

Ostrow, D. G., Beltran, E. D., Joseph, J. G., DiFranceisco, W., Wesch, J., & Chmiel, J. S. (1993). Recreational drugs and sexual behavior in the Chicano MACS/CCS cohort of homosexually active men. *Journal of Substance Abuse, 5,* 311–325.

Ostrow, D. G., DiFranceisco, W., & Kalichman, S. (1996). *Sexual adventurism, substance use and high risk sexual behavior: A structural model.* Manuscript submitted for publication.

Peterson, J. L., Coates, T. J., Catania, J. A., Middleton, L., Hilliard, B., & Hearst, N. (1992). High-risk sexual behavior and condom use among gay and bisexual African-American men. *American Journal of Public Health, 82,* 1490–1494.

Rofes, E. (1996). *Reviving the tribe: Regenerating gay men's sexuality and culture in the ongoing epidemic.* New York: Haworth Press.

Schoofs, M. (1995, January 31). Can you trust your lover? Gay couples weigh the risk of unprotected sex. *Village Voice,* 37–39.

Shidlo, A. (1994). Internalized homophobia: Conceptual and empirical issues in measurement. In B. Greene & G. M. Herek (Eds.), *Lesbian and gay psychology: Theory, research, and clinical applications: Vol. 1. Psychological perspectives on lesbian and gay issues* (176–205). Thousand Oaks, CA: Sage.

Victorian AIDS Council/Gay Men's Health Centre (1994). *Relationships: Your choice* [Poster]. South Yarra, Victoria, Australia: Author.

Yalom, I. D. (1995). *Theory and practice of group psychotherapy* (4th ed.). New York: Basic Books.

# 12 | Working with and for Children

## *Dottie Ward-Wimmer*

We sat together on his hospital bed. Beautiful dark eyes looked up at me and then at the picture he had just drawn. It was a six-year-old's typical rendition of a house. I asked, "Are you in this picture?" He pointed to the center of the paper and said quietly, "Sure I am . . . , but I'm so far in no one can see me."

Children with AIDS sometimes feel very alone.

More than anything else, he wanted to run and play with other kids. But he had hypertonic leg muscles. AIDS wasn't his problem; not being able to walk was. But physical therapy, a walker, and his indomitable spirit sustained him, and he won. He went to school, got messy, and made friends.

Children with AIDS sometimes just feel like children.

The petite eighteen-year-old and her three-year-old son, both HIV-positive, now live happily in their little apartment. At age sixteen she had decided that "when adults in the house don't treat you right, you just got to get out." So she packed up her infant son, went to a shelter (which she hated), and waited for housing to become available. She believes that "there's no one I can trust to raise him right," so she can't make a permanency plan to ensure the child's care after her death.

Children and teens with AIDS need support as they walk into the future.

"It's all right to fly now," they whispered. Hardly more than children themselves, the young parents sat next to their little boy's bed in the intensive care unit trying to find the words to help him die. "If you see a light, go to it because that's the safe place where you'll be loved." It was almost more than they could bear and they leaned back against the social worker and the medical intern who stood quietly waiting.

Children with AIDS, their families, and their caregivers deserve comfort as they embrace death.

Working with children and youth as they confront HIV is wonderful and exhausting, challenging and simple, unbelievably frustrating and totally satisfying.

First described in children in 1982, pediatric AIDS continues to be an ever-increasing statistic in terms of both infected and affected children. As early as 1988, HIV in children was recognized as a chronic illness (Power, DellOrto, & Gibbons, 1988). Yet, the majority of professional energy and fiscal resources had to be invested in its biomedical aspects rather than in its long term psychological impact.

## *Background Reading*

Although work with HIV-infected youngsters was based on models for working with children with cancer, HIV has brought unique issues into the healing arena (Hausher, 1989). Unlike cancer in children, HIV comes with profound stigma that drives families into deep holes of secrecy. Mary Tasker's book, *How Can I Tell You?* (1992), illustrates the dilemmas faced in revealing the diagnosis both within the family and to those outside. One dilemma is how and when to tell, a process unique to each family's story and circumstance. While the question of disclosure is often central in counseling children and families, there simply is no one absolute answer.

In *Children, Families, and HIV/AIDS* (Boyd-Franklin, Steiner, & Boland, 1995) we find a comprehensive look at the psychosocial issues of living with this virus. The model described is a multisystem, multigenerational meld that calls for a full range of coordinated services. Especially interesting, too, is their presentation of cultural subtleties that teach us that therapists need to be more than simply accepting of cultures other than their own. We must be knowledgeable about culturally accepted behaviors and, most important, about the culturally determined roles of children.

*Forgotten Children of the AIDS Epidemic* (Geballe, Gruendel, & Andiman, 1995) focuses squarely on the plight of affected children. It is estimated that by the year 2000 there will be between 82,000 and 125,000 children and adolescents left motherless by AIDS in the United States and Puerto Rico alone (Michaels & Levine, 1992). *Orphans of the HIV Epidemic* (Levine & Stein, 1994) outlines the issues and profiles work being done in six U.S. cities. It is clear that the children's futures demand that permanency planning and advocacy for appropriate placements after parents' deaths be priority action items.

And then there is writing for the children themselves. *Come Sit by Me* (Merrifield, 1990) tells the story of a preschool child who learns about HIV through her relationship with an HIV-positive classmate. The story describes the concerns of the parents of the other children and their need for information before they can feel comfortable having an infected child in the classroom. *Losing Uncle Tim* (Jordan, 1989), about a young boy who must come to terms with the knowledge that his favorite uncle is dying from AIDS, is of special value because it deals gently, yet clearly, with the youngster's initial fear and his subsequent ambivalence when he learns his uncle's diagnosis. In *Z's Gift* (Starkman, 1988), a youngster confronts his feelings when a favorite teacher tells the class that she has HIV. It presents a realistic alternative to turning one's back.

For infected children, who often feel profoundly isolated and different, there is *Be a Friend* (Wiener, Best, & Pizzo, 1994) and *Teens with AIDS Speak Out* (Kittredge, 1991), a compilation of the stories of infected children that can go a long way toward helping youngsters trapped in their secret to feel less alone.

Children's books are often useful as teaching tools for families. Their reading level makes complex material more comprehensible, and having the parent or an older sibling read to a youngster provides an opportunity for each to learn about the disease and about his or her own feelings.

While it is essential to stay abreast of the burgeoning literature, it is also essential that we don't get lost in theory. The ability to define clinical classifications and articulate theoretical frameworks must be balanced with deep respect for and awareness of the impact of HIV on clients' lives. Working with these youngsters and their families calls us to dare to be in touch with their very spirits as well as with their clinical issues. So, what should we do for the children? At the risk of oversimplifying, the best answer still is to walk with them.

## *My Clinical Work*

At the St. Francis Center, in Washington, D.C., we believe our job is to provide comfort and information and gently to invite clients to experience and honor their feelings. Our work includes individual therapy, group counseling, support for the caregivers, and education.

We offer a group for teens who are affected by HIV and a play therapy/support group, called the Hug Club, for younger children who are affected by the disease but may not know it. The club welcomes all children, whether or not they know the diagnosis. Although we've been criticized by those who say that keeping the secret perpetuates the stigma, we believe it is unethical to leave children unsupported while we argue about ethics. Thus, the Hug Club stands on our beliefs that all children deserve emotional support when confronting difficult situations and that each family has the right to determine its own ways and schedule for resolving issues.

It takes time for families to confront the painful realities of HIV infection. In the meantime, we negotiate with parents. We let the parents know that we never lie to a child. If the child asks, "Do I have AIDS?" we explore and deflect the question and let the parent know the child is asking so that plans about telling can be made. Experience has taught us that children can talk about feelings, learn about coping skills, and receive comfort without immediately being directly told, "Yes, you have AIDS."

To do so we often combine in our work psychodynamic developmental theories with Gestalt techniques (Axline, 1969; Oaklander, 1988; Polster & Polster, 1974). And we believe that ultimately, if we are patient, respectful, and creative, we can negotiate a comfortable and comforting path between the child's needs and questions and the family's decision on how and when to reply. Overall, the St. Francis program is built on the belief that the client truly has his or her own answers. Our job is to help each client discover that right path.

## *Barriers*

These are some of the barriers we face:

- *The complexities of issues.* HIV is simply not a singular event. Families rarely have only one HIV-positive member; in these families, dying and grieving are experienced simultaneously.

Many children in our grief groups are losing, or have already lost, both a parent and a sibling. Moreover, HIV disease in children is often found in the familial presence of drug abuse which, in itself, sets up complex and unhealthy intrafamily dynamics. Counselors must have at least a basic understanding of substance abuse and its impact within the family. In addition, we cannot forget to add the isolative social context within which families with HIV usually live.

- *Ethical/legal dilemmas.* It is simply impossible to work with HIV-infected children and teens without confronting myriad issues.

  Is it ethical to collude with the family in keeping an HIV diagnosis secret, or is this simply respecting the parents' right to make decisions on behalf of their children? Is it ethical to give a child the "truth" *and* the burden of keeping that truth a secret? Is disclosure always in the best interest of the child? If so, at what age? It is essential to consider the consequences of revealing the diagnosis. Think of the child who had been told about her younger sister's diagnosis (although the infected child herself was unaware). Think of how each must have felt when, in the midst of an argument, she yelled, "You're not so special. You only get away with stuff 'cause you got AIDS!"

  Disclosure issues are only one item on the list of ethical dilemmas. As we consider individuals' right to die, what are the rights of children? How do children gain access to treatment? The list seems endless.

## *Tools for Clinical Practice*

These guidelines are helpful in working with children in families affected by HIV/AIDS:

- *We must always start by looking inward.*

  Therapists must explore their own personal agendas, because our needs can strongly influence clinical judgments and expectations.

  Counselors must be regularly challenged to look within themselves and ask "why?" in reviewing therapeutic goals and actions. Recently, while working with a group of case managers around the issue of disclosure, I was reminded of how easy it is to blur the edges. In a role play the "counselor" repeatedly asked the "mother," who was considering telling her son about his HIV infection, "But how do *you* feel about this?" The role play was interrupted to explore the reason for the repeated question and it became clear that it was the "counselor's" feelings that really needed to be heard. The "mother" didn't need to talk about her feelings just then. She needed some practical guidance about talking to her child. But the counselor's need was getting in the way. These kinds of situations happen daily in this work, and it is a courageous therapist who is willing to see his or her own stuff and work on it.

- *Be sure you know who the client is — the parents, the child, or the family.*

  More than once you will find yourself caught in this quandary, and don't be surprised if the answer isn't always the same. In fact, the goal is not to find a consistent answer but, rather, to maintain a constant awareness of the question. You'll need to consider who really owns the problem. Is it the youth in front of you or the parent who doesn't see that the youngster is simply acting out the adult's issue?

  Rarely are the lines crystal clear. More often than not, families bring a bag of problems, which the counselor will help them to label as "yours," "mine," and "ours" before healing work can begin.

  In practice, I find it very useful to talk with the parents and the child together. If the topic is the child, then he or she has a right to hear it. Sometimes that process in itself is all that is really needed, because it sets up a forum for sharing what is happening. Each needs to be heard, but by each other, not just by the therapist.

- *It is imperative that counselors be cognizant of the parent's age and not automatically elevate to adulthood a young teen simply because she has given birth.*

  This becomes especially important when working with teenage mothers who must make decisions for their children, and it can be even more confusing when the mother is still a child herself living in her own mother's home. Time must be spent sifting out role expectations. Although the youngest child may be the designated patient, the teen caught in the middle is often the one who really needs your attention. She may also need you as an advocate so that her needs and decisions, not her mother's wishes or the therapist's expectations, are given primary attention.

- *A very large part of the work with clients is basic education.*

  All too often the medical information is daunting. It is imperative that the counselor understand the basic physiology of the disease so that he or she can communicate about it in simple terms, despite the fact that the immune system is most complex. A therapist must, for example, understand and be able to explain the fact that a newborn, though testing HIV-antibody-positive, is not actually infected. Though medical personnel may provide the information initially, it usually takes many discussions before clients integrate the information and fully understand it. Even the most knowledgeable person may experience diminished comprehension and memory during periods of crisis. So be sensitive to your clients' cognitive capabilities.

  Your working relationship with your client's physician will prove very useful here as you both work to keep the patient and the other family members in touch with their own realities, because that is the context within which the psychological work needs to be done.

- *In children, HIV disease can be manifested by developmental delays and regression.*

  Therapists must be alert to changes in the child's performance, which may signal a developmental change. In addition, it is important to remember that AIDS dementia occurs in children as well as adults, so affective and cognitive changes must be monitored. Pay attention to developmental milestones as well as to mood swings. You may be the first person to recognize subtle changes that signal a need for treatment, so be sure that written permission to exchange information with the child's physician is obtained early on and kept on file.

- *Children need more than comfort as they cope with life-threatening illness.*

  Children have a great deal of inner wisdom, but we must respect the fact that their internal capabilities are limited due to immaturity and lack of experience. We begin our therapeutic interventions with some emotional muscle building. We have found work in four areas to be essential for children who must face and deal with actual or anticipated loss. These building blocks are easily woven into the therapy hour as games and attitudes rather than time-consuming techniques.

1. *Ego boundary work.* The child must know where the edges are. Because sibling and/or parental death often occurs before the age at which the child would normally individuate, this becomes a very important part of the survivor's process. Children are concrete thinkers. Using their senses in tasting, touching, smelling, seeing, and hearing games and respecting their personal choices and space help to create a concrete sense of separate self. Body outline drawings and lists of "How I'm like (name of parent or sibling)" as well as "How I'm just like me" allows the child to experience his or her uniqueness.
2. *Mastery.* It stands to reason that a child must believe in his or her own potential to find the courage to move outward. First the boundaries are defined; then comes the sense of what is possible. The child again needs concrete experience, not just magical omnipotent thinking. Giving the child lots of choices and affirming the ability and right to choose is basic to this. Games in which they win are important. Kids often "cheat" because needing to win is important, so let them. When rules are turned around by the child, why not call it "creative"? Our work with these children is not about teaching social skills — it is about helping them to find the inner strength to cope with some really lousy circumstances.

   Manipulatable toys and art materials such as clay are useful in allowing the child to experience reshaping the world. "Do-overs" are fine. Children can learn that they don't have to like what's happening in their lives and that they can choose how they will respond to what they cannot change.
3. *Anger.* Now that the child sees who he or she is and feels capable, the youngster needs to harness the energy so often found as a core part of grief. I use the concept of anger here in the most positive context. Anger gets such a bad rap that children, and many therapists, are afraid of it. Adults tell themselves and the children that they need to find ways to "get rid of" their anger. Nonsense! We throw garbage away.

We keep the good stuff, and anger is part of the good stuff. It is the voice of the Self we work so hard to help the child discover. We need to learn to "have" our anger, to transform outrage into impetus.

Clay is great for hammering, throwing, or smooshing the object of our anger — the tumor, HIV, or drug pusher. Have the child use his or her voice to say, "I'm mad because . . ." or "I didn't like it when . . ." each time he or she throws the clay. Singing, drawing, and acting are other ways to discover what the anger looks like. Once the anger has form, it is no longer so scary. The child feels more in control of what he or she can see and thus more in control of him- or herself.

4. *Self-nurturing.* The ability to feel competent in caring for one's self is important to us all. It is especially useful for children who may not have much emotional support because the family is immersed in its own pain or because, simply, no one is there for the child. The ability to self-nurture is built on an ego with potential and energy.

   Drawing and imagery are very effective in learning this skill. For example, when a child asks for a hug, you may pause and invite the child to close her eyes and picture a person the youngster would really like to be hugged by. Let the child enjoy the picture and the feeling for a moment, then note that he or she can get that hug any time, just by closing his or her eyes. And don't forget to give the hug requested.

- *You cannot answer a child's questions honestly when the parent has forbidden you to do so.*

You can't always give a totally honest answer. But that doesn't mean you can't do effective work. Lying is unacceptable because it undermines the very foundation essential to a therapeutic relationship. So negotiating with the parent around disclosure is imperative. Negotiating does not mean convincing the parent to do it your way; it means that each of you lets the other know the boundaries. You must let the parent know exactly how you will respond to difficult questions if they arise.

Keep focused on what the child is really asking, rather than on what you think he or she ought to know. Questions about diagnosis are often more about fear than about clinical facts. When they first arise, it is usually more appropriate to reflect on them with the youngster, exploring the reason for asking as well as who else has been asked. Then plan with the child how to bring up the topic with Mom or Dad. Remember, disclosure is a process, and this give-and-take among the child, parents, and counselor is a part of that. On the rare occasion when a youngster absolutely demands to know if he or she has HIV, I've answered, "What if you do? What would it mean?" We then go quite naturally to all of the clinical and emotional questions needing to be asked without breaking the parents' directive. Kids know instinctively what they are allowed to ask. These are rules they've lived with all their lives. It's okay for kids to know that you are trying to help them within a prescribed set of rules. In fact, it usually works to your advantage because you're truly sharing a frustration.

Joey and his mom presented just such a dilemma. At age 8, he was in the final stages of AIDS. His mother refused to allow anyone to tell him his diagnosis, discuss the possibility of death, or mention God in any way. It was excruciatingly difficult to visit him because we all felt like hypocrites. Yet, we couldn't turn our backs on this child we had known for years.

One day he asked, "What happens when a kid gets tired of trying to get better?" The answer was simply, "Then he stops trying. It is okay to do that." We talked about how brave he was and how we all just do what we can do for as long as we can and when we can't, we can't. Some days later, the next question came: "What happens when you stop trying to get better?" The answer was, "Hmm, I wonder," and for several days after that we would touch on that question, wondering together. Finally, one day while drawing rainbows, a favorite activity of his, he said, "When you stop trying to get better, could you become purple in the rainbow?" I asked, "Would you like that?" He shook his head in the affirmative, and we both smiled.

We had followed all the rules and still found a way to comfort him and let him find answers for his questions. He died shortly after that last conversation. His mom was there, and we held his hands while talking softly about rainbows and always remembering Joey.

- *Everyone working with a family needs to be aware of the need for planning for the child's future.*

Laws regarding temporary and permanent guardianship vary.

Counselors ought not to attempt to be legal advisers, but they absolutely must know how to direct the parent to the legal service that most understands the difficulties that surround families affected by HIV/AIDS.

Your role may include supporting the parent through this process. Put yourself into the dilemma: You want to live, so you are focusing all your positive thoughts into taking care of yourself and being healthy. Your spiritual teachings tell you that God can make anything happen if you really believe. How can you say you "really believe" that you will be cured if you are planning for someone to care for your child after you die?

Maybe the language needs to be softened. Perhaps we would be better off talking about "life planning." The Child Welfare League of America has published an excellent guide, *Because You Love Them* (Merkel-Holguin, 1994). It is based directly on the lessons learned by listening to groups of HIV-infected parents talk about what they need to approach this tender subject.

- *Guilt and shame are issues that cannot be avoided.*

Once, I went to pick up a prescription for a child. Neither the mom nor I was known at the pharmacy, so it was assumed that I was the parent when I presented the Medicaid card asked for the medicine. The clerk had at first greeted me politely, but when she returned with the bag full of Retrovir (zidovudine) and antibiotics, her eyes were full of disgust. I wanted to scream, "It's not my baby, I'm just picking this up for a friend!" But instead I stood there and got a taste of what it's like for these mothers. Society overtly and covertly holds a mother responsible for the illness of her child, and the guilt experienced by the mother of an HIV-infected child can be enormous. As therapists, we must be cognizant of the fact that many HIV-infected women are wanting to have healthy babies — they are not intentionally passing HIV to their children.

Sooner or later the healthy child or teen in an AIDS-affected family knows guilt or shame, too, because of the diagnosis or because the child can't make the sick parent or sibling well. He or she may feel outrage and betrayed by a parent who didn't "practice what she preached," jealousy because the sibling is getting all the attention, or defeat when he or she wishes the sick person would "just die and get it over with" because the child wants a normal life for himself or herself. Few of the teens in our support group have told school friends about their infected parents, and they feel very guilty when their peers make "AIDS jokes" and they don't speak out in defense of the person they love.

The counselor can't erase the guilt and shame, but he or she can work to climb under the feelings and to help reframe and normalize them. Address the helplessness the child feels because he or she cannot make mommy better. Confront and allow the teen to experience outrage, and then move to help him or her to see the "betraying" parent as simply a person who made some really bad decisions. I sometimes find it useful to tell children about how I, too, at one time wished my mom would die because it was so hard to watch her battling an illness. I tell them how awful I felt as soon as I thought it, but after a while I realized that all I wanted was for mom not to be sick anymore. I was just a kid who was tired of having a sick mom. In understanding another's story, the youngster comes to understand, accept and forgive his own feelings.

- *Grieving is healing. It is multidimensional and belongs solely to the person journeying through it.*

Mourning progresses through multiple levels of shock, cognitive awareness, emotional experience and expression, and ultimately integration for all ages. But the journey down that road is different for children. It may be confusing and at times difficult for children, because they are only beginning to develop the coping skills needed to carry them through the experience. Often they feel alone as they struggle with these new feelings because the context within which children grieve is generally different from the world in which they experience other painful events. When death walks in, the parent is usually just as upset as the child. The child's support system is, therefore, generally unavailable. In addition, childhood grief is unique because:

— Developmental level and cognitive capacity influence the child's perception of the event. All children grieve, but young ones see death as life continuing elsewhere. For them, going to heaven may not be much different from going to Cleveland. If not told the truth, they wait for the deceased to return.

– Childhood bereavement has an intermittent rhythm. We've all seen children profoundly sad one moment and engrossed in play the next. That is their natural rhythm. The capacity to stay present to emotional pain increases with maturity.
– Children "regrieve" the event(s) as new coping and cognitive abilities emerge. Major life events such as birthdays and graduations often trigger a reworking of an early loss. This aspect of childhood grief is frequently overlooked by professionals who fail to connect a loss event occurring years ago with a presenting behavior.
– Children usually lack the vocabulary and the social skills needed to comprehend the reality of death and fully to experience mourning. Death is a secret so big we can't even talk about it, so it's frightening. For example, children learn about community helpers but never is the funeral director included on the list. How old were you when you understood what the difference was between embalming and autopsy? Cremation is the least expensive way of handling a dead body and is often done when funds are limited. Could you gently explain it to a child? If not, you need to visit a funeral parlor or a grief counseling center and become well acquainted with the vocabulary and the resources.

- *Children have survivor guilt.*
  "Why me?" is often turned into "Why not me?" Children need to hear over and over that it is not their fault. Therapists must be willing to enter with them into the "not knowing" rather than offer platitudes. The survivors need to find their own answers. One teen brought that point home with profound and crystalline clarity when, after listening to my rational answer to his truly unanswerable question, he put his face right up to mine and screamed, "When are you people going to learn? You can't stop the suffering!" Stunned, I swallowed and asked him, "What can we do?" He answered simply, "Just stay with us the way you've been doing."

When we turn our attention to supporting children in grief, we must respect the child's own grief process, the social context within which the child functions, and the inner world from which the child must draw the strength to cope and heal. In short, the therapist's role is to offer comfort, help find clear answers (that are acceptable to the family) for the child's asked and unasked questions, invite and witness the experience and the expression of feelings, and nurture hope.

- *As the parent watches the child's illness progress, he or she has to wonder about his or her own disease. It's that way for the child too.*

  "When will that happen to me?" each child asks. This becomes especially poignant and complicating when decisions around treatment need to be made. It is essential to remember that treatment decisions, especially those that will probably end in death, are a process. They cannot be made quickly, and the subject ought not be saved until the end is near. When the draft for *Caring at Home* (Ward-Wimmer & Riley, 1991), a handbook for parents of children with HIV, was sent out for review, the professional reviewers were aghast at the chapter entitled "Difficult Decisions," which introduced the subject of stopping treatment. Social workers across the country responded, "This is too frightening to be included in information for a family just coming to terms with the diagnosis." Parents who reviewed the draft, however, had an opposite reaction. The comments noted that while they didn't like to think about it, the thought that their child would die had been their first reaction when told the test results. It was good for them to know that if and when they had to face those decisions, therapists were willing to listen. They said they felt included and respected. The chapter stayed in.

- *Parents can consider ways to tell a comatose child that his or her respirator is about to be turned off.*

  It is very appropriate and healing for the parent and siblings to talk with a child who is comatose. We know that children, like adults, feel better when they understand what is happening (Evans, 1995), yet this ultimate moment in the youngster's life is all too often ignored. Working through this with family members is very helpful in allowing them to feel comfortable with the decision. One does not say to an unconscious child, "You're going to die now," but one can certainly say softly, "We know that the tube in your throat isn't comfortable, so we're going to let the doctor take it out and then we'll be able to hold you." Then, while the child is in the support of the parents' arms, he or she can be given permission to do whatever is desired. Like the child in the first vignette who heard his parents say, "It's all right to fly now," children may need to hear permission. And what sweeter words than "I love you" could a child hear as he leaves this world? Although difficult to speak in the moment, in retrospect words become primary comforters to the survivors who are not left burdened by "I wish I had said . . ."

When a child is dying, clear and open lines of communication between the therapists and the medical team is vital. Parents should never be allowed to make decisions alone that directly result in their child's death. Physicians need to approach parents with a willingness to bear the responsibility, to explain softly that the medicine and the machines aren't working anymore.

In truth, the outcome is out of mortal hands. When eleven-month-old Sean was removed from life support, he just kept breathing against all the odds. He was supposed to die that morning, but instead he lived to his fifth birthday. He taught us that human destiny is not always controlled by things we see and understand. Sean just wanted to live life and be an occasion of love for those he met along the way.

## *Conclusion*

The lessons of Sean and all the children pave the road that will carry us into caring in the twenty-first century. These children have taught us that this work demands the courage to embrace their anguish and offers, as reward, soft and gentle heart smiles as we share their joys. It's not easy. Little arms around our necks also wrap around our hearts, and sometimes we cry. But their courage and their ability to live hopefully is contagious. They are not only earth children but spirit children as well. So, if we find ourselves stumbling over some of the obstacles, it may serve us well to let those angels guide us as we turn fear into a reason for learning more, complexity of issues into an invitation truly to see each client as unique, and ethical dilemmas into a path wide enough for each of us — client, family, and therapist — to find our own "right way" while each helps the other along.

## REFERENCES


Axline, V. (1969). *Play therapy* (Rev. ed.). New York: Ballantine Books.

Boyd-Franklin, N., Steiner, G. L., & Boland, M. G. (Eds.). (1995). *Children, families, and HIV/AIDS*. New York: Guilford Press.

Evans, J. (1995). Are children competent to make decisions about their own deaths? *Behavioral Sciences and the Law, 13*, 27–41.

Geballe, S., Gruendel, J., & Andiman, W. (Eds.). (1995). *Forgotten children of the AIDS epidemic*. New Haven, CT: Yale University Press.

Hausher, R. (1989). *Children and the AIDS virus*. New York: Clarion Books.

Jordan, M. K. (1989). *Losing Uncle Tim*. Morton Grove, IL: Albert Whitman & Company.

Kittredge, M. (1991). *Teens with AIDS speak out*. New York: Julian Mesner.

Levine, C., & Stein, G. (1994). *Orphans of the HIV epidemic*. New York: The Orphan Project.

Merkel-Holguin, L. (1994). *Because you love them: A parent's planning guide*. Washington, DC: Child Welfare League of America.

Merrifield, M. (1990). *Come sit by me*. Toronto, Ontario, Canada: Women's Press.

Michaels, D., & Levine, C. (1992). Estimates of the number of motherless youth orphaned by AIDS in the United States. *Journal of the American Medical Association, 268*, 3456–3461.

Oaklander, V. (1988). *Windows to our children*. Highland, NY: Center for Gestalt Development.

Polster, E., & Polster, M. (1974). *Gestalt therapy integrated: Contours of theory and practice*. New York: Random House.

Power, P. W., DellOrto, A. E., & Gibbons, M. B. (Eds.) (1988). *Family interventions throughout chronic illness and disability*. New York: Springer.

Starkman, N. (1988). *Z's gift*. Seattle, WA: Comprehensive Health Education Foundation.

Tasker, M. (1992). *How can I tell you?* Bethesda, MD: Association for the Care of Children's Health.

Ward-Wimmer, D., & Riley, M. (1991). *Caring at home*. Washington, DC: Child Welfare League of America.

Wiener, L., Best, A., & Pizzo, P. (1994). *Be a friend*. Morton Grove, IL: Albert Whitman.

# III | Models of Clinical Care

# 13 | HIV Mental Health Services Integrated with Medical Care

*Barbara C. Kwasnik, Rosemary T. Moynihan, and Marjorie H. Royle*

HIV-affected clients in the inner city present with a Gordian knot of biopsychosocial and spiritual problems. For many, HIV is just one more strand in the knot that already includes medical problems such as diabetes, asthma, and hypertension; emotional disturbances; substance abuse and dependence; chaotic and violent living situations; and lack of resources (Gellin & Rodgers, 1992; Leukefeld, 1989; McKenzie, 1991).

For these individuals, medical needs most often take priority over mental health issues. Even if they recognize the need for mental health assistance, too many of them lack the energy to negotiate yet another treatment system and fail to get the help they need (Furstenberg & Meltzer Olson, 1984).

In this tangle, three issues stand out:

1. Like others struggling to cope with other catastrophic illnesses, HIV-infected individuals receiving medical care frequently do not view mental health services as a way to obtain help to cope with what is happening to them. Generally, they see themselves as being physically ill, not emotionally disturbed or mentally ill.

2. They fear being labeled "crazy," being condemned if their lifestyles are known, or being isolated and discriminated against if their diagnoses are disclosed.

3. The lack of stable housing, child care, transportation, and financial resources all act as barriers to care.

Women, who represent an increasing percentage of HIV-infected individuals, particularly among the urban poor (Altman, 1994), face additional barriers to mental health services. While they are more likely than men to use mental health services in general, HIV-infected women tend to avoid even medical treatment until late in the disease process, and they often do not access mental health treatment at all (HDI Projects, 1995, 60). As caretakers for their children and their partners, often they put themselves last (Wofsy, 1987). In our experience, other reasons for not seeking help are their feelings of shame and their lack of trust in the health care and the social service systems—they fear that they might be judged on their childbearing decisions or lose custody of their children if they admit that they have problems by seeking help. (See chapter 16 for additional information on care for women.)

People with substance abuse problems remain a treatment conundrum. They are caught in a fragmented system that supports their denial that their substance abuse creates or contributes to problems (Hazelden Foundation, 1993; Johnson, 1980). This denial may prevent them from seeking either mental health or substance abuse treatment. Mental health providers are hesitant to treat substance abusers because they feel unqualified and because they doubt the efficacy of mental health treatment undertaken before substance abuse problems have been addressed. Substance abuse treatment professionals prioritize substance abuse detoxification and rehabilitation as the basis for any other treatment (Evans & Sullivan, 1990), and medical care providers are frustrated by compliance issues.

## *Background Reading*

Through our experience treating HIV-infected people, we have come to a growing awareness of the interrelatedness of clients' problems and of the way that existing systems of care have failed to recognize this interrelatedness. Our clients have multiple medical appointments, multiple overlapping stressors, and limited energy. The need to negotiate multiple systems while facing the threat of fatal illness has been overwhelming for them. Service delivery systems have had to change to meet patient needs.

This change has already begun in related fields. In cancer treatment, a multimodal approach, including surgery, chemotherapy, radiation, nutrition, and mental health care, has become the standard treatment (DeVita,

Hellman, & Rosenberg, 1989). The emerging field of integrated mental illness and chemical abuse (MICA) treatment emphasizes the importance of using different perspectives and skills simultaneously to treat substance-abusing mentally ill individuals. The MICA approach highlights the need for common training and for appreciation of others' perspectives in managing overlapping treatment problems (Batki, Sorensen, Faltz, & Madover, 1988; Dilley, Shelp, & Batki, 1986; Evans & Sullivan, 1990; Hazelden Foundation, 1993; Minkoff, 1991). In the area of HIV mental health care, Winiarski (1993) described integrated mental health and primary care at community medical clinics.

In addition, national health policy documents such as *Healthy People 2000* (U.S. Dept. of Health and Human Services, 1991) and the *Latinas Partners for Health Partnership Plan* (HDI Projects, 1995, 59–60) provide an agenda for change, recommending increased integration of primary medical care and mental health services.

## *Our Clinical Practice*

How have we begun to unravel our patients' Gordian knots? At St. Joseph's Hospital and Medical Center, in Paterson, New Jersey, our tool is a program that integrates mental health services with HIV-related medical care, both in outpatient clinics and on inpatient units.

The concept of a multidisciplinary, integrated approach to care arose from a philosophy of understanding and meeting the needs of the residents of our community.

In Passaic County, HIV is primarily a family disease, with the most common transmission route being drug use or sexual contact with a drug-using partner. "The virus," as it is known on the streets, has touched families from all ethnic and cultural groups represented in the community, often with three generations affected. Our clients range from newborns to elderly grandparents who are now full-time caretakers of orphaned children. They include prostitutes, hard-core drug users, and prisoners, as well as working single parents with infected partners who are raising their children alone, gay and lesbian individuals who are frequently poor and substance-abusing, and suburban businessmen and their partners. The majority of the individuals on the clinic's active caseload are low-income African Americans or Latinos with few resources besides their families to help them to cope with their many and interrelated problems.

Our project to integrate care was funded in 1991 and again in 1994 by the Special Projects of National Significance program, created as part of Title II of the Ryan White C.A.R.E. Act. The project's mental health team comprises a coordinator, four social workers, a psychiatrist, and a psychologist, all of whom work along with the doctors, nurses, case managers, and other staff of St. Joseph's Comprehensive Care Center for HIV.

The center provides primary medical care and other ancillary services to people diagnosed with HIV and their families. Its current caseload is more than 1,000 clients from throughout Passaic County, New Jersey. Its offices are in the heart of the community, a block from City Hall. Pediatric and inpatient services are provided on the hospital campus nearby. Our project's mental health staff often work with patients in hospital rooms, medical clinic waiting rooms, the pediatric HIV clinic, the parole office, and drug treatment centers, as well as in their own offices, which are adjacent to the Comprehensive Care Center.

What is a multidisciplinary, integrated approach? Integrated care, as we define it, has the following four characteristics:

1. Professionals from many disciplines, including primary medical care, mental health, and other disciplines, must be located in close proximity, preferably in the same clinic.
2. These professionals must move beyond referrals and parallel treatment to sharing expertise and information about patients.
3. Treatment planning and ongoing clinical decision making must continuously incorporate understandings of a person's situation, needs, and experience that come from the insights and the expertise of each discipline.
4. Treatment must be responsive to events in patients' lives as they occur by being flexible in time, frequency, duration, modality, and place.

Integration of care, continuous throughout treatment, bridges gaps between essential services and addresses problems as people experience them. The case of Sherry is an example of how integrated care works.

Sherry is a thirty-two-year-old mother of four with a seventeen-year history of severe sexual abuse, heroin and cocaine use, and prostitution. After completing inpatient drug treatment, she was found to be HIV-positive. Faced with the full intensity of her problems without the help of drugs, she needed to negotiate medical care, ongoing drug treatment, and mental health services. Emotionally overwhelmed and unable to engage in either parallel or serial treatment by different disciplines, she needed a different model of treatment.

*Integrated Engagement*

In an integrated program, inpatient stays, medical visits, substance abuse treatment, and mental health visits are all used as opportunities for outreach and engagement for other needed services. Mental health staff members make rounds on inpatient units and do outreach in medical clinic waiting rooms and drug treatment programs, getting to know patients and staff and offering their services in an informal manner. Failed intake appointments are seen not as refusals of service but as challenges for more creative outreach efforts. Engagement is seen as a process that may take some time, as it did in Sherry's case.

Upon discharge from rehabilitation, Sherry asked for help to cope with her HIV diagnosis, her fears of death, and her deep desire to reconnect to her four daughters in a meaningful way before her death. But when she went to a community mental health program for recovering addicts, she was noncompliant and was discharged from the program. At a medical visit at St. Joseph's, Sherry requested mental health services but failed to keep her appointment. To help her overcome her barriers to accepting treatment, one of the program's mental health therapists met Sherry with her primary medical care provider, whom she trusted. For several weeks she was seen in therapy in a medical office, where she felt safe and secure, while waiting for her medical appointment. Only after a trusting relationship was established was she seen in the therapist's office nearby.

Other clients have somewhat different experiences in accessing care. Fred met his therapist in the infectious disease clinic waiting room, and Tiffany, a young mother, began to receive mental health services when she brought her child, Joshua, to the pediatric outpatient clinic for treatment. Ana met her therapist in a methadone maintenance program, while Max was first seen through outreach by a mental health provider in the parole office. His engagement with mental health services reduced his anxiety enough so that he was able to access medical care.

*Integrated Assessment and Treatment Planning*

Although all multidisciplinary treatment planning includes information from both medical and mental health perspectives, an integrated model uses more in-depth and varied information. Mental health staff are able to plan therapeutic interventions better when they understand the emotional impact of disease progression and medication. Similarly, medical staff benefit from knowledge of the patient's strengths, abilities to cope, and emotional responses to the progression of the disease and other concerns.

A commitment to work together from all care providers is fundamental. In an integrated model, treatment planning is ongoing. This is particularly important with a disease such as HIV/AIDS, which is characterized by rapid changes in physical and psychological manifestations. Regularly scheduled patient-care planning rounds on both inpatient and outpatient units, including mental health, medical, nursing and social work case management staff, provide a coordinating mechanism.

In Sherry's case, multidisciplinary rounds helped medical staff to understand her repeated psychiatric admissions and her problems keeping medical clinic appointments as resulting from fear, overwhelming problems, and limited coping abilities. Mental health staff began to understand the reality of rapidly decreasing T-helper (CD4) counts and laboratory results indicating serious underlying medical problems. This information helped each discipline plan more appropriate treatment.

### *Integrated Treatment*

Individual, couple, family, and group psychotherapy sessions are the building blocks of integrated care, just as they are of traditional care. In an integrated model, however, they may occur in a medical clinic office, in a hospital room, or on the telephone when clients are not strong enough to come to the therapist. Sessions may last for only fifteen minutes or for two hours, according to the client's need and tolerance. Rather than attending weekly, clients may come for therapy several times in one week during periods of crisis and then "check in" only every few weeks at other times. More time is spent in crisis intervention and psychiatric case management activities, such as accompanying a client to court or helping a demented client be admitted to the hospital, than is common in traditional models.

Because the psychiatrist is in the same location as the primary medical providers, they consult and share information quickly and easily while the patient is being seen. Also, we have found that a psychiatric medication record in the medical chart, providing a quickly accessible summary of dosage, frequency, and number prescribed, is a useful communication tool, especially for substance-abusing clients.

Throughout treatment, significant time is spent in consultation between mental health and primary medical care staff on the patient's progress and evolving needs and on assessment of the effectiveness of treatment. Multidisciplinary rounds provide structured opportunities for consultation, but consultation occurs between rounds as well, particularly during medical or mental health crises. Consistent with the integrated care concept, continuity of care is provided by having the same therapist and psychiatrist follow clients throughout their course of illness, on both an outpatient and an inpatient basis. Telephone contacts, letters, and home visits help maintain the project philosophy and keep people engaged in treatment.

Sherry's treatment included individual therapy either at the mental health clinic offices or at home by telephone when she was unable to get to the clinic, as well as a few crisis contacts. For a time, she was a regular attendee at a weekly drop-in therapy group for people diagnosed with HIV. Her medications were monitored by the psychiatrist. Her therapist worked closely with her primary care physician and nurse, including them in discussion of her concerns about her illness, especially when her anxiety was high or when she had ambiguous physical symptoms.

### *Integration of Children and Adolescents*

In addition to traditional services, mental health staff provide infected children and adolescents with more active interventions such as accompanying them to medical appointments, helping them to manage injections, or preparing them for hospital admissions through orientation visits. Children are seen at the pediatric outpatient clinic, on the inpatient unit, and in the mental health offices throughout the course of illness. As in traditional services, their parents are brought into mental health treatment whenever possible. In integrated care, special efforts are made to engage mothers and fathers in medical treatment as well.

Uninfected children and adolescents with infected parents are seen for individual and group therapy as early as possible before the parent's death. Hospital visits to sick parents provide important opportunities to facilitate parent-child communication to help children work through fears and conflicts related to their parents' illnesses.

Corey, Sherry's seven-year-old HIV-infected daughter, was removed from the home by protective services workers due to Sherry's substance abuse. The therapist helped Corey to manage her fears about needles and medications while addressing the pain of separation from her mother. From other families, Sacha and Dwight, both nine, worked through their grief for their parents in a weekly therapeutic play group, and fifteen-year-old Alysha visited her critically ill mother in the hospital with her therapist to deal with her questions and fears.

### *Integration with Substance Abuse Treatment*

As we saw the effectiveness of the integrated model for people with multiple diagnoses, the concept of integrated care grew to include drug treatment. At first, efforts were made to communicate with drug treatment professionals from other agencies on a case-by-case basis. Sherry's therapist, for example, reinforced her participation in Narcotics Anonymous, which had been part of her discharge plan, and coordinated her care with her NA program sponsor. As the program evolved, more formal referral and case management systems between mental health and area substance abuse treatment agencies developed. Ultimately, the success of this effort led to hospital-based mental health therapists providing services on-site at substance abuse treatment agencies.

## *Barriers to Integrated Care*

Any new program introduced into an existing organization is likely to encounter barriers. Problems are even more likely with a program that requires different disciplines and departments to work closely together for the first time. Potential barriers include the following:

- Especially in an area such as HIV care, staff may develop tightly knit teams "in the trenches." Staff members from the new program being integrated may need time to establish their credibility and their devotion to the client population. As in the beloved TV series *M.A.S.H.*, new staff are often accepted best when they produce under fire.
- Basic philosophical differences among medical, mental health and drug treatment professionals complicate communication. Integrated care introduces a new way of thinking about treatment, not just an easier way to make referrals or a different location of offices. Staff need modeling, practice, and time to understand that the new program entails assessing, evaluating, planning, and delivering treatment from varying perspectives.
- More interdisciplinary discussion means more rounds, staff meet-

ings, and time spent explaining, negotiating, and incorporating changes. This need for extensive communication, as well as the need for outreach efforts to engage clients, results in a higher percentage of unbillable time than is typical in traditional programs. Our experience with the program has shown, however, that the model may result in cost savings. It has been effective in decreasing psychiatric emergency room visits among heavy users of such services and in engaging hard-to-reach clients, especially substance abusers, who had not been engaged by traditional programs. Given the growth of managed-care approaches, cost/benefit analyses of the advantages of nontraditional activities in reaching vulnerable populations will be essential to justifying this approach.

## *Recommendations for Future Practice*

Providing mental health services integrated with primary medical care will be an effective way of delivering mental health services in the future, not only for the urban poor with HIV but also as a model for health service delivery in general. The model has implications for four other areas of practice:

1. *Other illnesses and other populations.* Although integrated care improves access for the traditionally marginalized, many middle-class patients with diseases other than HIV also define themselves as "sick, not crazy" and are emotionally distanced from accessing the mental health services they may need. Any major illness can be emotionally overwhelming. The necessity to choose among an array of complex and technical treatment options increases the stress. If mental health can be defined as one of a spectrum of services available to any patient, more of the people who need such services will receive them.

2. *Freestanding mental health services.* Integration with primary medical care may be easier for hospital-based mental health clinics than for freestanding facilities, but this model has implications for freestanding clinics as well. In an era of managed care, even free-standing clinics increasingly will have affiliations with medical facilities. These affiliations can become opportunities to integrate services and not just to expand referral networks. Freestanding facilities should consider providing some services onsite at affiliated agencies and allotting some staff time to communicate

with other health care professionals, both through formal consultations and less formal interactions.

3. *Mental health and substance abuse.* The need to provide medical, mental health, and substance abuse services to people with HIV has already broken down many of the traditional barriers between mental health and substance abuse treatment, and this trend can be expected to continue in the future. The collaborations that have been established, the networks formed, the trust developed will not disappear once a cure has been found for HIV. In many locations beyond Paterson, substance abuse and mental health treatment providers have learned that working together in joint treatment works far better than working separately.

4. *Managed care.* Finally, as more lives are covered by managed care and as primary-care physicians become treatment gatekeepers, the inclusion of mental health services will be particularly important in several ways. Mental health services can help people cope with catastrophic and chronic illnesses and can reduce the cost of medical care both by identifying those who use medical services when what they need are mental health services (Smith, Rost, & Kashner, 1995) and by helping people make necessary lifestyle changes in diet, exercise, or risky behaviors, such as smoking and unsafe sex, in order to prevent illness. Most of all, integration of mental health services with primary medical care may help primary care providers develop the holistic understanding of the patient on which managed care is based.

## *Tools for Clinical Practice*

After years of experience in promoting integrated care, we have made the following observations:

- *Educating medical staff about mental health problems extends their ability to deal with difficult cases more effectively.*

  Such education frequently requires considerable time, effort and tact, and includes:

  - Case-by-case demonstrations of effective approaches to deal with difficult or confusing behavior.
  - Participation in multidisciplinary rounds, sharing information and discussing cases. Stereotypes of the "difficult drug addict" or the "mental patient" are modified as staff more comprehensively understand patient problems. In addition, discussion of

the impact and the implications of disease progression and treatment helps all staff to think about and manage patients, especially difficult patients, in a less crisis-oriented, more consistent manner.

- *Physical proximity of mental health and health care staff decreases resistance to engaging in mental health care and makes referrals work.*

  Primary medical staff are more likely to make appropriate referrals when they know the people to whom they are referring. Clients are more likely to follow up on referrals when they first meet the new people in a familiar setting.
- *In an integrated program, both mental health and medical visits provide important opportunities for delivering the other service.*
  - Meeting patients informally while they wait for medical or mental health services makes accessing any new service less threatening.
  - Monitoring missed appointments in both clinics helps staff from either clinic to identify and address problems in compliance.
  - Continuing integrated care when clients are hospitalized for disease progression and intensive medical treatment or for psychiatric stabilization helps multidisciplinary staff collaborate to mitigate the patient's stress, prevent regression, and strengthen the ability to cope.
- *Clinical practice in an integrated model with HIV-infected individuals requires a flexible formula.*

  Flexibility can be achieved by:
  - Supplementing individual, family, and group treatment with outreach, brief psychotherapy, home visits, and telephone contacts (Boyd-Franklin & Boland, 1995; Nagler, Adnopoz, & Forsyth, 1995; see also chapters 2 and 3).
  - Taking an active, supportive role with an emphasis on the "here and now" to help people accomplish the social and psychological tasks related to their illness (Christ, 1991; Nagler, Adnopoz, & Forsyth, 1995).
  - Expecting interruptions in treatment. Dealing with chronic, fatal illness and treatment frequently requires periods of "time out" or rest. Substance abuse and recovery remains an ongo-

ing life struggle, often with episodic relapses and hiatuses in treatment. These are dealt with by keeping the cases open, maintaining connection with the clients, and accepting them back into treatment, using the same therapist and psychiatrist when they return. Clients who are organically impaired or who have histories of multiple traumas find relating to the same staff less confusing and frustrating.

- *A strong, effective support structure is required for clinical staff to be flexible and available to clients.*

  Both the program coordinator and the secretary/receptionist are crucial in making the program work. The program's secretary/receptionist serves as the communications hub of the group, keeping track of the whereabouts of the clinical staff as they meet clients in different locations. Pagers for all clinical staff help the secretary to locate them when needed by patients or other staff members.

  The program coordinator must allocate a significant portion of time to communicating with other disciplines as well as help all staff understand the integrated care model. Sufficient time should be allocated also to teaching staff members about integrated care and to supporting them as they deal with the enormous losses associated with HIV.
- *Adjust your expectations for clients' abstinence from drugs, while maintaining abstinence as a goal.*

  The rigid requirement of abstinence from drugs for mental health treatment in effect denies access to treatment for people with limited life expectancy. Current substance abuse treatment considers relapse part of the treatment process. HIV-infected person may be even more prone to relapse due to the increased social isolation and the constant stresses of this disease (Evans & Sullivan, 1990; Najavits & Weiss, 1994). Looking positively at the time off drugs and supporting the frequency of "clean" episodes can support a person's strengths and minimize feelings of failure (Orlin & Davis, 1993). This helps develop coping skills, supports limited ego strengths, and gives hope in the face of repeated medical and emotional crises.
- *To be multidisciplinary, you must engage in simultaneous translation into several "foreign languages" much of the time.*

You must spend the time to learn about the perspectives, knowledge bases, jargons, administrative structures, and formal and informal power structures in each of the other disciplines with which you work. Not only must you be able to communicate in the other disciplines' languages and cultures; you must do so as a matter of habit. Negotiating not one but several formal and informal organizational structures when changes need to be made or issues arise is time consuming but essential.

- *Commitment from staff of all disciplines to mutual availability is an essential component of this model.*

  Without this commitment, movement from parallel to integrated treatment probably will not occur. Making such a commitment is particularly difficult for professionals, however, because it means giving up some autonomy in practice, which requires trust, education, and a willingness to believe that the new approach can be an improvement. Modeling from leadership helps develop such a commitment, validates the efficacy of the new approach, and allows professionals to give up their autonomy with less anxiety. However, time and patience with oneself and others are needed for commitment to develop.

## *Conclusion*

Sherry is now drug free and active in Narcotics Anonymous, where she speaks publicly in its drug and HIV-prevention programs. She is slowly becoming more symptomatic but works closely with her health care team to maintain her health stability as long as possible. Since beginning mental health treatment, Sherry has moved from frequent psychiatric admissions to only one overnight psychiatric admission during the last year. She has reunited with her children in a warm and productive manner. She has coped effectively with multiple deaths of peers from HIV and drug use. While she continues to fear suffering and death, she uses weekly psychotherapy to work through her concerns. Due to her progress in reuniting with her family, her oldest daughter and her mother have helped her put aside her fears of abandonment by assuring her that they will care for her.

In our integrated program, health care professionals were able to understand the overwhelming complexity of Sherry's emotional life. Mental health staff were able to understand the physical and emotional stress related to her illness and treatment. Together they provided a supportive, integrated structure of care. Sherry was able to focus her energy and strengths to comply with treatment, work through her problems, and feel supported by the many disciplines endeavoring to help her.

## REFERENCES

This chapter was made possible by grant number BRH 970165–02-0 from the Health Resources and Services Administration. Its contents are solely the responsibility of the authors and do not necessarily represent the official views of HRSA.

Altman, L. K. (1994, March 11). AIDS cases increase among heterosexuals. *New York Times,* A-12.

Batki, S. L., Sorensen, J. L., Faltz, B., & Madover, S. (1988). Psychiatric aspects of treatment of IV drug abusers with AIDS. *Hospital and Community Psychiatry, 39,* 439–441.

Boyd-Franklin, N., & Boland, M. G. (1995). A multisystems approach to service delivery to HIV/AIDS families. In N. Boyd-Franklin, G. L. Steiner, & M. G. Boland (Eds.), *Children, families and HIV/AIDS* (199–215). New York: Guilford Press.

Christ, G. (1991). Principles of oncology social work. In A. Holleb, D. Fink, & G. Murphy (Eds.), *American Cancer Society textbook of clinical oncology* (594–605). Atlanta, GA: American Cancer Society.

DeVita, V. T., Hellman, S., & Rosenberg, S. A. (Eds.). (1989). *Cancer: principles and practice of oncology* (3rd ed.). Philadelphia: J. B. Lippincott.

Dilley, J. W., Shelp, E. E., & Batki, S. L. (1986). Psychiatric and ethical issues in the care of patients with AIDS. *Psychosomatics, 27,* 562–566.

Evans, K., & Sullivan, J. M. (1990). *Dual diagnoses: Counseling the mentally ill substance abuser.* New York: The Guilford Press.

Furstenberg, A., & Meltzer Olson, M. (1984). Social work and AIDS. *Social Work in Health Care, 9,* 45–62.

Gellin, B. G., & Rogers, D. E. (1992). Technical successes and social failures: Approaching the second decade of the AIDS epidemic. In V. T. DeVita, S. Hellman, & S. A. Rosenberg (Eds.), *AIDS: Etiology, diagnosis, treatment and prevention* (3rd. ed.) (497–502). Philadelphia: J. B. Lippincott.

Hazelden Foundation (1993). *The dual disorders recovery book.* Center City, MN: Author.

HDI Projects—National Hispanic Education and Communications Projects (1995, March). *Latinas partners for health partnership plan.* Washington, DC: Author.

Johnson, V. E. (1980). *I'll quit tomorrow: a practical guide to alcoholism treatment.* San Francisco: Harper & Row.

Leukefeld, C. G. (1989). Psychosocial issues in dealing with AIDS. *Hospital and Community Psychiatry, 40,* 454–455.

McKenzie, N. F. (Ed.). (1991). *The AIDS reader: Social, political, ethical issues.* New York: Penguin Books.

Minkoff, K. (1991). Program components of a comprehensive integrated care system for serious mentally ill patients with substance disorders. In K. Minkoff & R. E. Drake (Eds.), *Dual diagnosis of major mental illness and substance disorder* (13–27). San Francisco: Jossey-Bass.

Nagler, S. F., Adnopoz, J., & Forsyth, B. W. (1995). Uncertainty, stigma, and secrecy: Psychological aspects of AIDS for children and adolescents. In S. Geballe, J. Gruendel, & W. Andiman (Eds.), *Forgotten children of the AIDS epidemic* (71–82). New Haven, CT: Yale University Press.

Najavits, L. M., & Weiss, R. D. (1994). The role of psychotherapy in the treatment of substance-use disorders. *Harvard Review of Psychiatry, 2,* 81–96.

Orlin, L., & Davis, J. (1993). Assessment and intervention with drug and alcohol abusers in psychiatric settings. In S. Z. A. Strausner (Ed.), *Clinical work with substance abusing clients* (50–68). New York: Guilford Press.

Smith, G. R., Jr., Rost, K., & Kashner, T. M. (1995). A trial of the effect of a standardized psychiatric consultation on health outcomes and costs in somatizing patients. *Archives of General Psychiatry, 52,* 238–243.

Umbricht-Schneiter, A., Ginn, D. H., Pabst, K. M., & Bigelow, G. E. (1994). Providing medical care to methadone clinic patients: referral vs. on-site care. *American Journal of Public Health, 84,* 207–210.

U.S. Department of Health and Human Services (1991). *Healthy people 2000: National health promotion and disease prevention objectives* (DHHS Publication No. PHS 91–50212). Washington, DC: U.S. Government Printing Office.

Winiarski, M. G. (1993). Integrating mental health services with HIV primary care: The Bronx experience. *AIDS Patient Care, 7,* 322–326.

Wofsy, C. B. (1987). Human Immunodeficiency Virus infection in women [Editorial]. *Journal of the American Medical Association, 257,* 2074–2076.

# 14 | Delivering Mental Health Services to the Home

*Dennee Frey, Karen Oman, and William R. Wagner*

In the mid-1980s, when persons with AIDS first began to survive bouts of *pneumocystis carinii* pneumonia with the help of intravenous antibiotics, home infusion team nurses with the Visiting Nurse Association of Los Angeles (VNA-LA) began observing unusual behaviors in patients.

One field nurse remembers going into a patient's home to find that he had ripped open a line of sutures and pulled out his porta-catheter, a tube surgically inserted into a central blood vessel to provide medication. He then presented her with a basin full of blood, saying, with no emotional expression, "I want to die."

Another nurse recalls visiting a patient who was bedbound with wasting syndrome: "Here was this man who would never get out of bed again, would probably die within a few weeks, on SSI [Supplemental Security Income], and he just ordered a brand new, custom-made luxury car on the phone. He charged it! The crazy thing was the dealership actually delivered it to him!"

At the same time, field staff reported spending an extraordinary amount of time during the visits providing supportive counseling to their patients and to caregivers who presented with symptoms of depression, anxiety, or other emotional reactions to their situations. Because the majority of the patients were, in fact, homebound, they were unable to go to a psychiatrist's or psychotherapist's office or clinic.

It wasn't until the late 1980s that literature began to report the incidence and prevalence of psychiatric disorders in this population. First anecdotal, then more empirical literature began to describe the signs and symptoms of an AIDS-related dementia, or AIDS Dementia Complex (ADC) (see chapter 9 for additional information).

As more people with AIDS began to be treated at home rather than in acute-care hospitals, the VNA-LA field staff continued to notice and report difficulties in working with patients with ADC or other psychiatric symptoms. Many patients could not be responsible for their medication regimens because of the cognitive deficits associated with ADC. Others displayed dramatic personality changes that frightened their caregivers. Neuropathic pain, motor difficulties, and behavior management also required more in-home support than the IV (intravenous) field nurses could provide during their regular visits. In addition, because the disease process of HIV/AIDS is unstable and unpredictable, patients exhibiting these and other psychiatric problems posed a greater risk of more frequent hospital admissions and emergency room visits and were generally greater utilizers of health care resources (Hellinger, Fleishman, & Hsia, 1994).

In the late 1980s, there were few known programs available to provide the neuropsychiatric support required by these patients in their homes. Furthermore, no literature completely described the needs or possible treatments for homebound persons with neuropsychiatric difficulties. For patients unable to go to a clinician's office for psychotherapy, neuropsychiatric care, and psychotropic medication evaluation, treatment in the patient's home appeared to be the most viable option for effective care.

## *Our Clinical Work*

In 1991 the VNA-LA, in partnership with the National AIDS Fund, received Ryan White C.A.R.E. Act Title II Special Projects of National Significance funding from the Health Resources and Services Administration. The VNA-LA developed and implemented a three-year pilot program that would become a model for integrating in-home mental health and psychiatric care with primary medical care and that would be replicated in Detroit, Michigan, Cleveland, Ohio, and Washington, D.C. The objectives of our AIDS Psychiatric Homecare Program were threefold:

1. To maintain the patient at home and to reduce the risk for acute care or psychiatric hospitalization
2. To ameliorate, control, and manage neurological and psychiatric symptoms
3. To optimize the patient's quality of life

The first objective differentiates an in-home mental health care model from more traditional models of care. Homecare is often more effective in identifying and intervening in situations that might, if ignored, later require costlier care.

An interim evaluation of our effectiveness indicates that our project is "quite successful in easing patients' social and cognitive problems and in maintaining a satisfactory quality of life, despite deteriorating physical conditions" (National AIDS Fund, 1994, 15).

Several aspects of our program are noteworthy.

### *Interdisciplinary Model*

Most home health care psychiatric programs have been driven by Medicare or Medicaid reimbursement, but states have differed on which disciplines' services would be reimbursed. We believe that persons with AIDS, given their complex problems, required a multidisciplinary team with systematized interventions. Our program team now includes registered nurses and medical social workers with psychiatric training, a psychiatric social worker, a consulting psychiatrist, and a clinical pharmacist.

The team's registered nurses are responsible for education and management of medication issues, including teaching both patients and caregivers about the use, dosage, side effects, and schedule of each medication. Because many patients with neuropsychiatric problems cannot remember to take their medications, the psychiatric nurses develop a patient-friendly regimen to ensure that patients administer their medications properly and regularly.

The social worker offers psychotherapy and assistance with community resources. The pharmacist reviews the patient's medications for side effects, complications, and interactions and makes the appropriate recommendations to the primary medical doctor. The psychiatrist frequently makes home visits to evaluate for the use of psychotropic medications and for differential diagnoses. Both the pharmacist and the psychiatrist offer continuing education to the field staff about the ever-changing arena of HIV.

*Home-Based Services*

Because most of our patients have only limited ability to leave their places of residence for such activities as medical appointments, all program services are performed in the residence, whether it be a home, shelter, hospice, or other facility.

A key advantage of our model is that the field clinician actually witnesses the patient and his or her support systems functioning in the home. Many problems that impair a patient's functioning or activities of daily living are not immediately evident in a clinic or physician's office. In addition, regular supportive home visits often reveal crises such as inadequate home safety, caregiver inadequacy, substance abuse, and suicidality, which might not be presented to the patient's primary medical care provider or to a mental health provider in another setting.

*Seeing Caregivers as Clients*

A fundamental element of our care is the understanding that the "client" includes not only the patient but also the significant other, family, friends, and other formal or informal caregivers, including paid attendants. Because the patient's whole environment affects quality of life, all of it becomes an integral part of the treatment plan.

Often the team will work with the patient and his or her support system to define and develop treatment goals and a plan that will work in the patient's home. In one case, we worked with a thirty-six-year-old black woman living in a twelve-step residential facility for HIV-positive women and their children. She had been diagnosed with depression with psychotic features, and she had a history of alcohol and abuse of other substances. The facility's management felt that her HIV treatment should preclude her taking mood-altering drugs. Although the consulting psychiatrist had prescribed an antidepressant and an antipsychotic medication to manage her symptoms, the program managers required education to assure them that the therapeutic use of these medications did not interfere with the client's sober living goals. The psychiatric nurse and the social worker conferred with the facility's management and were able to work out a plan in which the client would take her medicine, which would be administered by the house mother. The plan was successful. Our client completed the drug treatment program, her depression resolved, and the psychotic features were eliminated.

### *Comprehensive Assessment*

The cornerstone of effective home-based mental health treatment is a comprehensive assessment to guide the care plan. Our assessment includes psychiatric and medical information; a description of the support system, including social service agencies involved in care; an evaluation of the patient's ability to perform activities of daily living, called "ADLs"; an understanding of all medications and the patient's ability to manage the regimen; and a description of the home, with special attention to physical safety issues.

In addition, we use a uniform assessment tool designed to assess specific areas of neuropsychiatric functioning and stages of ADC. The Neuropsychiatric AIDS Rating Scale (NARS) (Boccellari & Dilley, 1992) has subscales to rate cognitive, behavioral, and motor domains relating to the patient's orientation, memory, behavior, ability to problem-solve, and perform ADLs. The clinician rates the patient on the subscales, using information obtained during the home visit.

The NARS's advantages are its simplicity in staging the illness process, its usefulness in anticipating the need for ancillary support services like attendant care and hospice, and its service as a "common language" tool for team members to describe the patient's level of functioning and impairment.

While quality of life is, perhaps, subjective, having the patient assess quality of life can open up areas for the therapeutic process. In our experience, some of the factors that contribute to decreased quality of life include poor management of pain and symptoms such as diarrhea, depression and anxiety, and concern over finances. Once these issues are identified, appropriate interventions are initiated, and an improvement in the patient's perception of quality of life should result.

The assessment leads to development of a problem list that targets specific needs. A regular review of the problem list is helpful in monitoring progress toward goals and in maintaining the focus of the treatment plan.

### *Reinforcement of Existing Support Systems*

Since most patients can be maintained at home with adequate support (Hellinger, Fleishman, & Hsia, 1994; Reitmeijer, Davidson, Foster, & Cohn, 1993), all of the team's interventions are designed to reinforce the patient's existing support systems.

We may introduce the patient to ancillary community resources as a critical beginning both to ensure that basic needs are met for housing, food, and finances and to "jump start" the therapeutic rapport through immediate, active, anxiety-reducing interventions.

### *Psychotherapy*

Psychotherapy and counseling, both for the patient and caregivers, typically focus on adjustment to the illness process and dealing with the multiplicity of losses: past, present, and anticipated.

### *Education*

Education regarding the illness process, especially when dealing with ADC, helps patients and caregivers understand the limitations of the illness, retain a sense of control, relieve real and imagined fears, and anticipate their future needs.

An illustrative case: The parents of a thirty-year-old Latino patient were angry and frustrated because, they said, their daughter was always lying and trying to manipulate them. "In the hospital, she kept saying that the nurses wouldn't feed her. I'd get mad and yell at the nurses. They told me that they gave her dinner, but she wouldn't eat it. I don't know why she's lying so much. She just wants to start trouble." Our project social worker assessed cognitive symptoms of a moderate stage of ADC causing severe impairment of short-term memory—an inability to store new information. She educated the parents about the signs and symptoms of ADC as well as counseled them to assist with their frustration. On the next home visit, the patient's mother told the social worker: "Now it makes sense . . . what she does. If the nurses in the hospital would have explained it to me, I would have felt better."

### *Crisis Anticipation*

There is no place to better identify a crisis than in the patient's residence. Early assessment and intervention are the best tools for averting crises, which can include anything that might jeopardize the objectives of the program, such as inability to maintain the patient at home, risk of hospitalization, and/or the exacerbation of acute psychiatric symptoms. Changes in the caregiver's ability to continue providing care, patient suicidality or substance abuse, neglect, inadequate care provision, and safety risks are just a few of the potential crises that can develop in the home. These issues need to be assessed during each home visit and the appropriate intervention implemented.

Moreover, working in the patient's home permits immediate access to crises that often cannot wait for the next scheduled clinic appointment.

A forty-three-year-old man with AIDS was referred by his physician for evaluation and treatment of "paranoia." The team assessed moderate AIDS Dementia Complex, bipolar disorder, and severe schizoid personality disorder. Because of the patient's psychiatric condition, he could tolerate only the team's psychiatric nurse and social worker. No home health nurse could visit to manage his physical needs. After some weeks passed in which the patient either did not return team phone calls for visits or refused visits, the psychiatric nurse "stopped by" unannounced, finding the patient gasping for air and with extremely low blood pressure, able to say only, "Don't send me to the hospital." After consulting with the physician, she was able to secure liquid oxygen and agreement from the infusion team to administer intravenous antibiotics in the patient's home. Our team members increased visits for a while to assist the patient in coping with another home health worker in his home and to maintain his care at home.

## *Barriers to In-Home Care*

Some of the barriers to in-home mental health care are:

- Lack of knowledge of the effectiveness of this type of program and its critical role in the continuum of care. Our program has demonstrated the critical role of psychiatric homecare in integrating comprehensive services for people with AIDS. There continue to be few published data to document the beneficial effects of this model of care, but we are in the process of documenting the benefits of our program. This underscores the need for good evaluation and publication of findings (see chapters 17 and 18).
- Limitations on financial support for in-home care. The current managed care environment challenges providers' continued ability to respond to the growing need for psychiatric homecare services. Most Medicaid programs provide only very limited coverage for in-home mental health care. Private insurance carriers

offer even fewer benefits. The challenge in the next decade will be to demonstrate empirically the cost-effectiveness of home-based mental health care in preventing acute-care hospitalizations.

- The tradition of office-based psychiatry and psychotherapy. Home delivery of mental health care introduces a new concept of practice. As a new clinical resource for HIV/AIDS care, there does not yet exist the wealth of "how-to" information available, for example, on working within a changing frame, fees, transferences, countertransferences, that is available for other modalities.
- Lack of government support. Because traditional providers lobby for governmental funds for their practices, governmental agencies are less likely to fund novel approaches to care provision.

## *Tools for Clinical Practice*

After five years of providing mental health services to persons with AIDS (PWAs) in their homes, we've learned a few lessons. What follows are some of the more salient features of the work that differentiate psychiatric homecare from more traditional office or clinic models of mental health care.

- *The patient's home is his or her castle. Its walls protect secrets.*

  A forty-five-year-old Latino male with AIDS was referred for evaluation and psychosocial treatment of ADC, depression, and anxiety. He lived with his wife of twenty-five years and their four children: two sons, ages twenty-three and twenty-one, and two daughters, seventeen and nine. Although the wife was present during each of the interviews, she was mostly silent. The older daughter assumed all responsibility for managing her father's needs, including changing diapers and bathing. During the course of treatment, the patient's wife explosively admitted that her husband had been sexually molesting the elder daughter since she was ten. When the local reporting agency was notified, both patient and daughter denied the allegations, and the workers were unable to intervene. Immediately after the patient died, the team's social worker needed to involuntarily hospitalize the daughter in a psychiatric facility for treatment of acute psychotic depression.

In another case, a twenty-nine-year-old single male was referred for evaluation of early signs and symptoms of ADC. He was living with his parents. Fearful of sharing with them his AIDS diagnosis as well as his homosexuality, he had said he had a brain tumor. He shared with us his fears of abandonment and rejection should he divulge his sexual orientation and diagnosis. His parents accepted his false diagnosis and provided excellent care for him at home, assisting with infusions and personal care. Because it was necessary to educate the parents about universal precautions, which requires barriers when handling blood and body fluids, the patient needed to address his fears of anticipated loss and rejection by his parents in order for the team to educate them to safety issues. Through counseling, the team provided the support necessary for the patient to share his diagnosis and lifestyle with his parents for the first time. The team was then available to provide the necessary support to the parents to assist them in dealing with these issues.

Secrets abound in homes. It is important that the clinician deeply respect the patient's and the caregiver's needs for privacy. Only those secrets that clearly pose a threat to the treatment, the patient and/or others need to be addressed and worked through — delicately.

- *To be . . . or not to be? If suicide's the question, what's the answer?*

John, a single, fifty-eight-year-old with AIDS, was referred for community resources to assist with homemaking, meals, and other functions. He presented as an upbeat, intelligent, positive-thinking man. He was pleasant to be around, conversational, flattering, with a hearty sense of humor. Because of the patient's apparent positive outlook on life, a complete mental status evaluation was never done at intake.

The visits were enjoyable, with the patient complimenting the worker on his excellent skills at helping people, sharing laughs, and making certain the patient followed through with the referrals. On the fifth visit, our project staff member noted that the patient had been quieter than on prior visits. After a long silence, the patient quietly asked: "Do you know the California policy on assisted suicide?" He had been thinking about suicide for more than a year. He had a stockpile of unused morphine and sleeping pills stored up "just in case."

Suicidal ideation is no alien thought to people with AIDS (Dilley, Ochitill, Perl, & Volberding, 1985; Dilley, Shelp, & Batki, 1986; Marzuk, Tierney, & Tardiff, 1988). It may, however, be one of the most easily overlooked symptoms. The social worker working with John had been "fooled," along with his physicians, into believing that the patient was doing well.

The therapeutic rapport between patient and worker in the home provides, perhaps, a better opportunity to assess and intervene with suicidal patients than do meetings in the clinic. This may be due to the transference that the patient feels toward the homecare worker. As noted earlier, the boundaries get blurred in the home: There may not be any starched white lab coats, and the setting is often far from sterile. It is, again, the patient's home, offering him or her safety and comfort. The patient has already allowed the worker in the door and has control over the situation; the rapport seems to develop rapidly, making it easier for the patient to reveal his or her "secrets." Uncovering consequent suicidal plans and often the intended means flows easily after assessment of suicidal ideation.

- *The risk of suicide must be assessed during each home visit.*

Because of the volatile nature of the disease itself, persons with AIDS are often confronted with unexpected and unwelcome news of another infection or change in prognosis, which challenges their ability to cope. The clinician's regular visits provide the opportunity to assess the nature of the risk and to intervene appropriately and in a timely manner to reduce the risk of suicide.

There is presently much debate on the issue of "rational suicide" — when the patient makes a well-informed, conscious decision to end his or her life (see Kain, 1996; Motto, 1994). This kind of decision should not be confused with the patient's wish to limit or discontinue aggressive therapies in favor of palliative care only. Our responsibility as clinicians with people considering suicide is to assist them in clarifying their wishes, desires, and needs. For most of our patients considering this option, the authors uncovered the patients' need to regain some control, the wish not to have pain and discomfort, and the desire to live and die with dignity.

- *The medical model emphasizes "medication compliance." Our profes-*

*sional values make us advocates for every person's right to self-determination.*

One of the more frequent comments cited by physicians referring someone to our project is "The patient is not compliant with medications." This usually means that, for whatever reasons, the patient is not taking his or her medications as ordered and as scheduled, if at all. The issue is a complex one.

A thirty-three-year-old male accountant, living with his significant other of six years, was referred for evaluation and treatment of depression. During the initial assessment, the nurse logged nineteen different medications. While he initially presented with blunted affect and slightly depressed mood, his symptoms did not meet the criteria for a depressive disorder. He stated, "I take my medicine, but it's so confusing." On further evaluation, the patient was assessed with early-stage ADC. The nurse helped to organize a weekly medication planner and educated the patient and his caregiver about dosing schedules. In addition, the pharmacist discovered that the interactions of some of his medications could be contributing to his depressed mood. The patient became "med compliant," and his physician reevaluated his regimen for side effects and interactions.

Often, the patient will make a conscious decision to discontinue some or all medications. Because such decisions have critical repercussions, it is the clinician's role to provide the support needed for the patient to make an educated, informed choice. Our professional values make us advocates for every person's right to self-determination. Decisions against further medical treatment should thus be made with full knowledge and understanding of the ramifications of this choice, including their impact on prognosis and quality of life, and not as a result of hopelessness stemming from depression, suicidal ideation, or other psychiatric symptoms.

A thirty-two-year-old single male with AIDS was referred by his physician for treatment of depression and "noncompliance with medical regimen." The patient was first diagnosed with AIDS five years ago. Last year, he built himself a new home. After his latest bout with *pneumocystis* pneumonia, his mother came to stay with him from the East Coast to assist with his care. During her stay, her son became progressively weaker and more depressed. The associated feelings of hopelessness, coupled with the weakness, impaired the patient's desire to take his many prophylactic medications. He agreed to antidepressant therapy with adjunctive supportive psychotherapy with the goal of relieving his depression. After about a month, the symptoms of depression had abated, but weakness, nausea, vomiting, and diarrhea persisted. He had done some research into the medications he was taking and realized that some of them were contributing to these physical symptoms. He told the social worker, "I don't want to die, but I don't want to live this way either. I feel like it's time to choose between all of these meds and some quality in my life. I don't know what to do. I feel like I'm taking them for my mom." We explored options with the patient, his physician, and his mother, including the immediate and the long-term effects of discontinuing all but pain and antinausea medications. The patient opted for control. He chose to take only "comfort" — or palliative — medications, hoping that with the weeks or months he had left, he could feel well enough to accomplish what he wanted to. The team helped the patient's mother understand and support her son's difficult decision.

- *Home treatment raises new transference and countertransference issues regarding maintaining professional boundaries.*

  In a clinician's office setting, the boundaries between client and therapist are fairly well defined by the furniture, decor, and seating and by the traditional medical model in which the patient actually goes to the healer's office. In home mental health care, the clinician is the guest of the patient and his or her caregiver and family. The home is the seat from which the patient controls his or her world. It is designed for the patient's comfort and maintained in accordance with the person's own individuality, tastes, and chosen lifestyle. It is the patient's home, and the patient ultimately maintains control over its comings and goings.

  Because it is easy for professional boundaries to get blurred in the patient's home, frequent self- and supervisory reminders that the visit is more than a social call are required to maintain therapeutic integrity, especially when working with patients and their families over a long period of time. The patient may feel that he or she was developed a good friend, sibling, or parent figure in the clinician. The family or caregiver may feel the same way or may develop a more negative transference because of the perceived intimacy between the patient and the worker. While it is often unproductive to engage in an in-depth analytic exploration of the patient's or caregiver's transference in this setting, it is important to recognize it and to help them to interpret the underlying need behind their feelings. Nurturance, safety, security, a decreased sense of isolation, association, and self-esteem and self-value are common needs associated with positive transferences. Negative transferences need to be confronted and resolved quickly in order to protect the integrity of the treatment. Interpreting the transference then becomes a clinical tool where appropriate interventions can be made on the basis of the patient's need.

The clinician's countertransference falls into two categories: those issues we bring with us that are based on our own personal and professional life experiences, including our deepest needs, biases, and prejudices, and the empathy we experience as clinical containers for the patient's and caregiver's emotions (Cohen, 1952/1988; Ferenczi & Rank, 1923/1988; Orr, 1954/1988; Racker, 1957/1988; Reik, 1949/1988). Both need to be carefully monitored and checked by the individual with clinical and team supervision.

Working with persons who have life-threatening or terminal illnesses, who are facing the ultimate loss, may kick up many of our own feelings about loss, life, and death. Doing clinical work in an office setting, in some ways, protects us from the intensity of witnessing the whole life of the patient. In homecare, everything about the patient's life, lifestyle, and illness process is right there to see in abundant detail, replete with the direct effects of the illness on the patient's daily life. It is therefore easy to be not only overwhelmed but also overextended. Setting firm professional limits on working hours, frequency, time, and duration of visits, and times available for phone consultation and recognizing the boundaries of our own discipline are valuable tools in maintaining an effective "therapeutic closeness," if not distance. Anytime we consider working outside these established limits, we should examine the reasons and be aware of the risks to ourselves and to the relationship.

Paying close attention to our personal reactions to the patient's body, surroundings, smells, and neediness is a good place to begin. Each member of the team needs constantly to examine areas of intense curiosity to determine whether the patient's needs or the team member's are being met. The key to maintaining healthy personal and professional boundaries in psychiatric homecare is to manage a well-balanced life of work, rest, and leisure, including the generous use of a network for social support.

- *Clinical work in the field can be isolating and overwhelming.*

  Psychiatric homecare requires the field clinician to make several home visits each day. Usually, the social worker or the nurse travels alone, although joint visits are sometimes indicated and helpful to coordinate and maintain the care plan. This aspect of the work can leave the clinician feeling alone and isolated from peers. These feelings are especially evident during the initial home visits, during which the clinician may assess a seemingly overwhelming mountain of problems and needs. A frequent sentiment mirroring these feelings is, "There are so many problems, I can't seem to find a place to start."

  Because these feelings are so common, clinicians need to have an available connection to peers and colleagues who understand the work and can assist them with prioritizing the patient's needs and focusing the treatment goals. The interdisciplinary team approach is an invaluable resource to manage the sense of isolation as well as to maintain quality care. Staying within the clinical realm of our respective disciplines and referring to other team members for more specialized evaluation and intervention is critical in both managing feelings of being overwhelmed and maximizing good patient care. Regularly scheduled team conferences and the frequent use of informal consultations provide built-in support. Another important resource is the use of clinical supervision and peer support, whether formally scheduled or obtained through informal, but regular contacts.

- *Homecare mental health providers face dogs, gangs, unsafe neighborhoods, weapons, darkness, and other threats.*

  There are times when field clinicians may long to work a fifty-minute hour session in an office setting. In the microcosm of a clinical office, safety and security are pretty much assured by the layout of the space, accessible doors, comfort-controlled temperatures, pleasant lighting, possibly panic or alarm buttons, and privacy. Working in the field, uncertainty abounds. We never know what situations we're going to confront until we get to the patient's home.

On a recent visit, one social worker was bitten by the patient's seemingly docile dog. The threats of gang violence in "unsafe" neighborhoods is always a concern. People hanging out in the streets are curious about the increased presence of doctors, nurses, and other clinicians. Many of our field staff have been approached by people hoping to score drugs or money.

In unsafe neighborhoods, it is not unusual for patients and their caregivers to have guns or other weapons used for self-protection. It is important to assess the presence of any potentially violent weapons and their perceived purpose during the initial evaluation visit. An appropriate time for this is usually during the assessment of the patient's psychiatric history and suicidality.

Staff safety must be a priority. No clinician should be forced into a situation where he or she does not feel safe. In areas where safety is at risk, the policy about after-dark visits should be stated clearly with the patient during the initial assessment visit. The field staff should feel comfortable in asking the patient and the caregiver to accommodate safety concerns by placing pets in another room, putting away unconcealed weapons, or even having someone meet workers at the curb when they arrive. Most patients want and desperately need the in-home services and are usually more than willing to work with the homecare staff.

## *Conclusion*

Fifteen years after the first case was reported, AIDS has become a fact of life that will continue to challenge patients, caregivers, and health care professionals well beyond the year 2001. As our understanding of the disease and its psychosocial effects advances, we must develop treatment options that are innovative, cost-effective, and directly responsive to the needs of our patients. These options must include service provision in the patient's home. Care that maximizes quality of life can be accomplished by comprehensive, patient-centered services. And, sometimes, as Dorothy Gayle of Kansas said, "There's no place like home" to provide these services.

## REFERENCES

The project described was supported by grant number BRH970015-03-3 from the Health Resources and Services Administration. The contents of this chapter are solely the responsibility of the authors and do not necessarily represent the official views of HRSA.

The authors are listed in alphabetical order and each contributed equally in the preparation, research, and writing of this chapter.

The authors acknowledge with appreciation the support of Elaine Brown for her assistance with the preparation and editing of this work.

Boccellari, A., & Dilley, J. W. (1992). Management and residential placement problems of patients with HIV-related cognitive impairment. *Hospital and Community Psychiatry, 43,* 32–37.

Boccellari, A., Dilley, J. W., & Shore, M. D. (1988). Neuropsychiatric aspects of AIDS dementia complex: A report on a clinical series. *Neurotoxicology, 9,* 381–390.

Cohen, M. B. (1988). Countertransference and anxiety. In B. Wolstein (Ed.), *Essential papers on countertransference* (64–83). New York: New York University Press. (Original work published 1952.)

Dilley, J. W., Ochitill, H., Perl, M., & Volberding, P. A. (1985). Findings in psychiatric consultations with patients with AIDS. *American Journal of Psychiatry, 142,* 82–86.

Dilley, J. W., Shelp, E., & Batki, S. (1986). Psychiatric and ethical issues in the care of patients with AIDS. *Psychosomatics, 27,* 562–566.

Ferenczi, S., & Rank, O. (1988). The development of psychoanalysis: A historical critical retrospect. In B. Wolstein (Ed.), *Essential papers on countertransference* (25–35). New York: New York University Press. (Original work published 1923.)

Hellinger, F. J., Fleishman, J. A., & Hsia, D. C. (1994). AIDS treatment costs during the last months of life: Evidence from the ACSUS. *Health Services Research, 29,* 569–581.

Kain, C. D. (1996). *Positive: HIV affirmative counseling.* Alexandria, VA: American Counseling Association.

Maj, M., Janssen, R., Starace, F., Zaudig, M., Satz, P., Sughondhabiron, B., Luabeya, M., Reidel, R., Ndetei, D., Calil, H., Bing, E., St. Louis, M., & Sartorius, N. (1994). WHO neuropsychiatric AIDS study, cross-sectional phase I. *Archives of General Psychiatry, 51,* 39–49.

Marzuk, P., Tierney, H., & Tardiff, K. (1988). Increased suicide risk in persons with AIDS. *Journal of the American Medical Association, 259,* 1333–1337.

Motto, J. A. (1994). Rational suicide: then and now, when and how. *Focus: A Guide to Aids Research and Counseling, 9(5),* 1–4.

National AIDS Fund (1994). *Evaluation report for second year of the AIDS Psychiatric Homecare Project.* Unpublished manuscript.

Navia, B. A., Cho, E. S., Petito, C. K., & Price, R. W. (1986). The AIDS dementia complex: II. Neuropathology. *Annals of Neurology, 19,* 525–535.

Navia, B. A., Jordan, B. D., & Price, R. W. (1986). The AIDS dementia complex: I. Clinical features. *Annals of Neurology, 19,* 517–524.

Orr, D. W. (1988). Transference and countertransference: a historical survey. In B. Wolstein (Ed.), *Essential papers on countertransference* (91–110). New York: New York University Press. (Original work published 1954.)

Perry, S., & Tross, S. (1984). Psychiatric problems of AIDS inpatients at the New York Hospital. *Public Health Reports, 99,* 201–205.

Racker, H. (1988). The meanings and uses of countertransference. In B. Wolstein (Ed.), *Essential papers on countertransference* (158–201). New York: New York University Press. (Original work published 1957.)

Reik, T. (1988). The surprised psychoanalyst. In B. Wolstein (Ed.), *Essential papers on countertransference* (51–63). New York University Press: New York. (Original work published 1948).

Reitmeijer, C. A., Davidson, A., Foster, C., & Cohn, D. L. (1993). Cost of care for patients with human immunodeficiency virus infection. *Archives of Internal Medicine, 153,* 219–225.

Tross, S., & Hirsch, S. (1988). Psychological distress and neuropsychological complications of HIV infection and AIDS. *American Psychologist, 43,* 929–934.

# 15 | Case Management: Coordination of Service Delivery for HIV-Infected Individuals

*David D. Barney and Betty E. S. Duran*

My name is Bobby, and I want to tell you about the Ahalaya Project in Oklahoma City. I was referred to Ahalaya after being diagnosed with HIV in 1992. The day my results came back, the HIV counselor with the health maintenance clinic of the Oklahoma City-County Health Department suggested I meet someone from an American Indian organization that provided HIV/AIDS case management. That same evening I was introduced to Gloria Bellymule, project manager for Ahalaya, and she invited me to visit their offices.

Gloria, my case manager, helped me get services that I needed and may not have received without her help. These included referrals to a homeless shelter when I left my partner, a food pantry for food when I ran out of food stamps, and to Salvation Army for clothing. She also helped me apply for jobs and housing. I needed help with making doctor appointments and getting my medications. Staff provided counseling and helped with other personal stuff like taxes.

When I first learned I was HIV-positive, I felt afraid, alone, and angry, but after attending client support group, I realized I was not alone. I have been a participant in recording a prevention education video on HIV/AIDS and have volunteered as a PWA speaker at conferences and workshops in Oklahoma, New Mexico, and California. I have also been temporarily employed by the project to conduct surveys.

I have participated in sweat lodge and other Indian ceremonies that have helped me in connecting with my American Indian heritage. I believe that all the services and healing ceremonies have helped me build self-esteem and obtain independence. Through the encouragement and support of staff, I have obtained employment as a teaching assistant at a local university.

Above all, the staff at Ahalaya have been really wonderful to me. They have also been inspirational. I remember a time about a year and a half ago when I was still with my partner and having a difficult time personally, psychologically, and monetarily as a result of this relationship. My caseworker counseled with me, supported me in my decisions, and a member of the staff reached into their own pocket and gave me some money to tide me over. I will never in my life forget the staff for their gestures of caring, love, understanding, and sharing. The Ahalaya Project has been like a second family to me because I know I can always count on them to come through when I need them.

— An Ahalaya client

Case management is an essential component of HIV care because most individuals living with HIV/AIDS have complex needs that exceed those caused by medical or health conditions. Individuals with HIV infection are likely to require additional assistance with emotional, financial, legal, and social problems throughout different stages of their HIV-disease progression (Sonsel, 1989).

## *Background Reading*

While there is no one standardized definition of case management, it can usually be agreed that the primary function of case management for HIV-infected persons is to coordinate care (Sierra Health Foundation, 1991). Piette, Thompson, Fleishman, and Mor (1993) have identified two dominant goals for case management:

- Case management links clients with appropriate services to improve the quality of the client's life.
- Case management should reduce the use of expensive inpatient care, thereby ensuring that more resources are available for a greater number of needy individuals.

The definition and goals, however, should not be taken as literal or exclusive, since a key aspect of effective case management is flexibility and responsiveness to the particular needs of the client. Indeed, case management practice does vary greatly depending on the types of clients served and the agency providing the case management services.

Even though case management can vary greatly, two dominant types of approaches have been identified in the literature (Piette, Thompson, Fleishman, & Mor, 1993), depending on the organizational setting where the case management is practiced. The first is hospital or medical-based case management, and the second is case management offered by a community-based agency. Each type of setting offers advantages and disadvantages from a client's perspective. Hospital-based caseworkers are usually better able to acquire public entitlement benefits, whereas community-based caseworkers have increased flexibility to work directly with clients in field settings (Indyk, Belville, Lachapelle, Gordon, & Dewart, 1993; Piette, Fleishman, Mor, & Dill, 1990).

The process of case management for HIV-infected individuals has been identified by Piette, Fleishman, Mor, and Thompson (1992) from the experience of twenty HIV-care case management sites. These five steps include:

1. *Assessment.* During the intake process, clients should receive a comprehensive case assessment that identifies their personal life situations from a holistic perspective, including strengths and weaknesses that the clients can emphasize in their treatment or care plans.

2. *Care plan.* A written care plan, with goals and objectives related to each client's status, needs to be developed with the client's participation. The plan should identify who will be responsible for each activity stated in the plan.

3. *Referral.* Referral of clients to social and medical services is a foundation of the actual implementation of the care plan. The core of case management activities usually includes, but is not limited to, coordination of service delivery, counseling, and advocacy functions.

4. *Monitoring.* Monitoring includes frequent checking to ensure that services are actually being provided to the client and that the case plan is being followed. It is also important to conduct regularly scheduled reassessments of the plan.

5. *Advocacy.* Throughout case management services, advocacy is necessary to ensure that entitlements are received and services are delivered. The purpose of advocacy is to eliminate barriers that limit access to the needed support services. Caseworkers can be advocates at the client level,

by advocating for the individual needs of a particular client, or at the systems level, by promoting the interests of a group of the agency's clients.

## *Our Clinical Work*

The Ahalaya Project in Oklahoma City is a case management agency that serves American Indian clients throughout the state of Oklahoma. The staff is, for the most part, American Indian. The director of client services is from Pojoaque Pueblo where she has served as governor of her tribe and as a tribal council member. The project manager and one case manager are Cheyenne, one case manager is Cheyenne/Kiowa, one case manager is Cherokee, and the administrative assistant is Pawnee. Staff are professional social workers, registered nurses, and alcohol and substance abuse counselors. All are committed to working with American Indians and the multiple social issues they are confronted with, especially in the area of HIV prevention and direct care.

When working with American Indians, a culturally unique population, it is essential to determine the cultural barriers that affect clients when they are accessing medical and social services. Community needs and culturally sensitive approaches to offering services also need to be determined. This requires input from clients and community representatives in the development of case management services and in the selection of staff to be employed by the agency. At our agency, the goal, in addition to providing the best case management services possible, has been to determine what constitutes effective case management for American Indian clients.

In the development of culturally relevant services for a specific population of persons, it is important to conduct a thorough review of existing professional literature that may assist the provider in identifying specific cultural differences, values, social and psychological issues, and past response to Western therapies, medical treatments, and social services. The literature reports that due to historical oppression and to their distrust of Western culture, American Indians do not use Western medicine or mental health services and seek assistance through social service programs at lower rates than the general population.

In addition, the literature on Indian spirituality and traditional healing suggests that a blending of Western medicine and Indian traditional healing has increased receptivity to treatment by American Indians receiving psychological and medical care. Tribal ritual and ceremonial practices provide a code for ethical behavior and a social organization that contribute to a meaning of life. It also provides a means for intervening in individual and social dysfunction. Information from existing literature and the participation of American Indian representatives in the development of culturally relevant services have aided in the development of services that are responsive to American Indians living with HIV.

At the Ahalaya Project, we have started with the traditional model of case management, a model built on the belief that clients' needs are too great to be met by any one agency. Accessing multiple agencies to meet client needs is thought of as a "horizontal" orientation to case management. We have also addressed the reality that American Indians and persons living with HIV are often confronted with multiple problems and personal needs. These clients are dealing with social stigma and discrimination arising from one or more of the following factors: homosexuality, HIV infection, racial and ethnic heritage, poverty, illiteracy, homelessness, and poor mental health. Many of our clients have experienced working with social service systems that have complex eligibility criteria, are perceived as nonsupportive, and treat human beings as numbers or cases. It has therefore become important at Ahalaya to assign a primary caseworker who assumes all responsibility for providing and coordinating services for an individual client. This enables the client to develop a close working relationship with the caseworker, enhances trust and increases client compliance with the mutually agreed-on care plan. The one-on-one working relationship also allows the caseworker to become well informed about the client's life (problems, needs, and personal goals), and the caseworker becomes recognized as the person on whom the client can rely on for services and support. Ultimately, this traditional model of case management means that if the client's needs are not adequately addressed, then only the caseworker can be held accountable, and blame cannot be placed on another agency or person.

At the Ahalaya Project, we created an office environment that strengthened cultural identity, supported confidentiality, and provided clients with a dayroom for personal space and a kitchen for their use. We've also made strong efforts to include clients in community education projects. This effort empowers clients by allowing them to invest in the Ahalaya Project's case management services. This sense of ownership increases clients' self-esteem in a nonjudgmental, supportive environment and leads to the development of client support groups and to increased interaction with persons with similar problems and backgrounds.

An important element in creating this environment has been the practice of employing staff who are culturally sensitive, professional, and committed to working with our American Indian clients. Because of the safe and relaxed environment created, as well as the close working relationship between clients and staff, Ahalaya staff members are often identified by clients and their families as extended family members. Ethically, this type of relationship is discouraged in professional settings, but when working with American Indians it is important to recognize that interference from outsiders is unacceptable. Establishing an identity with the client as a person from the family or community enhances the caseworker's ability to recommend services and behavior changes with success.

After starting with the traditional model as our foundation for case management services, we knew that our clients would have unique programming needs because of their cultural heritage as American Indian people. So we added new concepts and components to the case management program. From a design perspective, we built in the opportunity for our caseworkers to do much of their work with clients in the field. This means that our caseworkers have the ability to work beyond their office doors – to be in hospitals, medical offices, public entitlement programs, clients' homes, and places where the client is located and needs the caseworker's support or guidance. This also allows caseworkers to provide education on HIV transmission, disease progression, and care of an HIV-infected person to family and community members; work on issues of family and community reunification (important for clients who have severed family ties due to their sexual orientation or other personal issues), and assist the client in identifying resources and supports within the community.

An important component of the Ahalaya Project is traditional spirituality and healing services. Although our clients come from different tribal backgrounds and have varying degrees of American Indian identity, many of the clients wish to participate in American Indian spirituality and traditional healing. This aspect of the project allows caseworkers to aid clients in learning more about themselves and their tribal backgrounds, sharing their knowledge base with other clients, and actively participating in traditional ceremonies. We have found that this practice increases clients' senses of personal identity, enhances self-esteem, and increases their desire to interact with other clients. It also provides opportunities to teach clients stress management, health care practices, nutrition, and use of natural/herbal medicines.

In American Indian culture, there is a belief that a person is subject to illness caused by natural and supernatural causes. Through traditional spirituality, clients are able to work out many personal issues that they believe are not related to their physical health. (Under the American Indian belief system, there are three causes for illness, both mental and physical. These are natural illness, such as broken bones and cuts; disease caused by the supernatural, such as curses; and non-Indian disease associated with contact with non-Indian culture. Illnesses also fall into three categories: illness only traditional healers can treat; illness only Western medicine can treat, and illness both methods can treat, comprising the majority of all illness [Baines, 1992].) Through ceremony, clients may seek the support of their ancestors through healing, seeking guidance, or releasing a recently departed into the care of the ancestors and their creator.

Death and dying are significant issues in clients' lives. These topics are discussed in therapeutic interventions and in client support group discussions. Traditional Indian elders are often invited to teach on the topic of death and dying and to conduct ceremonies for clients and staff. A common ceremony is the spirit-releasing ceremony conducted after the death of a client. This ceremony allows clients and staff to reach closure with the deceased while providing support for each other.

It is important to remember that these supports are important not only for clients but for staff as well. Caseworkers and other staff develop close ties to the agency's clients. We experience frustration with the lack of available services and the social stigma attached to HIV, stress from work demands, and anxiety from working with clients faced with incurable disease. We suffer exhaustion from long hours worked and feel personal grief over the dying process of our clients. We at Ahalaya therefore also provide a therapeutic group for staff to address these issues and to encourage staff to participate in spiritual and healing ceremonies with or in behalf of clients.

In addition to the more obvious medical needs related to HIV infection, clients also have substantial needs for mental health services. Among our case management clients at the Ahalaya Project, 26 percent have been or are presently receiving mental health treatment. Eighteen percent have a long-term history of mental illness; 19 percent have a history of homelessness; 64 percent have a history of abuse of alcohol or other substances or both. Despite these substantial social barriers and the disadvantaged backgrounds of most of our clients, we have found that our agency's case management services actually improved their quality of life. By using a pre- and posttest instrument, we found that the improvement in the quality of life to be statistically significant ($p = .01$). (For more on evaluation, see chapters 17 and 18.)

Since the development of the traditional model of case management, in which one individual is assigned complete responsibility for a case, a newer model has arisen. This alternative model provides case management services through an HIV-care team. HIV-care teams are usually composed of a combination of staff from social services and medical care programs. A typical team is likely to have a case manager from the social service department, a mental health specialist, a nurse, a physician, and many others. Each team member is responsible for ensuring that the client gets services related to the area of that member's specialty. HIV-care teams represent a "vertical" approach to brokering services, with almost all services being offered within one agency, rather than multiple agencies. Teams can, however, include staff from several agencies, depending on the structure of the local social and medical service delivery system. In large part, the type of agency that serves the client will determine whether a team approach or an individual caseworker is more appropriate. Larger programs which have medical providers, such as medical clinics and hospitals, can benefit from the team approach. This approach is more difficult to implement in smaller agencies with limited staff or with programs that don't provide health or medical services.

## *Barriers to Case Management*

Case managers may face the following barriers:

- *Large caseloads.* Perhaps the most common problem associated with providing case management services is that of large caseloads. The majority of community-based agencies that provide case management services are funded under Title I or Title II of the Ryan White C.A.R.E. Act. These agencies usually have caseloads that range anywhere from a low of fifty to four hundred clients, an often-unmanageable size, given the high level of neediness of HIV-infected individuals.

  One way to address the problem of high caseloads has been to use case aides, persons with a strong sense of personal commitment to the affected community, to supplement caseworkers' activities. While this is clearly beneficial to the caseworker, there are quality-of-care issues to consider; if the coordination between the caseworker (who holds primary responsibility for the client's case) and the case aides is not adequate, then the quality of care provided by case management services will diminish. Additional concern and planning are necessary when using case aides as substitutes for caseworkers. In general, if caseloads are too high, it is necessary to evaluate if enough case activity is actually being provided to properly call it case management.

- *Inappropriate case mix.* Another barrier to providing quality case management services is an inappropriate case mix. By case mix we refer to the range of different types of clients in a caseload. The concern in HIV case management is that individuals in the symptomatic end stages of HIV infection require substantially more caseworker time than do those with early, asymptomatic HIV infection. If by chance a caseworker were to have a majority of clients in the final stages of the disease, then that caseload would need to be reduced. On the other hand, if a caseworker were to have predominately asymptomatic HIV cases, then he or she could be assigned a larger number of clients. The effect of having a caseload made up predominately of AIDS clients, or of having a high caseload, is a caseworker whose activities shift into a "crisis mode" in which the caseworker spends the majority of his or her time responding only to the most critical situations that the most vociferous clients may be encountering. This type of crisis-oriented case management is usually inadequate to qualify conceptually as actual case management, since the caseworker has little time to conduct prevention-oriented activities mostly for HIV-asymptomatic clients. Prevention-oriented activities, such as good nutrition or early response to an infection, are essential to prolonging clients' life expectancies.
- *Inadequate resources.* Social and medical services can often be nearly impossible to locate and access. HIV-infected individuals have substantial needs for a wide variety of social and medical services, including, but not limited to, low-cost housing, medical care, affordable prescriptions, and an income adequate to pay for necessities such as utilities and food when the clients are disabled in the advanced stages of AIDS. Unfortunately, many of the social service and medical service delivery systems are poorly designed and lack adequate resources to respond to all of the

clients' needs. An experienced caseworker will be able to acquire more benefits for clients; however, it is likely that many client needs will be unfulfilled. Even though it is in some circumstances considered unprofessional, it is not unusual for a caseworker to subsidize a client's prescription purchases. Caring for the client's well-being has become one important expression of what case management is about.

- *Difficulty in making referrals.* The cornerstone of case management activity is the ability to make referrals to other agencies to satisfy client needs. Even though this sounds simple, in reality it can be one of the more difficult and time-consuming activities for the caseworker. A successful referral is one in which contact is made with the secondary agency, the agency agrees that the client meets its criteria for eligibility for services, and the client is actually able to follow through with the intake appointment. After those steps, it is essential that follow-up be completed. This entails contacting either the referred-to agency or the client to ensure that the referral actually happened and that the referral will meet the client's needs. In general, a successful referral means crossing bureaucratic lines and negotiating a jungle of complicated eligibility rules. As the caseworker becomes more familiar with the social and medical services community, referrals may become easier but only after the caseworker has put in a lot of time in the field.
- *Transportation difficulties.* Convenient transportation is essential and often difficult to access. For many caseworkers, transportation issues related to getting clients to appointments are critical. Often caseworkers find themselves conducting client interviews while driving the clients to medical or counseling appointments. The transportation issue is one reason that case management services tend to be more effective in urban areas, which usually have public transportation that can be accessed by a majority of clients. When an agency is located in a rural area, however, and many of its clients do not have access to personal or public transportation, then accessing social and medical services becomes nearly impossible. Most agencies located in rural areas struggle to provide case management services. Their budgets and caseloads need to be modified to represent the concerns of increased costs and time required for transportation. At present,

there are few models of case management services that effectively serve rural populations.

## *Tools for Clinical Practice*

Drawing on our project's experience, we have made these observations:

- *Case management services need to be targeted to a diverse client base.*
  Even though HIV-infected individuals share a strong bond based on the common experience of their HIV status, caseworkers must be aware that their caseloads will be very heterogeneous. About 50 to 70 percent of our caseloads are gay men, with the remainder a mix of intravenous drug users, those infected through heterosexual transmission, hemophiliacs, and infants and children. Over time, it is also reasonable to expect that the composition of caseloads will change as the HIV virus targets different groups. Caseworkers need to be flexible in addressing client needs in the context of a particular group's values. Even within a group, such as gay men, there is much diversity. Caseworkers therefore should not emphasize one population too much in their activities and should be careful not to respond to group stereotypes.
- *Client mental health and medical needs should be monitored regularly.*
  Acquiring HIV disease is a major life experience that requires attention to all the details of a client's life. Clearly, physical, emotional, and spiritual needs should be continuously reassessed to ensure that none of the spheres of a client's life are overlooked. Practitioners must be sure to consider their clients' needs in ways that exceed the boundaries of their disciplines.

  In particular, it is essential that the mental health needs of clients not be overshadowed by medical issues. After the first diagnosis of HIV infection, some clients become clinically depressed. This is to be expected, given the associated consequences of being infected with HIV. Medications have been successfully prescribed that help clients with the initial depression. Suicide risk and dangerousness to others need to be assessed and reassessed. Clients' mental health changes continuously in response to both life situations and advancing stages of HIV progression.

  At the Ahalaya Project, our evaluation efforts have indicated that the most important mental health-related goal of case management, from our clients' perspective, is to reduce stress. Clients believe that good case management is a service that reduces stress in their lives. Careful attention should therefore be placed on stress reduction activities.

One area of controversy in HIV case management has been whether caseworkers should be responsible for monitoring the health status of their clients. We recommend to caseworkers that they accept this responsibility, since this is a critical part of a client's life that cannot be overlooked. (See chapter 1 for related information.)

- *Positive self-esteem must be built into the care plan for successful case management outcomes.*

It is important to recognize that many clients come from backgrounds that have negatively affected their self-esteem. It therefore becomes crucial for the agency environment, the agency staff, and the primary caseworker to be cognizant of the need to enhance their clients' self-esteem. The care plan and service delivery should focus on clients' strengths. In therapy it may be necessary to discuss clients' deficiencies, but it is important to use the deficiencies as learning tools by discussing them as life experiences that were not productive but that were ultimately beneficial because they allowed the clients to learn from them.

In developing the care plan, the caseworker begins by assigning the client simple tasks, but over time the client's responsibilities increase to the point where the client is achieving most of the results independently. The caseworker should provide recognition throughout to the client for all achievements, regardless of their significance. In addition, the client should feel comfortable asking the caseworker for assistance with issues that are perceived as difficult or intimidating. The important point is that development of improved self-esteem leads to positive life changes. Positive self-esteem is necessary before we can effectively ask clients to make radical changes in their health and social behaviors.

- *Clinicians must be sure that their case management programs offer clients the opportunity to interact with others of similar background who are also HIV-infected.*

Many clients are isolated due to their sexual orientation, poor health, and other social issues. The agency needs to develop support services that allow clients to meet other persons with similar needs and problems. Client therapeutic groups, talking circles, group discussions, social activities, and community meetings need to be available. Our clients say that through these opportunities their stress and anxiety are reduced, they are made to feel less alone, personal fears are reduced, they come to realize that others share their feelings and concerns, and they learn about other community resources—all while making new friends. Through the sharing of personal life experiences, some clients may come to seek additional therapy to resolve pending life issues. Peer support often results in positive life changes.

- *Permanency planning on behalf of the clients who are parents is an essential activity of case management.*

  Caseworkers in future years are likely to find increasing numbers of dependent children in clients' families. This can be mostly attributed to escalating number of HIV-infected women on caseloads. It is critical, however, that caseworkers be aware that men are increasingly becoming the exclusive caretakers for children. When an HIV-infected client has minor children for whom he or she is the sole provider, the caseworker will need to have permanency planning as an important component of the case management services. By permanency planning, we are referring to the creation of a plan whereby the children will have a permanent home available to them after the death of the primary caretaker. In case management programs it is known that this is the service that caseworkers like least to provide, if they did actually provide the service. It is difficult to talk with a mother or father about the care of children after the parent's death. There is no easy way to do this, but it is imperative for the welfare of the children that a well-constructed plan be developed as soon as possible, ideally during the early stages of asymptomatic HIV infection. This will reduce or perhaps prevent custody disputes after the death of the parent. Even if there are not competing divisions of the extended family likely to vie for custody, permanency planning will designate an appropriate family for the children.

  In addition to the difficulty of discussing death with a parent, permanency planning includes another difficult task. The caseworker will probably need to contact individuals and family members and, in the process of discussing the children's needs, reveal the client's HIV status. This comes after the caseworker skillfully negotiates confidentiality concerns, balancing the parent's right to confidentiality against the best interests of the children. As a rule, clients approve the release of HIV status to friends and family members on a "need-to-know basis."

- *Secondary prevention education is another essential part of case managing those individuals who are HIV-infected.*

  HIV prevention is a ongoing activity. It will never be enough just to educate the current young adult and adult populations without considering that younger persons are continuously maturing and entering higher-risk age groups. HIV education is necessary for our clients as well. It is insufficient to assume that once an individual becomes HIV-infected, he or she no longer needs to be educated about the risk of spreading HIV. Once an individual becomes HIV-infected, that person moves from being at risk to being a potential risk to others. Clients need education to help them prevent the spread of HIV to others. One of a caseworker's professional roles is to be an agent of social control. Social institutions will hold workers responsible, in some part, for guaranteeing that their clients have the requisite knowledge to aid them in not infecting others. HIV-infected clients also have the potential to reinfect other HIV-positive individuals with different strains of the virus. (For secondary prevention information, see chapter 8).

- *Death and dying and burnout are all interrelated issues that must be regularly addressed in the practice setting.*

  When working with HIV-infected individuals, caseworkers must be continuously aware of their clients' concern with death and dying. Some clients may feel comfortable about the issue of death, as this is often regarded as a natural process. One event that increases a client's anxiety about death is the death from AIDS of another client. The caseworker and the agency need to be prepared to bring clients together at times when another client dies. Support and therapy should be provided to them as individuals or as a group.

  The process of dying causes a great deal of stress and anxiety for all clients. When diagnosed with a terminal disease, the natural response is, "I will die before my time." Clients are faced with thinking about how much time they have left, what they want to achieve before they die, and, most important, whether their disease process will involve long periods of illness and hospitalization. Issues of dependency, financial obligations, family, and other concerns continuously confront clients. It is important for caseworkers to aid in the development of supportive forums where individual clients or groups of clients can address these concerns. If cultural or spiritual methods of addressing these issues are available, caseworkers can encourage clients to access these services as well.

It is important to remember also that staff must deal with death and dying and burnout. Staff burnout among caseworkers is very common. The agency must provide support to staff in addressing the issues of client death and dying, as well as providing therapy for staff members. Staff should develop groups to discuss work issues related to stresses and problems encountered in working with terminally ill clients. Flex-time for caseworkers may also be approved by the agency. Supervisors need to encourage staff to take leave on a regular basis and continuing education and training on HIV need to be made available to staff and clients.

## REFERENCES

This chapter was supported in part by grant number BRH-970167 from the Health Resources and Service Administration. Its contents are solely the responsibility of the authors and do not necessarily represent the official views of HRSA.

Baines, D. (1992). Issues in cultural sensitivity: Examples from the Indian peoples. In D. Becker (Ed.), *Health behavior research in minority populations*. Washington, DC: National Institutes of Health.

Indyk, D., Belville, R., Lachapelle, S., Gordon, G., & Dewart, T. (1993). A community-based approach to HIV case management: Systematizing the unmanageable. *Social Work, 38,* 380–387.

Piette, J., Fleishman, J. A., Mor, V., & Dill, A. (1990). A comparison of hospital and community case management programs for persons with AIDS. *Medical Care, 28,* 746–755.

Piette, J., Fleishman, J. A., Mor, V., & Thompson, B. (1992). The structure and process of AIDS case management. *Health and Social Work, 17,* 47–56.

Piette, J. D., Thompson, B. J., Fleishman, J. A., & Mor, V. (1993). The organization and delivery of AIDS case management. In V. J. Lynch, G. A. Lloyd, & M. Fimbres (Eds.), *The changing face of AIDS: Implications for social work practice* (39–62). Westport, CT: Auburn House.

Sierra Health Foundation (1991). *Challenges for the future: Coordinating HIV/AIDS care and services in the next decade.* Rancho Cordova, CA: Author.

Sonsel, G. (1989). Case management in a community-based AIDS agency. *QRB: Quality Review Bulletin, 15,* 31–36.

# 16 | A Comprehensive Center for Women with HIV

*Karen Meredith and Rebecca Bathon*

People who make me feel like a normal person, who are not afraid of me because I have HIV, who treat me with respect, who give me love, support, and friendship.

— Common responses to a survey that asked fifty women, enrolled at the Helena Hatch Special Care Center, what they need from a center for women who have HIV

For HIV-infected women, HIV/AIDS is at the nexus of who they are in society—daughter, mother and mate—how they are positioned in society—in terms of power and control over their own lives—and who they are within themselves. To care for them cannot simply be a biomedical task. HIV/AIDS caregivers must care for the entirety of a woman's being.

While programs of the early epidemic focused primarily on white gay males (Novello, 1993; Rosser, 1991), the increasing impact of HIV disease on women has necessitated a rethinking of our response to the disease (Health Resources and Services Administration, 1995).

Through June 1996, the Centers for Disease Control and Prevention reported 78,654 AIDS cases in adolescent and adult females in the United States. This represents 14.5 percent of this country's cumulative total of AIDS cases in these age groups (Centers for Disease Control and Prevention, 1996). It is among the leading causes of morbidity and mortality in women, especially those of childbearing age (Centers for Disease Control and Prevention, 1995; Quinn, 1995).

## Background Reading

HIV disease has disproportionately affected minority and disenfranchised women, many of whom are unmarried mothers and poor, with low educational levels (Chatters, 1993; Quinn, 1993; Schneider & Stoller, 1995; Shayne & Kaplan, 1991; Shelton et al., 1993; Ward, 1993; Ybarra, 1991). Many engaged in high-risk behaviors such as injection drug use or unprotected sex with multiple partners. Others, however, were not aware of the risk of infection, having had sex only with a partner or spouse who had not disclosed, or denied, being HIV positive (Novello, 1993).

Our experience corroborates the literature on the counseling needs of women in general, as well as those that are specific to women with HIV. Because of the demands of women's multiple roles, as daughters, mothers, and mates, women often overlook their own mental and physical health requirements (Minkoff & DeHovitz, 1991). Numerous authors have shown that women have a need for connection and intimacy with others in order to feel their own sense of value (Gilligan, 1982; Jordan, Kaplan, Miller, Stiver, & Surrey, 1991; Miller, 1986). Preserving a relationship, even an abusive one, may be a primary concern, with consequent subjugation of the woman's own sense of self and personal needs.

The stigma attached to having HIV can make disclosure difficult for women, particularly because they fear rejection by people who provide important relationships. On the other hand, keeping their serostatus a secret can lead to a torturous form of isolation (Miller & Goldman, 1993; Pizzi, 1992). A woman's self-image can be destroyed by the diagnosis; she may feel "sexually dirty and unloved" and, as a result, may withdraw from future relationships (Ybarra, 1991).

The issues surrounding reproductive decisions are significantly complicated by HIV. Giving birth to a child can meet biological, social, and self-esteem needs, foster a relationship, and offer a sense of future to the mother (Lee, 1995). Despite this, there can be great psychological conflict over the chance of transmitting the virus to her child and her partner. Although recent findings of the study known as ACTG 076 (Centers for Disease Control and Prevention, 1995) showed a reduced risk of perinatal transmission when pregnant women and their newborns took zidovudine (ZDV, also called AZT or Retrovir), women face the sobering fact that their children still may be infected and that the children may be motherless at a young age. In addition, women must consider how they will be able to manage the daily demands of motherhood as they become more ill

(Armistead & Forehand, 1995; Arras, 1990; Bradley-Springer, 1994; Shelton et al., 1993).

In addition, women have to face providers who may be confounded and angry at an HIV-positive woman's decision to get pregnant, resulting in unavailable or inadequate counseling and support (Ward, 1993). Finally, the woman faces depersonalized and unwieldy health care and social services systems, compounding her lack of control over her care and fate.

Several panels of experts have defined the need for providing accessible, coordinated, comprehensive, family-centered, and culturally sensitive care for women infected with HIV (Health Resources and Services Administration, 1995; Shelton et al., 1993). Several such projects have been created, including ours, and as of this writing the HIV/AIDS literature has just begun to report their practice (Harris & Williams, 1995).

## *Our Clinical Practice*

The Helena Hatch Special Care Center serves HIV-infected women who reside in metropolitan St. Louis, a twelve-county area within eastern Missouri and southwestern Illinois. At least three quarters of our enrolled clients are African American and unmarried and live in poor, urban settings. The majority fall in the twenty-one- to thirty-year-old category, and 43 percent care for at least one child.

Our center offers primary and specialty medical care as well as psychosocial support and case management in a one-stop-shopping environment, meaning all services are available at one site. Less than nine months after we opened, our enrollment had increased from 43 to 106.

Before the individual attends clinic for the first time, our social worker meets with her and conducts a psychosocial assessment. Usually this meeting takes place in a nonclinical setting of the client's choosing, such as the home, a restaurant, or even a street corner.

When the client arrives at the center, the social worker is there to meet with her, helping to establish a sense of trust and continuity. The social worker also serves as a Ryan White services coordinator, providing access to community resources that might not be available at the center. Women may present with symptoms of depression such as sleeplessness, lack of appetite, or feelings of inadequacy. The clinical social worker addresses mental health needs by making an assessment; the social worker and nurses then provide basic ongoing psychosocial support. If the woman's psychiatric situation is sufficiently serious, referral is made to various community mental health programs and, if necessary, inpatient psychiatric services. Unfortunately, compliance with referrals off-site is low; patients seem to prefer services that are provided within the center, and that fact increases our staff's sense of responsibility in caring for the woman *in toto*.

The center's nurses provide clinical management of the client, which includes providing education about the condition and its treatment, offering reminders about upcoming appointments, and allaying fears at the various transition points of the illness. The entire interdisciplinary team, including physicians, social worker, nurses, dietitian, chaplain, and OB/GYN nurse practitioner, meets regularly to share information and recommendations about each client.

In working with women, we find it important to understand whom they identify as their families. Issues regarding children and role responsibilities must be addressed before we can tackle areas regarding HIV/AIDS. In other words, if a client is most concerned about how to get formula for her infant, while the clinician is addressing safer sex issues, both parties will end up frustrated. Women usually put their families first before they attempt to meet any other needs. Our providers strive to hear the woman's messages about what comes first in her life, thus meeting her "where she is," through family-centered, coordinated care.

We invite consumer suggestions so that we can tailor the program and policy decisions to client needs. We have involved clients in focus groups, interviews, and surveys. Our center also has a community advisory board, which meets quarterly to provide input into programmatic decisions. Our clients tell us we must address the issues of confidentiality, safety, child care, and transportation.

Our mental health services are illustrated by our work with Mary, a young mother of five boys. She has known of her HIV infection for four years and likely was infected by her first husband, who died four years ago. None of her children is infected. Mary is undergoing divorce proceedings with her second husband, who is not the father of any of the children. He is seronegative and has had difficulty accepting her HIV diagnosis. He also is feeling overwhelmed by the thought of taking responsibility for her children after she dies.

The center's social worker has followed this family since the birth of Mary's fifth child. She provided emotional support and counseling to Mary during the anxious months of waiting to learn the child's HIV serostatus. During that six-month period, Mary dealt with her feelings of guilt about possibly infecting her child. She expressed constant fear about how she would be able to care for herself as well as for a sick child.

Mary has had symptoms of depression for the past five years. Despite numerous referrals for psychiatric treatment, she has not sought outside services. Yet, she has attempted suicide twice and continues to struggle with guilt about her infection and "leaving her five boys."

Our social worker has provided counseling sessions to Mary and her husband to help them consider the various issues surrounding their marital conflict and their parenting roles. She assisted Mary in permanency planning for her five children, since they will be orphaned after her death. She also served as liaison with legal aid services in the divorce action and in arranging legal guardianship for the children.

Permanency planning is an issue addressed with all women followed by the center. The process may take years for many women and days for some. Regardless of symptoms, women are encouraged to address this issue with their support systems and eventually to follow up with community-based legal services. The agencies will assist with and file the legal paperwork necessary for a women to complete this process.

At our center, Mary has completed an eight-week Steps to Living educational support group program where she developed relationships with other women in similar circumstances. We worked with the local chapter of the American Red Cross to bring to the center this program, which provides the structured environment needed for a sense of security and purpose and the camaraderie so needed by HIV-impacted women and their families.

The program offers a series of speakers who provide information about coping with issues related to HIV, such as contraception, HIV prevention, legal services, and spirituality. Most of the facilitators and speakers and many of the issues addressed are Afrocentric, since the majority of participants are African American. Participants include not only the women but also their caregivers (e.g., their mothers or partners). Following each educational session, there is an hour of support group interaction, one for the clients, another for the caregivers. Our center addressed barriers to participation by scheduling the program at a convenient time, offering a free dinner to attendees, arranging transportation, and providing on-site child care.

Mary continues to see the other women by attending biweekly support group sessions for program "graduates."

## *Barriers to Dealing with HIV in Women*

Barriers we have encountered include:

- *Denial of HIV infection or avoidance of discussion related to it.* This can occur early in the disease process when the client has few or no physical symptoms. The concept of being infected is too terrible and intangible to accept. To many women, being diagnosed with HIV, regardless of symptoms, means that they are going to die.

  Some feel the infection doesn't exist if they don't acknowledge it and therefore are noncompliant with medical care or do not make long-term plans. A few women have reported that seeing the members of the center is a constant reminder of having HIV. Long-term planning is very difficult when the client is in this stage. When timely, such planning may include such topics as permanency planning for children, setting up a will, establishing a durable power of attorney, and securing basic adequate housing and entitlements.
- *Fear of disclosure.* Most women show care and deliberation before revealing their HIV status. Because of this, they may avoid attending clinic or support groups that are openly for persons with HIV or where staff are members of their own community.
- *Poverty and chaotic lifestyles.* Many women we serve are poor, homeless, and engaged in substance abuse and/or prostitution. Meeting basic physical concerns takes precedence over entering into therapeutic relationships and focusing constructively on psychosocial needs.
- *Conflicting interpersonal demands.* Women, regardless of their HIV statuses, often have difficulty sorting out their own needs from those of others, such as their children, parents, partner, and peers. This can create problems when they need to allocate time and resources. It can also interfere with making difficult decisions, such as planning for the future, deciding to practice safer sex (Rosser, 1991), or choosing whether to get pregnant.
- *Low self-esteem.* Often women who engage in risky behaviors do so because of low self-esteem. Learning that they have HIV infection reinforces their sense of worthlessness and adds to their feelings of isolation and rejection. A history of abuse can be a

cofactor in this situation. In a recent survey of sixty-nine women, predominantly African American and white, at our center, 53 percent reported some form of sexual or physical abuse.

- *Entering into care late in the disease process.* A client may not realize that she is positive until she experiences the symptoms of AIDS, or she may have been tested earlier but chose to deny the infection because she was feeling healthy. Regardless of the reason, seeing a new client late in the disease can be challenging to the counselor if the physical demands overshadow the emotional needs. In addition, the client may be experiencing AIDS Dementia Complex, making it difficult for the counselor to understand her baseline personality.
- *External locus of control* (deCharms, 1980; Deci, 1980). If the client is impoverished and has lived within the realm of the welfare system, she may have little sense of internal power and control. She may not be accustomed to making her own decisions and to thinking far into the future. Rather, she may merely follow the directions given to her by those who make "the rules." She also may be unable to negotiate safer sex with a demanding partner or to work through the difficult decisions of making terminal care plans.

## *Tools for Clinical Practice*

We follow these principles in our work with HIV-infected women:

- *Self-empowerment must be a theme when counseling the HIV-infected woman.*

  HIV infection can force the individual to prioritize her personal goals. Ironically, this may provide her with a major impetus to take some control over her life. With the proper assistance, she may learn to make decisions that are best for herself, take charge of what will happen to her children, and learn skills that otherwise might not have been gained. Many clients are able to find a new inner strength and an appreciation for the essential beauty of life. The provider can facilitate this process through careful assessment, guidance, and concrete opportunities for the client's growth.

  We have found three components to be helpful in promoting our clients' sense of self-efficacy:

1. *Education.* The client must have adequate information in order to be able feel in control of her own decisions. To optimize the experience, the provider should regularly assess the client's stage of acceptance and personal informational needs. This can occur using a formalized assessment instrument, as we are using, or informally, by asking the client, "What questions do you have at this time?" or "Are there specific skills that might help you work through this situation?" It is critical that the counselor take into consideration the literacy, educational level, and learning-style preferences of the client to properly tailor the interventions. For one individual, videotapes along with one-on-one counseling may be the best course of action. For another, it might be group skill-building sessions with take-home written materials. We have found *AIDS: A Self-Care Manual* (AIDS Project Los Angeles, 1989) a useful reference for our clients. Family members and caretakers should be included in the educational process for reinforcement and to ensure continuity if the client becomes too ill to care for herself.

   In some cases the education might take place in the home setting, which can enhance the level of comfort. Most important, the best education occurs when the messages are repeated and provided in a multidimensional fashion.
2. *Networking.* No matter how skilled the professionals involved, the affected woman seems to gain the most understanding by interacting with someone else experiencing the same situation. Many women with HIV/AIDS find it beneficial to meet others who have the same condition. This can occur through the development of a "buddy system" whereby two women get together in person or by telephone or more openly in a social or support group. The latter works best if there is at least one trained professional or peer facilitator who can watch for signs of severe discomfort or uncontrolled negativity in the group process. Women with similar problems can work together towards a positive synergy, thereby fostering a sense of power in resolving their own personal issues.
3. *Consumer advocacy and self-efficacy.* A real sense of empowerment can be fostered by involving the client in all phases of a program's implementation. At the most basic level, this

means including the client when her clinical and psychosocial care plans are being developed. This can occur by having the client (and if she wishes, family members) sit around the table with members of the care team to discuss her health status and treatment options. Regardless of the venue, it is important that the client have an opportunity to ask questions and receive honest answers about her condition. When decisions are to be made, the client should have enough information and support to make them for herself, knowing that the team will endorse her wishes.

- *Treat the woman within the context of her family unit.*

Rarely does a client present herself as a separate entity. Most are involved in a personal relationship, some more permanent than others. Often when it comes to coping with a life-threatening illness, the affected person returns home, where there is a greater sense of acceptance and security. In many of our women's cases, this often means taking up residence with her mother, who may end up caring for her grandchildren when the mother is no longer able to do so. Sometimes, if the individual is married or in a long-term relationship, she and her partner may hold the information about HIV to themselves, fearing that they might in some way burden their family members with the news.

It is important for the counselor to understand the composition of the family and the dynamics of the relationships. Sometimes it is helpful to use a genogram in order to work with the client in identifying who knows about the diagnosis and how prepared each is to assist with her or her children's care. This analysis is never static and must be reconsidered frequently. It is important to realize that family member roles may be nontraditional. For example, a lesbian lover may care for her sick partner's children, or a distant aunt may provide home care (such as giving injections or changing dressings) for the woman who is ill, while the mother may want to prepare the meals.

In some situations, the male partner or husband may decide to take full responsibility for caring for both the infected mother and any children. In such a scenario, this might mean taking a leave of absence from his work, which might require enrolling in Medicaid.

- *Because women often place their care needs last, encourage a client to "listen to her body and her psyche."*

  One client explained that she had to be the strong one in the family as her husband was having difficulty coping with AIDS-related symptoms. She had grown up with a physical disability and said she was accustomed to dealing with this type of adversity. At the same time, she expressed a certain weariness at not being able to care for herself fully in this relationship. It is important for the counselor to offer the woman encouragement to listen to her body and her psyche and to help her sort out her needs from those of others. Concrete suggestions might be helpful, such as providing the client with an attractive blank book in which she can keep a journal. *The Woman's Comfort Book: A Self-Nurturing Guide for Restoring Balance in Your Life* (Louden, 1992) provides a variety of innovative, individualized ways for women to care for themselves. We have several copies on our reference shelf for loan and have used its ideas when working with our women.
- *Understand the client's culture.*

  Regardless of the ethnic, socioeconomic, or other group to which a client belongs, she exists within a particular culture that has its own context for understanding HIV/AIDS (Bevier, Chiasson, Hefferman, & Castro, 1995; Flaskerud & Rush, 1989; Randall-David, 1995, 1989; Wofsy, 1995). The counselor should understand the nature of that environment from the standpoint of how the client receives information, what has value, and how certain actions by herself and by her care providers are perceived. This requires patience, sensitivity, and observation on the part of the counselor (see chapter 6).

  Culture is identified not only by race or religion but by how the family unit uses that information within its context. An example is the topic of spirituality. Most of our women believe in a higher power. Delivering services effectively means that the clinician needs to identify the woman's spiritual belief even if that clinician does not personally share that same religion or philosophy (see chapter 4). Prayer after support groups and disclosure at church are issues for many HIV/AIDS-affected women.
- *Use the "stages of behavior change" model to understand and intervene with clients who continue risky behaviors.*

It can be frustrating for the counselor to work with clients who continue behaviors that put themselves and others at risk for infection. Thinking about the client in terms of "stages of behavior change" can be helpful to practitioners (see Prochaska, DiClemente, & Norcross, 1992; McConnaughy, DiClemente, Prochaska, & Velicer, 1989). The authors categorize clients into one of several stages: precontemplative, contemplative, ready for action, action, and maintenance. Each stage describes how the client views a "problem" and requires a different response and intervention. A client in the precontemplative stage, for example, believes she has no problem, although the clinician may think otherwise. A clinician's response to a precontemplative client may be simple assurance that she may return for counseling anytime. A provider who fails to perceive that a client is precontemplative and continues to pressure her for a change only ends up feeling impotent and frustrated.

When the client shows readiness, the counselor can then provide interventions that are consistent with the client's stage of behavior change. Someone in the contemplative stage may need further nudging regarding the problem; a client in the action stage requires concrete helping steps to resolve the situation.

- *Reproductive issues are a major issue when working with women.*

Many women discover their HIV status during pregnancy. HIV-positive serostatus usually comes as an enormous shock and brings subsequent feelings of guilt and fear that the unborn child may become HIV-positive. Other women, not yet pregnant, may desire to bear a child even if they already have an infected child.

Despite new scientific information regarding the use of zidovudine, reproductive issues are always complex. Without special antiretroviral intervention, the rate of vertical transmission, from mother to fetus, is between 13 percent and 30 percent. In AIDS Clinical Trials Group (ACTG) 076, zidovudine therapy was given to women with T-helper cell counts greater than 200 after the fourteenth week of pregnancy, during labor and delivery, and to infants after delivery. In the group that received the therapy, vertical transmission was 8 percent compared to 25 percent in a placebo group (Centers for Disease Control and Prevention, 1995; Kurth, 1995). How effective the therapy will be in the general HIV-infected population, in women with different levels of adherence, and especially in women with advanced disease, remains to be learned.

We see a couple in which the wife is infected but the husband is not. They have a child who is terminally ill with HIV/AIDS. After careful consideration, they decided to conceive another child because the husband would like to have a healthy child after his wife and his first child are gone. They are using artificial insemination to protect him from infection. This and other complicated situations regarding childbearing are quite common among women with HIV.

The counselor can play a pivotal role in assisting the client in making an active and informed decision about whether she wants to have a child (Hutchison & Shannon, 1993). The provider can discuss the advantages and disadvantages, the risks and benefits. Issues to discuss are:

1. Reasons for having the child. Sometimes the client herself is unable to clarify this.
2. Plans for care of the child when the mother is too ill and after her death.
3. Personal behaviors that can decrease risk of transmission and contribute to having a healthy baby.

These discussions must be done in a nonjudgmental, nondirective manner, with respect and assurance of continuation of care regardless of the decision. This is easily said but may be difficult in that the provider may have a certain opinion on the subject at hand. Our judgments are best kept to ourselves, lest we recapitulate a situation that women have faced all their lives: someone else attempting to be in control and to force decisions on them. Our task is to care for women and their families, not to direct their lives.

## *Conclusion*

At the Helena Hatch Special Care Center we feel we succeed in building relationships when the women return for care. And for us, care extends beyond the biomedical. Women may seek our assistance in resolving housing issues or obtaining food. We have created a nonjudgmental, accepting atmosphere in which the women feel welcome, where issues can be discussed by the women without their feeling ridiculed or embarrassed by their lack of knowledge. Women come to the center for clinical care and take much more than that home with them.

## REFERENCES

This chapter was supported by Grant Number BRH 900125–02 from the Health Resources and Services Administration. The opinions expressed are those of the authors and do not represent those of HRSA.

AIDS Project Los Angeles (1989). *AIDS: A self-care manual* (3d Ed.). Santa Monica: IBS Press.

Armistead, L., & Forehand, R. (1995). For whom the bell tolls: Parenting decisions and challenges faced by mothers who are HIV seropositive. *Clinical Psychology: Science and Practice, 2,* 239–249.

Arras, J. D. (1990). AIDS and reproductive decisions: Having children in fear and trembling. *Millbank Quarterly, 68,* 353–382.

Bevier, P. J., Chiasson, M. A., Hefferman, R. T., & Castro, K. G. (1995). Women at a sexually transmitted disease clinic who reported same-sex contact: Their HIV seroprevalence and risk behaviors. *American Journal of Public Health, 85,* 1366–1371.

Bradley-Springer, L. A. (1994). Reproductive decision-making in the age of AIDS. *IMAGE: Journal of Nursing Scholarship, 26,* 241–246.

Centers for Disease Control and Prevention (1995). U.S. Public Health Service recommendations for human immunodeficiency virus counseling and voluntary testing for pregnant women. *Morbidity and Mortality Weekly Report, 44(RR-7),* 1–14.

Centers for Disease Control and Prevention (1996). *HIV/AIDS Surveillance Report, 8(1).*

Chatters, L. M. (1993). HIV/AIDS within the African American communities: Diversity and interdependence. A commentary on AIDS and the African American woman: The triple burden of race, class, and gender. *Health Education Quarterly, 20,* 321–326.

deCharms, R. (1980). Personal causation and locus of control: Two different traditions and two uncorrelated measures. In H. M. Lefcourt (Ed.), *Advances and innovations in locus of control research* (337–358). New York: Academy Press.

Deci, E. L. (1980). *The psychology of self-determination.* Lexington, MA: Heath.

Flaskerud, J. H., & Rush, C. E. (1989). AIDS and traditional health beliefs and practices. *Nursing Research, 38,* 210–215.

Gilligan, C. (1982). *In a different voice: Psychological theory and women's development.* Cambridge, MA: Harvard University Press.

Grimes, R. M., & Grimes, D. E. (1995). Psychological states in HIV disease and the nursing response. *Journal of the Association of Nurses in AIDS Care, 6(2),* 25–32.

Harris, K., & Williams, L. D. (1995). Communities of caring: Integrating mental health and medical care for HIV-infected women. *Focus: A Guide to AIDS Research and Counseling, 10(12),* 1–4.

Health Resources and Services Administration (1993). *HIV/AIDS work group on health care access issues for African Americans.* (DHHS Publication No. HRSA-94–023). Rockville, MD: Author.

Health Resources and Services Administration. (1995). *HIV/AIDS work group on health care access issues for women.* (DHHS Publication No. HRSA-RD-SP-93–7). Rockville, MD: Author.

Hutchison, M., & Shannon, M. (1993). Reproductive health and counseling. In A. Kurth (Ed.), *Until the cure: Caring for women with AIDS* (47–65). New Haven: Yale University Press.

Jordan, J. V., Kaplan, A. G., Miller, J. B., Stiver, I. P., & Surrey, J. L. (1991). *Women's growth in connection: Writings from the Stone Center.* New York: Guilford Press.

Kurth, A. (1995). HIV disease and reproductive counseling. *Focus: A guide to AIDS research and counseling, 10(7),* 1–4.

Lee, F. R. (1995, May 9). For women with AIDS, anguish of having babies. *New York Times,* A-1, B-6.

Louden, J. (1992). *The woman's comfort book: A self-nurturing guide for restoring balance in your life.* New York: HarperCollins.

McConnaughy, E. A., DiClemente, C. C., Prochaska, J. O., & Velicer, W. R. (1989). Stages of change in psychotherapy: A follow-up report. *Psychotherapy, 26,* 494–503.

Merkel-Holguin, L. A. (1994). *Because you love them: A parent's planning guide.* Washington, DC: Child Welfare League of America.

Miller, J. B. (1986). *Toward a new psychology of women* (2d ed.). Boston: Beacon Press.

Miller, R., & Goldman, E. (1993). Counseling HIV-infected women and families. In M. A. Johnson, & F. D. Johnstone (Eds.), *HIV infection in women* (37–48). London: Churchill Livingstone.

Minkoff, H. L., & DeHovitz, J. A. (1991). Care of women infected with the Human Immunodeficiency Virus. *Journal of the American Medical Association, 266,* 2253–2258.

Novello, A. C. (1993). The HIV/AIDS epidemic: A current picture. *Journal of Acquired Immune Deficiency Syndromes, 6,* 645–654.

Pizzi, M. (1992). Women, HIV infection, and AIDS: Tapestries of life, death, and empowerment. *American Journal of Occupational Therapy, 46,* 1021–1027.

Prochaska, J. O., DiClemente, C. C., & Norcross, J. C. (1992). In search of how people change. *American Psychologist, 47,* 1102–1114.

Quinn, S. C. (1993). Perspective: AIDS and the African-American woman: The triple burden of race, class, and gender. *Health Education Quarterly, 20,* 305–320.

Quinn, T. C. (1995). The epidemiology of the acquired immunodeficiency syndrome in the 1990's. *Emergency Medicine Clinics of North America, 13(1),* 1–25.

Randall-David, E. (1989). *Strategies for working with culturally diverse communities and clients.* Washington, DC: Association for the Care of Children's Health.

Randall-David, E. (1995). *Culturally competent HIV counseling and education.* Rockville, MD: National Hemophilia Program, Maternal and Child Health Bureau, Health Resources and Services Administration.

Rosser, S. V. (1991). Perspective: AIDS and women. *AIDS Education and Prevention, 3,* 230–240.

Schneider, B. E., & Stoller, N. E. (1995). *Women resisting AIDS: Feminist strategies of empowerment.* Philadelphia: Temple University Press.

Shayne, V. T., & Kaplan, B. J. (1991). Double victims: Poor women and AIDS. *Women and Health, 17(1),* 21–37.

Shelton, D., Marconi, K., Pounds, M., Scopetta, M., O'Sullivan, M. J., & Szapocznik, J. (1993). Medical adherence among prenatal, HIV seropositive, African American women: Family issues. *Family Systems Medicine, 11,* 343–355.

Ward, W. C. (1993). A different disease: HIV/AIDS and health care for women in poverty. *Culture, Medicine and Psychiatry, 17,* 423–430.

Wofsy, C. B. (1995). Gender-specific issues in HIV disease. In M. Sande & P. Volberding (Eds.), *The Medical Management of AIDS* (649–664). Philadelphia: W. B. Saunders.

Ybarra, S. (1991). Women and AIDS: Implications for counseling. *Journal of Counseling and Development, 69,* 265–287.

# IV How Do We Know It Works?

# 17 | How Do We Know It Works? Quantitative Evaluation

*Michael Mulvihill*

In these times of shrinking resources and cost containment, funders and providers of HIV-related services want more than ever to know that they get results for dollars spent. In fact, the pressures to demonstrate whether health service programs have a measurable effect are probably greater than at any other time in recent memory. Until the political pendulum swings back to the days of "The Great Society," budget cuts will most likely affect those service areas that fail to demonstrate that they make a difference.

Government funding agencies and foundations now require that sophisticated evaluations be conducted to determine whether mental health and other program dollars are well spent and whether new models of care being tested or "piloted" through grants should receive additional attention.

Ethical providers of HIV-related services ask similar questions: "I know that people like our mental health clinic. But does our psychotherapy, or our psychiatric service, really improve people's lives?" and "Are there ways of finding out how we can improve our services?"

Program administrators who seek quality and patient satisfaction rely more and more on evaluations. For them, evaluations feed back information to service providers so that they can improve their programs. Evaluations also help define which services work better than others and provide guidelines on how to make service packages most effective. For programs, a good evaluation creates an information loop, informing administrators and clinicians, who then modify the service package, which is again evaluated.

Not too long ago, many evaluations were based simply on surveys of either a program's providers or its clients at one or several points in time, asking them questions about the program's effects. This strategy is weak for many reasons. It is based on subjective notions about what works or doesn't work, and it fails to provide concrete evidence for its conclusions. It does not consider how things were before the new program began, or even at different stages of the program, and it does not consider that respondents may have many reasons to praise a program, only some of which may have to do with real effects. Employees may say wonderful things about a program, for example, so that they can keep their jobs, or clients may praise a program so that they don't risk angering their service providers.

These types of evaluations are no longer considered sufficient. The field has become much more sophisticated: A profession of evaluation now exists, and professional societies have sprung up. Many consulting firms offer evaluation services, and some academic departments have evaluation experts on staff.

This chapter, and the next, provide basic information about evaluation, with an emphasis on HIV-related issues, so that readers can enter the mental health field knowing the questions it is asking itself and how it is attempting to find the answers. If any reader ever becomes involved in requesting money from governments or foundations, this information will be a start toward understanding what must be included in a viable application for grant funds.

This chapter focuses on quantitative evaluations, that is, those done with numbers and statistics; I illustrate my points with an actual federally funded HIV mental health project. The next chapter discusses qualitative evaluations.

## *What Is Evaluation?*

In brief, an evaluation seeks to answer questions about a program's processes and outcomes. Typical process questions, broadly stated, are: Are we reaching the service population(s) we hope to serve? Is the full array of psychosocial problems being addressed? Qualitative evaluations are more likely to deal with process, whereas quantitative evaluations typically deal with outcome questions, including these concerns: "Does the program make a difference?" and "Is the program cost-effective?"

Many evaluations are concerned with outcomes that can affect local or national health care policies, since many governmental and foundation grantors want applicants' projects to be generalizable and replicable. *Generalizability* means that findings determined at one agency can be applied at—are generalizable to—others. Federal agencies often fund tests of new programs not because they want to assist one agency but because the findings are potentially useful to hundreds of agencies. *Replicability* means that the structure of the program being studied, if successful, can be adopted at other institutions and will provide the same results. Programs that are very idiosyncratic, and hence not replicable elsewhere, are not likely to receive funding.

Going from these broadly stated questions and concepts to meaningful specific questions and answers is a very rigorous process that requires evaluation expertise and involves labor, time, and a willingness to tolerate the possibilities of nonflattering results. If you learn nothing else, learn that you need to seek the assistance of experts before you plan the program. The program and evaluation should be built together.

CASE EXAMPLE: Congress, in passing the Ryan White Comprehensive AIDS Resources Emergency (C.A.R.E.) Act, created the Special Projects of National Significance (SPNS, pronounced "spins") program to support development and evaluation of cutting-edge programs in HIV services. SPNS programs were created at Montefiore Medical Center in the Bronx, New York, and at St. Joseph's Hospital and Medical Center, in Paterson, New Jersey, to integrate HIV-related mental health services with primary medical care. My task, and that of my colleagues in the research division of the Department of Family Medicine, Albert Einstein College of Medicine, was to evaluate those HIV-related mental health programs.

## *How to Think about Quantitative Evaluation*

A quantitative evaluation can best be described as a comparison or, more accurately, as a whole host of comparisons.

The most common comparisons to consider for a new program are:

- The old way of doing things versus the new program.
- The new program versus a "control" program. A control pro-

gram is one that appears very much like the new program but is absent the "active ingredients" — those that are believed to make the difference — contained in the new program.

For a quantitative evaluation of a mental health program, patients are generally assessed in some way both before and after being exposed to the program. This comparison is called pretest versus posttest. The program manager's hope is, of course, that the programs will be found to have made a difference in the client's life.

Another comparison that can be made is one made across time. The scores of tests taken in January, April, July, and October, for example, may be compared to see if there is a pattern of change. This is called a time series and is really just an extension of the pretest-posttest idea but with multiple measurement points.

*Those Confounding "Confounds"*

If these comparisons were a simple matter, experts (and this chapter) would be unnecessary. Unfortunately, making comparisons that stand up to scrutiny can be devilishly tricky.

Confounds (some people call them confounders) are factors that undermine the comparisons made in the evaluation process. Here are some confounds (there are many others):

- Regression to the mean. This concept refers to the fact that individuals usually enter treatment at personal low points (e.g., when severely depressed or anxious). Since these emotional states are variable within individuals, a reassessment later will, on average, simply measure a natural rebounding of the mental state. This rebound would be expected to occur naturally whether or not the person received treatment. This is referred to as "regression to the mean" because it is a measure of a return to an average (mean) mental state.
- Other changes that occur during the course of the program that have an effect, independent of the treatment itself, on the desired outcomes. The person being treated for depression, for example, may lose a partner or be evicted from an apartment. His or her depression scores may then worsen, despite the clinician's best treatment efforts.
- Participation in multiple programs. A client may attend several

different treatment programs in the community so that it cannot be ascertained that one program alone was responsible for improvements.
- Changes in treatment agent. A patient's therapist may leave the program, for example, negatively affecting the client.

In evaluation, these are referred to as "historic" or "contextual" biases. Campbell and Stanley (1963) list many other confounds, which they term threats to a research design's internal or external validity.

A successful evaluation requires that as many of the confounds as possible be eliminated through the study design or controlled for in the analyses by an examinination of their independent effects. If serious confounds cannot be eliminated, it may not be possible to learn whether a program makes a difference, and funders may respond negatively to an application for funds.

## *What Do I Evaluate?*

One of the most challenging aspects of creating an evaluation plan is deciding what aspects of a program should be assessed. The best way for you as the researcher to think about this is to reflect on these considerations:

- What groups do you want to affect? "Clients" may be your immediate answer. But do you want the program also to change the practice of clinicians? Do you want the program to change the institution or agency in some way? If so, then you need to evaluate whether these changes occurred.
- For each group, what change do you want to occur as a result of and only as a result of your program? For clients, you may want to determine whether your services affected their depression. For a clinic, you may want to increase physicians' referrals to mental health specialists.

CASE EXAMPLE: In the Montefiore and the St. Joseph's programs, providers felt that patients receiving mental health services would generally feel better, that they would have better coping skills, that they might not show up in the emergency room as often, and that their feelings of stress would be reduced. It was also felt that in those clinics with integrated mental health care, a greater number of patients with HIV would avail themselves of those services since they would be available on site. This arrangement would surmount the barrier of traditional reliance on referral to another agency or provider at another location. The program developers also believed that medical providers might feel better about their work if they could make quick mental health referrals and receive quick consultations.

## *How Do I Measure These Things?*

Once you decide what aspects you want to measure as part of the evaluation, you will want to consider how to measure the attributes. Some would say you have to "operationalize" those aspects — to give them concrete, measurable meaning. That concreteness generally is stated in the phrase "as measured by [name of instrument]." Instruments use numbers to express the concept being measured. These numbers are likely to include raw scores (the client's score without any statistical massage); corrected scores, which are raw scores massaged, for example, to correct for response omissions; and scale scores, which are a measure of how the patient performed relative to a group. We call what we do quantitative evaluation simply because we use numbers — scores — as the bases for our comparisons.

The first task is to conduct a literature search of how others have measured the phenomena you want to measure. Many published scales exist that may suit your purposes, but the literature may indicate a preference for the use of one particular instrument. You may also want to consult the latest edition of what is familiarly called *Buros' Mental Measurements Yearbook* but is officially *The 11th Mental Measurements Yearbook* (Kramer & Conoley, 1992), which reprints reviews of psychological instruments.

You will want to find an instrument that has proven *validity* and *reliability*. These words have special meaning to evaluators:

- A scale is *valid* when it has been proven to measure what it claims to measure.
- The scale is *reliable* when it has been shown to produce results that are the same when confronted with the same amount of the phenomenon. An instrument scale is reliable when the same results are obtained from the same individuals, provided they have not changed, in repeat administration of the instrument. Your bathroom scale is reliable if it is always ten pounds off, because the amount of error is always the same.

> To ensure reliability, often those who administer the assessment instruments have to be specially trained to a certain standard, which is statistically checked, and they are rechecked over the course of the project. If you decide to use instruments that are administered by someone or several someones, such as psychologists, you will have to spend the time and money to train these individuals to a certain standard and to check them occasionally to ensure that the reliability is maintained.

Another important term is *construct validity,* which refers to the degree to which question items that measure different aspects of a construct "hang together" in a meaningful way. If, for example, you wish to measure a particular attitude, it is often important to have several questionnaire items that are intended to measure different aspects of the same attitude. The degree to which individual responses to the varied items follow the same response pattern is a reflection of the validity of the scale.

It is beyond the scope of this chapter to undertake a thorough discussion of the ways that the validity of an instrument is assessed, but a psychometrician should be consulted when planning an evaluation that uses assessment instruments. See also Campbell and Stanley (1963) for a discussion of different concepts of validity.

A major concern of those who work in the inner city is whether instruments are available that have been validated with minority culture groups, including groups that cannot read English. Unfortunately, even major publishers of assessment instruments have merely translated instruments into, for example, Spanish, without conducting new validation studies to determine whether the instrument really measures the desired phenomenon in the responding group. Issues of validity for personality assessment and psychopathology are well reviewed by Rogler, Malgady, and Rodriguez (1989) and by Marin and VanOss Marin (1991). Rogler, Malgady, and Rodriguez (1989) suggest that we should assume that there is cultural bias in instruments, unless proven otherwise. Certainly, an evaluator should be able to defend his or her choice of instruments as consistent with the American Psychological Association's *Standards for Educational and Psychological Tests* (1985), which offers many warnings to consider in work with cultural minorities.

In the event that the literature search does not produce an instrument with adequate reliability or validity, you might wish to produce a scale tailored to the particular issues of your evaluation. This can be a laborious process, but it can be quite enlightening as well.

One approach might be to conduct a focus group, in which a group of professionals gathers to discuss the meaning of a concept and to suggest the components of how it should be evaluated. The members of the group might suggest items to be used in instrument development. The rationale for having several participants is to make sure that many perspectives are included and that a sharper definition of the concept will result. It may even be worthwhile to have a focus group with the recipients of care to discuss how and in what ways they value the services. This may identify issues that weren't thought about by the providers. A more complete discussion of this process of evaluation can be found in Chapter 18.

CASE EXAMPLE: In the evaluation of the integrated mental health services at Montefiore and at St. Joseph's, several informal focus group sessions took place to discuss the qualities that should be included in the evaluation plan. We decided that patients' sense of well-being, levels of depression and anxiety, dependence on emergency room visits as a result of crises in their lives, and levels of physical and social functioning might all be affected in a positive sense if they received mental health counseling in a timely and appropriate manner. A literature review was conducted to ascertain what instruments were already available to assess these issues. We uncovered two instruments that dealt with many of the psychosocial and physical functioning dimensions. These were the Medical Outcomes Survey (MOS) short-form questionnaire (SF-36) (McHorney, Ware, Lu, & Sherbourne, 1994; Ware & Sherbourne, 1992) and the Brief Symptom Inventory (BSI) (Derogatis, 1992; Derogatis & Melisaratos, 1983). Both scales have been used extensively and have been extensively assessed for their reliability and validity.

Another area we felt was important to include was the degree to which barriers to obtaining care would be altered. For this we found an instrument titled "Primary Care Physicians and AIDS Scale" (Gerbert, Maguire, Bleecker, Coates, & McPhee, 1991), which addresses this issue. Last, we thought that if mental health services were readily available to the health team, the program staff itself would feel a reduction in job stress. For this we located the Work Environment Scale (Abraham & Foley, 1984), which includes items that address how people feel about their jobs and the level of stress they perceive. All of these scales were available and finding them obviated the need to reinvent them. Figures for the other issues we felt to be important—severity of illness, use of the emergency room, the number of medical and mental health visits, etc.—were all obtained by reviewing patients' medical records.

## *How Do I Structure the Evaluation?*

One of the most vexing issues in doing a credible evaluation is deciding how to structure the evaluation or how to pick the most appropriate design for an accurate comparison. The best structure is one that eliminates all confounds and allows for an unambiguous response to the question "Did our program, and our program alone, make the difference?"

Scientific research methods have informed quantitative evaluations on ways to eliminate, as much as possible, confounds. The main strategies are these:

- *When making comparisons, compare your program with a control program, that is, a concurrently studied control group.*

  It may seem unethical to have a control group of severely depressed or anxious clients from whom you withhold treatment in order to obtain a "cleaner" measure of the effects of treatment. If so, then you are thinking good ethics. Whenever we deal with a clinical condition for which there is a known treatment that has evidence of a therapeutic benefit, it is unethical to have an untreated control group. We have to create a comparison of one treatment approach (the accepted standard) to another, the experimental approach. In this way, the regression-to-the-mean problem is handled because it presumably operates in both groups to the same degree.
- *When possible, randomly assign patients to your program and to a control program.*

  A design based on a random assignment to two or more groups is the ideal. This is the classic randomized clinical trial. In this design, patients in need of mental health services are randomly assigned to an experimental approach to treatment or to a traditional approach. Although this represents the standard one should always strive to approach, it is rarely done because of logistical issues. This approach has the best chance of overcoming all the problems or confounds inherent in other approaches because it assumes that confounding aspects are equally spread over each group. The nature and the severity of the health problems are similar in the two treatment groups, the historical factors that might have an impact on the outcomes are similar, and the regression-to-the-mean issues are theoretically equal. In other words, by the randomization process, one has the greatest likelihood of creating two comparable groups in order to isolate the impact of one treatment approach relative to another.

CASE EXAMPLE: In the Montefiore evaluation, the goal was to assess the relative effects of a new delivery system of mental health services to HIV-infected individuals in the context of primary medical care. This new approach is called "integrated delivery of mental health services" because the mental health worker became a regular member of the health care team and participated on an equal footing with the other members of the team. The need for a mental health referral to another agency at another time was therefore eliminated. This modality of delivery of care was to be evaluated relative to the traditional model, which was based on referrals to other agencies or departments, all of which were at other locations. There were sufficient funds to develop an integrated service model in four of the eight Montefiore Ambulatory Care Network (MACN) sites. The remaining four, which would not be exposed to the integrated model, would be available to serve as control sites. In this manner, a "natural" experiment was possible in which an innovative approach to delivery of mental health services could be measured against a traditional model of care. This was not a randomized clinical trial because patients were not randomly assigned to one system or another, nor was the selection of sites for the integrated model made on a random basis. The best name for this design is probably a "cohort" model, because two cohorts were to be followed: the patients served by one of the two systems, the integrated mental health service model or the traditional delivery system.

We became aware of a potential problem relating to the regression-to-the-mean phenomenon. In the integrated model, patients would presumably more easily gain access to mental health services on average than they would in the traditional model based on physician referral. This might mean that at the outset of receiving services, those in the traditional model might be in worse states than those in the integrated model. In the reassessment of these patients at some later date, it would therefore appear that the patients in the traditional model had improved more, if only because they started at a different, lower point. To overcome this potential problem, we adopted an approach called an "intent-to-treat" model in which we evaluated mental and social functioning of HIV patients who entered both systems of care irrespective of whether they received mental health services. In this way we were able to address the issues of whether patients entering one system of care fared better relative to patients entering another system of care. Furthermore, we were able to assess the degree to which mental health services were delivered to more patients and whether the severity of patients' mental health problems was different at the point the patients received services. The effects of care were assessed by comparing, in the broadest sense, whether patients who entered one system of care fared better at some later point than did patients entering another system of care.

## *Compiling the Numbers*

You realize now that you will be doing a lot of measuring and that many numbers will result. In addition, you will compile a host of information on the clients themselves, including age, race, ethnic identification, sex, sexual preference, route of infection, and other demographic information you deem important. This descriptive information is important because the reader of your evaluation report will want to know if your findings will be applicable to his or her service population.

All these numbers have to be stored somewhere. This requires two components: a database software package and a computer with enough capacity to run the program. It is important also that you realize that compiling and maintaining a database are very labor-intensive and require a person willing to give a lot of attention to detail. Throughout the project, the database manager has to ensure that the information entered into the database is accurate and complete. Failure to attend to this jeopardizes the entire evaluation.

## *How Do I Analyze My Findings?*

This is not a chapter on statistics, which are uniquely complex in and of themselves. To satisfy statistical requirements, for example, you must have a sufficient number of clients in a quantitative analysis to be able to find meaningful differences, if they exist. You must also determine what you mean, statistically, by "difference." And you must determine what parameters of error should be built into statistical equations. These and other issues require the assistance of someone knowledgeable in statistics.

For purposes of introducing you to quantitative analyses, we introduced the concepts of comparison and measurement. It is in the analyses that these concepts interact and produce results. While statistics can do many tasks, including making predictions, we will discuss only comparisons.

### *Comparing Group Means*

We discussed evaluative comparisons, broadly speaking, and then the narrowing of these issues into operationalized, measured concepts. We now have a computer disk full of numbers, arranged correctly in designated rows and columns. We turn this disk over to a statistician who uses software, such as Statistical Package for the Social Sciences (SPSS) and Statistical Analysis System (SAS), which will compile the numbers into meaningful chunks. The statistician will have decided, on the basis of your initial proposal, what family of statistical tests he or she will use. Nonparametric statistics are used when certain kinds of data are used (e.g., frequencies), for example, and parametric tests are used when other types of data are examined (e.g., group means).

For evaluation purposes, perhaps the most typical comparison is that of group averages or means. The statistical program will compute the mean depression score of the group of patients enrolled in your new program and the group mean of all patients in the traditional program. The statistical software will also compute a measure of "score spread" for each of the groups. Then, the computer will take other orders — such as what you determined was a statistically significant difference and the error tolerance you will accept. Using these factors and the measurement data, the software will tell you if there is a significant difference between the group mean of your treatment patients and the group mean of your controls. This is the simplest comparison.

More complex comparisons are possible. Group means for many groups, or for multiple measurements of individuals in each group, can be compared using statistical processes such as analysis of variance (ANOVA). If you wanted to take many different scores — depression, anxiety, and sense of well-being, for example — and make multiple comparisons, the statistician might decide to use multivariate (multiple variable) statistics. A printout of a multivariate analysis might indicate that there were differences between the group means on some variables and not on others or on all variables or that no differences were evident, which would mean that your program functioned just like the program you compared it with.

Multivariate analyses are the minimum statistical analyses done in evaluation, because studies have to concern themselves with many variables that aren't even the target of our programs. These variables include gender, age, race, ethnic identification, and marital status, among many others. If you want to learn if individuals in a certain age group or sex responded better to your program than did comparable individuals in the control program, then multivariate statistics are what you will use.

CASE EXAMPLE: The Montefiore and the St. Joseph's data, as compiled by the database software, are placed on a disk. Then statistical experts program SAS to respond with different analyses. One simple group comparison is whether patients at St. Joseph's Hospital use the emergency room fewer times than subjects in the control program, at another Paterson institution. A more complex analysis would be to compare use of the emergency room by Latinos or blacks in both study groups.

## *HIV-Specific Issues in Evaluation*

When planning an evaluation of an HIV-related program, you need to take into account the following special concerns:

- Many inner-city clients are overwhelmed with myriad psychosocial and medical issues, and they tend not to put an agency's evaluation project on the top of their priority lists. Because they are unlikely to remain in a study that extends over several months, ensuring their continued involvement tends to be labor-intensive and expensive. Fowler et al. (1992), reporting on a longitudinal survey of persons with AIDS, noted that every facet of their work posed challenges; they suggested solutions to problems in identification and recruitment of subjects, consent, and data collection.

  More and more, evaluators and researchers are offering financial incentives to persons to induce them to complete assessment forms.

  CASE EXAMPLE: The Montefiore project research assistants spend significant time attempting to track clients so that they can complete additional assessment forms. Despite our efforts, there is a significant attrition between the first assessment and subsequent assessments. This requires that we enroll many extra patients, to compensate for the dropout factor. Also, we provided patients $10 apiece for each of three assessment sessions. They indicated that the money was a major factor in their participation.

- In evaluating services, you will likely need to include in your list of independent variables each patient's stage of illness. When considering issues of depression and anxiety, for example, it may be that persons with more symptoms or in later stages of the illness have different levels of anxiety (perhaps more, perhaps less) than persons who are asymptomatic.

CASE EXAMPLE: We used the Centers for Disease Control (1987) staging system for HIV, which has four stages, with five substages in Stage IV.

## *Common Barriers to Evaluation*

Before an evaluation can be considered, it has to be valued by administration and the service providers. If it is seen as an "extra"—something of limited importance—then the likelihood of its being treated as a serious activity or having a real impact on the program is doubtful. The mechanisms of how the results of the evaluation are to be used should be spelled out early in the planning process.

The value of early planning cannot be underestimated. Very often an evaluation is called for well after the program has started and when it is too late to measure things that were going on at baseline. This tends to render good evaluation designs less feasible.

I have found that behavioral scientists (e.g., psychologists, social workers) tend to resist using standardized instruments because, they feel, they limit their autonomy and expressiveness in conducting their clinical assessments. They also resent the "overly structured" feeling they get when they are asked to fill out standardized assessments. The problem the researcher faces is that different clinicians emphasize different aspects of a case, thus making it difficult to use narrative notes as a means to develop uniform measures of how patients are doing and what degree of change has taken place. One way to handle this common situation is to attempt to reach a compromise, often by conducting a focus group session with the clinical staff to identify the critical areas that all service providers should be addressing, and then adopting instruments for those areas and relying on narrative comments for the remainder of the clinical assessment.

If you don't have the expertise to conduct a carefully designed evaluation, it may be worth contacting a local university or medical center to obtain help. For relatively affordable consultation fees, you may get the guidance you require, if not the assistance you need to develop a grant to support a major evaluation effort. The academic community often welcomes the development of partnerships with service programs because such partnerships bring them into the "real world" to see whether their theories hold up.

Last, the evaluation process usually requires extra funding. Services are often covered by third-party payers, and the costs of the evaluation are not usually part of that package. Grant support, increasingly more difficult to obtain, is usually required. Many federal or state programs that fund clinical services, however, increasingly require evaluation activities to demonstrate the value of the services. In this case, it is appropriate to include the costs of evaluation in the program grant application. Even in cases in which the program announcement doesn't specifically call for an evaluation, it is worth building in an evaluation component. It serves to remind the agency that you value evaluation and that competing renewals are more easily defended when there is good evaluation evidence of the program's impact.

## REFERENCES

This chapter was made possible by grant number BRH 970165-02-0 from the Health Resources and Services Administration. Its contents are solely the responsibility of the author and do not necessarily represent the official views of HRSA.

Abraham, I. L., & Foley, T. S. (1984). The Work Environment Scale and the Ward Atmosphere Scale (short forms): Psychometric data. *Perceptual & Motor Skills, 58,* 319–322.

American Psychological Association (1985). *Standards for educational and psychological testing.* Washington, DC: Author.

Campbell, D. T., & Stanley, J. C. (1963). *Experimental and quasi-experimental designs for research.* Boston: Houghton Mifflin.

Centers for Disease Control (1987). Revision of the CDC surveillance case definition for acquired immunodeficiency syndrome. *Morbidity and Mortality Weekly Report, 36,* 3–18.

Derogatis, L. R. (1992). *BSI administration, scoring & procedures manual—II.* Riderwood, MD: Clinical Psychometric Research Inc.

Derogatis, L. R., & Melisaratos, N. (1983). The Brief Symptom Inventory: an introductory report. *Psychological Medicine, 13,* 595–605.

Fowler, F. J., Jr., Massagli, M. P., Weissman, J., Seage, G. R., III, Cleary, P. D., & Epstein, A. (1992). Some methodological lessons for surveys of persons with AIDS. *Medical Care, 30,* 1059–1066.

Gerbert, B., Maguire, B. T., Bleecker, T., Coates, T. J., & McPhee, S. J. (1991). Primary care physicians and AIDS: Attitudinal and structural barriers to care. *Journal of the American Medical Association, 266,* 2837–2842.

Kramer, J. & Conoley, J. (Eds.) (1992). *The 11th mental measurements yearbook.* Lincoln, NE: Buros Institute of Mental Measurements, University of Nebraska, Lincoln.

Marin, G., & VanOss Marin, B. (1991). Research with Hispanic populations. *Applied Social Research Methods Series, 23.* Thousand Oaks, CA: Sage.

McHorney, C. A., Ware, J. E., Jr., Lu, J. F., & Sherbourne C. D. (1994). The MOS 36-item Short-Form Health Survey (SF-36): Tests of data quality, scaling assumptions, and reliability across diverse patient groups. *Medical Care, 32,* 40–66.

Rogler, L. H., Malgady, R. G., & Rodriguez, O. (1989). *Hispanics and mental health: A framework for research.* Malabar, FL: Robert E. Krieger.

Ware, J. E., Jr., & Sherbourne, C. D. (1992). The MOS 36-item short-form health survey (SF-36): Conceptual framework and item selection. *Medical Care, 30,* 473–483.

# 18 | Qualitative Approaches to Evaluation

*Martha Ann Carey*

Qualitative evaluation is a much underused and underappreciated tool that can help mental health professionals answer questions that quantitative techniques cannot address. Questions that qualitative techniques can answer include these: Why do adolescents engage in behaviors that put them at risk for HIV infection? What are the psychosocial concerns of women who live with injection drug users?

With the answers to these questions, one can create relevant and specific intervention programs. Then, when the programs are operating, qualitative techniques can help determine if they are meeting their goals.

Government agencies and foundations appreciate needs assessments as bases for program development. And these funding sources require evaluations for most programs. Qualitative methods are especially useful for exploring new topics, replicating work with new populations, and developing hypotheses. Moreover, evaluation studies can examine:

- Why and how programs work. This information is important to agencies that fund programs, to program planners, and to administrators, who may want to improve an existing program or recreate an existing program in another setting.
- Client issues and themes, especially in populations that are unfamiliar to providers or scarcely researched.

- How to make surveys relevant and in the natural vocabulary of respondents.
- Rich and deep details about causal relationships, beyond the statistical information provided by quantitative work.

Quantitative approaches, which use numeric assessments such as scores from assessment instruments and which are described in the previous chapter, are inadequate to explore these and similar questions.

Qualitative studies can help researchers explore the essence of experience in its natural setting. Because an experimental context is not imposed, qualitative work preserves the real world setting. And the resulting well-told story, with rich, well-grounded details, can have a greater impact than pages of statistical results.

Some people mistakenly believe that qualitative study is restricted to descriptive work or to the preliminary phase in research or evaluation. In fact, sophisticated qualitative work goes beyond description and can effectively be used alone or in combination with quantitative methods to assist researchers with many crucial questions.

Although there were sharp disagreements in the past, today most evaluators and researchers acknowledge the value of qualitative evaluation when used appropriately. Like quantitative evaluation, qualitative evaluation requires expertise, the use of known and accepted theory and practice, and the ability to make the results meaningful to a larger audience, such as public policymakers.

Qualitative research is based on a very different paradigm from that of quantitative work. Its essence is a belief that there is not one single reality. Rather, the qualitatively based evaluator accepts that different individuals and different groups have different realities, based on their personal, idiosyncratic interpretations. Those interpretations are what is described as meaning, according to qualitative evaluators.

Qualitative evaluators try to understand the meaning of each person's experience, which may be unique with respect to time, place, and personal history. By time we mean not necessarily the hour or day but rather a socially defined period, such as an era or epoch or, perhaps, an epidemic. A person who has sex in the age of HIV/AIDS, for example, lives in a different time than one who was sexually active in the 1950s. By place, we mean not a geographic location but a psychological space—"where the person is at psychologically." This psychological place can, of course, be affected by physical surroundings and geography. The person in the inner city is affected differently by his or her geography than is a person in a wealthy suburb. Finally, the concept of personal history is something we all know intuitively. If someone has a history of having parents die in a hospital, then that person is likely to have specific feelings about being hospitalized.

The task of the qualitative evaluator is to capture the *meaning* of a situation or condition to a person or a specific group of persons. Qualitative methods of data collection and analysis, which have as their goal the exploration of an issue or experience in a natural setting as contrasted with an experimental condition, follow from these understandings.

There is no single agreed-upon way to do qualitative work, nor even a standard within each of the qualitative fields. Miles and Huberman (1994) provide a comprehensive approach that is easily readable, particularly for researchers trained in quantitative methods.

## *Major Theoretical Frameworks*

Paradigms — understandings of how we do science — differ in qualitative and quantitative approaches, and within the qualitative approach. Our paradigms guide how we think about data and how we develop useful information from the data. The major frameworks that underlie most qualitative techniques are grounded theory (Glaser & Strauss, 1967) and phenomenology (Cohen & Omery, 1994).

### *Grounded Theory*

Grounded theory developed from the symbolic interaction school (Blumer, 1969; Mead, 1934/1964), which understands everyday life as based on shared meanings. Through interactions with others, meanings are continuously modified, and behaviors derive meaning and can become appropriate in the person's social group. An example of a shared meaning in the area of mental health is the experience of the stigma attached to severe mental illness and its consequences for the patient and family.

Looking for understanding of basic processes or meanings and how they relate to each other, the evaluator who uses grounded theory begins with few or no hypotheses. Then, by gathering information in several possible ways, the evaluator develops and tests hypotheses and refines "theory" in an ongoing process.

In this context, *theory* means an understanding of experiences of the participants from their perspective. Data collection and analyses occur jointly in a "constant comparative" process, as analysis of the initial data collection provides some understanding, or preliminary hypothesis, that is to be tested in the next data collection and analysis step. Using this ongoing process, the evaluator continues to develop and refine the theory.

An application of grounded theory is Swanson's (1993) study of her clients with *herpes simplex*. She began by reading the available literature and used her clinical experience as a public health nurse to plan her study. Then, using interviews, Swanson explored the meaning of this chronic infection in the lives of middle-class young people. While she had some knowledge of this disease and some professional experience with it, she developed her "theory," or her understanding from the perspective of the patient, from the data collected and analyzed in her study. She found that the psychological consequences of herpes are enormous and had critical impact on patients' adherence to treatment. These results served as the basis for a psychological intervention with herpes patients to help them regain their self-worth and to manage their disease.

### *Phenomenology*

Work guided by the second major framework, phenomenology, also begins with no formal hypotheses. Phenomenologists generally believe that there is no *one* reality to discover, in contrast to quantitative researchers. The phenomenologist seeks to understand the deeper meanings in the clients' statements and actions by reflecting on the data to infer meaning. What does it mean for a mother to have an HIV-infected child with uncontrollable diarrhea admitted to the pediatric ward, for example? What experience does this mother have with hospitals? Do all people who come to the hospital die? Did a neighborhood child recently die? Is she a bad mother if she cannot prevent her child from being sick? This approach of logical insight and heightened awareness (of the researcher) based on careful consideration of all information can bring to light the essence of the experience.

Because this approach uses a high level of inference, evaluations based on phenomenology have been criticized as more subjective than those based on grounded theory. Some say phenomenology is more an art than a science. This perception has limited funding by government agencies and private foundations, and hence this approach is used relatively less often.

Evaluation using this approach generally focuses on needs assessment or on the description of implementation of a service program, as contrasted with studies to demonstrate the effectiveness of a service program. See van Manen (1990) and Patton (1990) for further descriptions.

One researcher whose work in this area is especially compelling is Jan Morse, who, in the tradition of nursing, has studied the phenomena of enduring and suffering as well as comfort (Morse, Bottorff, & Hutchinson, 1995). As part of a larger program of study, Morse used information from interviews to identify stages in the process of coping with major personal loss. She and her colleagues found that initially the person may be just barely hanging on to reality, using all available mental energy just to "endure." Later the person may be able to process the tragic event and work through the process of "suffering." Understanding where a person is in coping is crucial to the nursing process.

By now it should be evident that qualitative evaluation can assist mental health providers in two areas. The first responds to the question, "What is the meaning of a specific experience to clients?" which leads to program development. The second area grows out of the question, "How does the program work?" The techniques described can be applied to various questions, including program evaluation. The chapter concludes with a discussion of concerns specific to program evaluation and some thoughts on combining qualitative and quantitative techniques.

## *Qualitative Evaluation for Program Development*

Too often, when program administrators learn that funding is available for mental health services for HIV-infected persons, providers create service programs without much consultation with the community regarding what is actually needed. A better, and stronger, approach in competitive funding is to have a qualitative evaluator actually ask those with a stake in the situation (stakeholders) questions that can lead to development of a responsive program. Stakeholders typically include clients, program staff, local program administrators, and policy decision makers.

The evaluator, then, does a literature search to determine what others have reported about similar issues. Using this information, the evaluator plans to explore these issues with the community through the use of focus groups and interviews.

*Focus Groups*

Use of focus groups is a recently popular approach that provides insight into complex behaviors and that is useful in learning why people think or feel the way they do. Although there is not a single definition of focus groups, there is a general consensus that they use a semistructured format, are moderated by one or two leaders, are held in an informal session, and have the purpose of collecting information on a designated topic. Although group sessions may provide group members with useful information and some moral support, the intent of this data collection technique is information gathering. This section briefly describes the basics of the focus group technique. For additional information see Krueger (1994) and Carey (1994); for some advanced topics see Morgan (1993).

To prepare to run a focus group, researchers explore what is known about the designated topic and then formulate three or four general questions that provide the structure for the session. Group size varies with the experience of the group members and the nature of the topic. For people who are not used to being in groups, when the topic is very sensitive, when the group interaction is expected to require extra attention from the leaders, or when the leaders are inexperienced, four to six people are suggested—a smaller group than the usually recommended five to twelve.

The group leader guides the discussion and probes for depth and range of specific personal experiences and for inconsistencies in description. After a group member describes his or her experience in response to the leader's general question, another person will respond, providing a more-detailed story. This group interaction is what brings out the depth and richness of data. For topics that may elicit emotionally laden responses, the leader must constantly monitor the group for the level of comfort and intercede to prevent injury. For this type of session, it is important for the leader to have clinical expertise.

The research purpose of a focus group can range from an in-depth exploration of the experience of foster parents caring for a child with HIV to the identification of issues and natural vocabulary for the development of an instrument. The chemistry of the group will affect what people say, and the evaluator will need to consider this factor when analyzing the data. The group interaction both enhances the collection of rich data and may inhibit some participants' description (i.e., as they seek to fit in with the group) (Carey, 1994).

After focus groups are conducted, the evaluator may use the information gathered to further refine the questions asked and then revisit the groups to seek further depth and detail.

### *Interviews*

There are many possible ways of structuring interviews. The evaluator may have well-defined questions, use a highly structured format for asking questions, and have specific instructions for asking follow-up questions. This approach permits the collection of quantitative data, similar to an oral version of a questionnaire.

In contrast, an open-ended approach may be appropriate for some purposes, such as when clients' concerns are not known. Broad topics with general instructions for follow-up questions permit a wider range of possible responses but are more time-consuming to analyze. An example of a broad topic is: What services are most useful in helping you cope with a positive HIV-test result?

The advantages and disadvantages of each approach to interviewing have been well discussed in the literature. The classic reference on interviewing is Kahn and Cannell (1957), and an informative discussion is provided in Pedhazur and Schmelkin (1991).

### *Data Saturation*

Generally speaking, the process of conducting focus groups or interviews ends when "data saturation" occurs, that is, when additional interviews or focus group sessions yield no new information. Saturation refers to the richness and detail, not to the amount of data (Morse, 1995). Data saturation is actually more a conceptual goal than an actual occurrence.

Often the resources limit the amount of data collection. The evaluator should, however, feel comfortable with the data collected for the purpose of the study. It may be necessary to narrow the goals of the study, to focus on a narrower population, or on only one aspect of the experience.

## *Data Analysis*

Qualitative approaches can be intuitively appealing and, deceptively, can appear easy. A clear and well-articulated plan of analysis is crucial to credibility and therefore to the usefulness of the results. Planning for analysis should be done before data are collected.

Qualitative data analysis is quite different from quantitative analysis, which analyzes the numbers obtained from different instruments and uses statistical methods to determine whether statistically significant differences have been found between groups. Qualitative analysis may use one of several different approaches to discover commonalities and variations in the data and try to understand the meanings.

One useful approach in analysis is the process of condensing, clustering, sorting, and linking data as described by Miles and Huberman (1994). Basically, the first step is developing categories in the data (condensing). The researcher then tries to discern one or more themes (clustering). The process of sorting helps the researchers determine who said what; for example, African Americans across focus groups may have responded one way to a question and Asians, another way. Linking data is the process of connecting themes to the responses across sites or groups.

The purpose of the first step in the analysis of data — called first-level coding — is to develop general categories. For example, reading through the transcripts of focus groups sessions, I would note concerns that may be similar to the planned questions that were asked in the session; often, however, other issues arise. For many evaluators, the initial categories are fairly concrete and factual. Next, in second-level coding, as I looked across these initial codes, I would look for broader themes such as distrust/trust of the medical system. I would then explore similarities and variations in relation to subgroups in the sample. Do clients follow medical advice better when they can be seen by medical personnel of the same ethnic group? Results would then be "recontextualized," which means that I would go back to the data to verify that the themes noted and their relation to appropriate subgroups were accurate. Identifying examples of themes and relationships may lead to further analysis.

Appropriate documenting of each step of the analysis process is necessary if the results are to have credibility. A reasonable person should reach the same conclusion as the evaluator. In a study of health care personnel who provide care in settings with a high risk for HIV transmission, for example, Duffy (1994) reviewed her analysis of interviews with a team of both qualitatively and quantitatively trained researchers. Each step in the analysis was examined for logical consistence and appropriateness.

## *Evaluation of Existing Programs*

### *Evaluability*

Not every program can, or should, be evaluated. Program developers, and those writing grant applications, can create significantly stronger — and more fundable — programs by designing programs that combine services with the requirements of evaluation. Before evaluation can occur, one must have a clear understanding of the program's target population and its purpose. Only then can evaluation determine if the program's goals are being met for the specific population.

Evaluation takes staff time and costs money. If an evaluation is conducted, the practical limits on the usefulness of the evaluation results should be known. If the goal of the program is a particular long-term effect of service, for example, other factors may also affect clients and therefore restrict the cause-and-effect statements possible regarding the program impact. Also, one should know if the program will actually be modified based on the evaluation results.

To be "evaluable," a program must have common goals and a common description. This is important in designing a new program, and particularly important for evaluating an existing program. Because clients, staff, managers, policymakers, and evaluators probably have different perspectives and values, developing a common definition of the program is the first step. This can be done through focus groups and interviews. If program planners and staff have difficulty in identifying goals and program effects (summative evaluation) or the important processes in delivering the program (formative evaluation), the evaluator may ask how they would know if their program worked well or have them describe how an ideal program would work (O'Sullivan & O'Sullivan, 1994).

Wholey (1994) describes criteria to consider in determining whether to evaluate a program. They are the existence of well-defined program goals and information needs, plausible program goals, availability of program information, and agreement on the uses of evaluation results. Programs that cannot meet these criteria or that cannot be modified to do so probably should not use limited resources to evaluate.

After performing an evaluability assessment, the researcher can make a decision on the relative importance of evaluation for the program in question. With adequate resources, the needed expertise can be obtained or personnel trained. Evaluation techniques are usually the enlightened application of good research methods. Computer software is now available to make coding and analysis much easier, permitting a more thorough examination. See Weitzman and Miles (1995) for a review of software.

When a new program is designed to be evaluable, or an ongoing program is found through an assessment to be evaluable, administrators need to consider resources, sampling, and design issues.

### *Resources*

Adequate resources — people, expertise, money, equipment, data systems — must be available and the time frame for the evaluation must be realistic. Without a requirement for evaluation or recognition of its importance, the usually scarce resources will be spent on services and not on evaluation.

### *Sampling*

An important life experience is often perceived differently by various groups. An evaluator will, therefore, have to consider important characteristics when creating the sample group. Segmenting the target population in meaningful ways and purposely sampling within relevant categories will enhance the likelihood of collecting an appropriate range of data. If the effects of the program are expected to vary for men and women and for ethnic minorities, for example, it will be useful to plan to have adequate numbers of research participants representing each of these groups.

In the final report, the evaluator will likely mention how the sample was recruited. This will assist readers in understanding how the people actually recruited represent the population that is the target of the study. This information is necessary in interpreting how well the study results can apply to people beyond the sample (external validity). Miles and Huberman (1994) provide an excellent discussion of sampling and offer sound advice for the novice evaluator.

### *Design*

Statements of program effects are limited by the design of the evaluation. To say confidently that a service program leads to client improvements and that results are not influenced by nonprogrammatic factors such as employment or peer supports, the design of the evaluation must be rigorous.

This is the same concern that surfaced with regard to confounds in the previous chapter. One must be able to determine that the program made the difference or to what extent it contributed to the outcome. As a result, qualitative evaluators seek to understand the program in its natural context — what is actually happening in the world of the client and what other events and treatments might have had an effect on the program outcomes. For all types of studies, the focus is on ruling out other potentially relevant causes — "rival hypotheses" — not ruling out *all* possible causes.

Due to ethical considerations and practical logistics, most service programs are not able to use rigorous experimental conditions with random assignment of subjects. Evaluation therefore requires that the experimental design be modified. Most qualitative evaluations are not true experiments with control groups; consequently, cause-and-effect statements will be arrived at by comparing program results with those from a comparable group.

Descriptions can provide useful information about service effects. In a new program that provides mental health services to persons with HIV/AIDS, for example, quality of life and level of stress may be assessed at entry to service and six months after services have been provided. By describing the program, the clients, the barriers to care, and the costs of care, such a program evaluation can provide useful information for program planners in terms of feasibility and acceptability of the new service delivery model. This type of evaluation is not intended to provide cause-and-effect statements; it is preliminary to further evaluation of effectiveness.

## *Combining Qualitative and Quantitative Approaches*

Many studies use a combination of qualitative and quantitative approaches. The not uncommon practice of adding a few quotes to the statistical results does not really take advantage of the potential of qualitative data. Planning for the best use of each approach should consider the purposes and strengths of each, and any combination should take advantage of their complementary strengths. The purposes of combination include:

1. *Expansion: Going beyond the limitations of each method.* An example of expansion is O'Brien's (1993) use of qualitative technique in the develop-

ment of a questionnaire in HIV/AIDS research. She used focus groups to explore issues and problems in the lives of adult males. By so doing, she identified major areas that then became the basis of the questionnaire items. Natural vocabulary for questionnaire phrasing was also obtained.

2. *Explanation: Understanding data and results.* A common approach uses quantitative data to inform the development of a qualitative study. Epidemiological data regarding substance abuse, for example, can be used to target populations for a qualitative study of coping with stresses of living with HIV infection. On the other hand, focus groups or interviews may help in understanding quantitative results that are unexpected and not readily interpretable. This approach can provide the evaluator with new insights and avenues to explore.

3. *Reinforcement: Enhancing credibility.* The process of reinforcement increases believability when data from two sources, using different collection methods, produce the same results. When questionnaire data may be regarded as underreporting the occurrence of a phenomenon, such as substance abuse, or when the generalizability of focus group data is limited by logistic issues, the concurrence of data allows the evaluator to weigh the results more effectively.

In work with HIV patients in the military, Carey and Smith (1992) used qualitative data to improve the overall program of research. Input from a protocol adviser who is a former military person and who is HIV-positive, a patient advisory panel, and focus groups was used to improve the research program. The researchers began by focusing on the validity of the psychosocial instruments, which had not previously been used with a military population. It was quickly apparent that the validity of the research process was in question. The logistics of scheduling appointments for medical and research purposes and the burden of the lengthy questionnaires led the researchers to reconsider the research experience for the participants and to revise the protocol. They reduced the number of questionnaires and coordinated the scheduling for the convenience of the participants.

### *Case Study and Ethnography*

Two approaches that combine qualitative and quantitative methods are case study and ethnography. Both approaches can be helpful and may, in selected cases, be useful in outcomes evaluation.

Although often thought of as solely a qualitative methodology, the case study approach actually uses all relevant information. Without using many cases (and in contrast to a typical quantitative approach, which has enough subjects to permit the appropriate statistical analysis), a case study examines one unit, such as one community. Here "case study" does not mean the discussion of a single client or patient, the term *case* refers to that unit of the study's focus, which is generally at an aggregate level. Using multiple cases can increase confidence in the results, and this technique can be used to explore a topic more broadly (e.g., examining a program's effects on different ethnic populations).

The second approach that combines qualitative and quantitative approaches is ethnography. Focusing on structure, ritual, or symbols, the researcher uses all relevant data to study a population from the perspective of its culture. The drug culture of an inner city, for example, might best be studied with an ethnographic approach.

## *Conclusion*

With the increasing emphasis on program development and evaluation, qualitative methods will have a significant role in assessing HIV mental health programs. Personnel who are comfortable with qualitative evaluation and understand its potential usefulness will more likely receive funding, create and administer quality programs, and take a leadership position in the next century.

### REFERENCES

Blumer, H. (1969). *Symbolic interactionism.* Englewood Cliffs, NJ: Prentice-Hall.

Carey, M. A. (1994). The group effect in focus groups: Planning, implementing, and interpreting focus group research. In J. Morse (Ed.), *Critical issues in qualitative research methods* (225–241). Newbury Park, CA: Sage.

Carey, M. A., & Smith, M. W. (1992). Enhancement of validity through qualitative approaches: Incorporating the patient's perspective. *Evaluation and the Health Professions, 15,* 107–114.

Chen, H. (1990). *Theory-driven evaluations.* Newbury Park, CA: Sage.

Cohen, M. Z., & Omery, A. (1994). Schools of phenomenology: Implications for research. In J. Morse (Ed.), *Critical issues in qualitative research methods* (136–156). Newbury Park, CA: Sage.

Duffy, P. R. (1994). How mental health providers can help manage the threat of occupational exposure to HIV. *Psychosocial Rehabilitation Journal, 17(4),* 117–144.

Glaser, B., & Strauss, A. (1967). *The discovery of grounded theory.* Hawthorne, NY: Aldine.

Hofstede, C. (1984). *Culture's consequences.* Beverly Hills, CA: Sage.

Kahn, R. L., & Cannell, C. F. (1957). *The dynamics of interviewing: Theory, technique, and cases.* New York: Wiley.

Krueger, R. (1994). *Focus groups: practical guide for applied research* (2d ed.). Newbury Park, CA: Sage.

Mead, G. H. (1964). *George Herbert Mead on social psychology* (Rev. ed.). Chicago, IL: University of Chicago Press. (Original work published 1934.)

Miles, M., & Huberman, A. (1994). *Qualitative data analysis: An expanded sourcebook* (2d ed.). Thousands Oaks, CA: Sage.

Morgan, D. (1993). *Successful focus groups: Advancing the state of the art.* Newbury Park, CA: Sage.

Morse, J. (1995). The significance of saturation. *Qualitative Health Research, 5,* 147–149.

Morse, J., Bottorff, J. L., & Hutchinson, S. (1995). The paradox of comfort. *Nursing Research, 44(1),* 14–19.

O'Brien, K. (1993). Improving survey questionnaire through focus groups. In D. Morgan (Ed.), *Successful focus groups: Advancing the state of the art* (105–117). Newbury Park, CA: Sage.

O'Sullivan, R., & O'Sullivan, J. (1994, May). *Evaluation voices: Promoting cluster evaluations from within programs.* Paper presented at the annual meeting of the Canadian Evaluation Society, Quebec, Canada.

Patton, M. Q. (1990). *Qualitative evaluation and research methods* (2d ed.). Newbury Park, CA: Sage.

Pedhazur, E. J., & Schmelkin, L. P. (1991). *Measurement, design, and analysis: An integrated approach.* Hillsdale, NJ: Lawrence Erlbaum.

Rossi, P., & Freeman, H. (1993). *Evaluation: A systematic approach.* Newbury Park, CA: Sage.

Russon, C., Wentling, T., & Zuloaga, A. (1995). The persuasive impact of two evaluation reports on agricultural extension administrators from two countries. *Evaluation Review, 19,* 374–388.

Silverman, J. (1993). *Interpreting qualitative data: Methods for analyzing talk, text, and interaction.* Thousand Oaks, CA: Sage.

Swanson, J. (1993). Regaining a valued self: Young adults adaptation to living with genital herpes. *Qualitative Health Research, 3,* 270–297.

van Manen, M. (1990). *Researching the lived experience.* London, Ontario, Canada: Althouse.

Weitzman, M., & Miles, M. (1995). *Computer programs for qualitative data.* Thousand Oaks, CA: Sage.

Wholey, J. (1994). Assessing the feasibility and likely usefulness of evaluation. In J. S. Wholey, H. P. Hatry, & K. E. Newcomer (Eds.), *Handbook of practical program evaluation* (13–39). San Francisco: Jossey-Bass.

# V HIV Mental Health Policy and Programs

# 19 | HIV/AIDS Mental Health Care: Politics, Public Policy, and Funding Decisions

*Douglas A. Wirth*

Most HIV/AIDS mental health providers — and certainly almost all who work in institutions such as hospitals or community health and mental health centers — provide services that are paid for by federal programs. Two federal programs in particular have significantly shaped that care — the Ryan White Comprehensive AIDS Resources Emergency (C.A.R.E.) Act of 1990, reauthorized with modifications in 1996, and Medicaid.

The Ryan White C.A.R.E. Act was passed in 1990 to provide funding for HIV-related primary health care and support services. With other funding streams such as Medicaid supporting a variety of AIDS services, this legislation was designed to fill gaps and provide emergency assistance, to facilitate and engage new clients into care, and to foster "the development, organization, coordination and operation of more effective and cost efficient systems for the delivery of essential services to individuals and families with HIV disease," in the words of the 1990 legislation.

The C.A.R.E. Act has enabled the creation of thousands of programs, including many HIV mental health programs, throughout the United States. Many of the programs described in this book came into existence because of these Ryan White funds, and the book's foreword was written by the man who administered these funds until his retirement from government service in 1996.

The other major federal funding stream for HIV-infected persons is Medicaid (Title XIX of the Social Security Act Amendments of 1965). Medicaid annually pays for six times the amount of services funded by Ryan White.

While many working and middle-class persons with HIV disease may begin paying their mental health and medical bills with private insurance, toward the later stages of the illness they may choose or need to turn to Medicaid for assistance. Many persons with HIV/AIDS never had private insurance and have been entirely dependent on Medicaid to pay their medical and mental health costs. Medicaid covers 40 percent of all people with HIV, as many as 60 percent of adults living with AIDS, and 90 percent of all children with AIDS. In fiscal year 1994, Medicaid served approximately 56,000 persons with full-blown AIDS.

## *Why a Chapter on These Issues?*

HIV/AIDS mental health care in the twenty-first century may be funded wholly differently than it has been in the early 1990s. Funding may be extremely limited, funding policies may be very constrictive, and policy debate may pit the needs of persons with AIDS against persons with other diseases. In contrast to the early 1990s, very lean times may be ahead.

As the epidemic shifts from one affecting primarily gay men to one striking substance abusers and, more generally, poor people in urban centers, these funding issues will be compounded by the pervasive media disinterest in AIDS and by the political contempt for poor people and urban centers.

This chapter is important because many readers of this book will be hoping to practice HIV/AIDS-related care as we approach and enter the twenty-first century. As you will discover, no practitioner can afford to ignore federal and state policy-making; the costs to your clients but also to you as a provider are too great!

This chapter examines the two major funding streams: Ryan White and Medicaid. In the section on Medicaid, the government program likely to be most transformed in the next decade, I extensively describe possible changes, including managed care and block grants, and their ramifications. In the last section, I suggest survival strategies on your part.

I write as a professional social worker, a gay man active in HIV/AIDS issues, a former director of five homeless shelters, a senior public policy analyst, and someone who has been active in federal and state policy-making as the director of government relations for an organization that represents more than 100 community mental health agencies. I urge you to know what may be ahead, and to act on it. Denial and/or avoidance are not adaptive coping mechanisms for today's — and tomorrow's — challenges.

## *The Ryan White C.A.R.E. Act*

### *Understanding Ryan White*

In 1990 Congress passed landmark AIDS/HIV legislation, the Ryan White Comprehensive AIDS Resources Emergency Act, which created a five-year federal program that eventually spent more than $2 billion for HIV-related services.

The results of the Ryan White stream were invaluable. With Ryan White support, states and localities have developed medical, mental health, and support services that promote early treatment and cost-effective care to individuals and families with HIV/AIDS. A recent study found that many Ryan White-funded programs in New York City were successful in engaging clients who would otherwise not have received care (Warren, Fullwood, Lee, & Salitan, 1995).

The initial authorization of the Ryan White legislation expired in September 1995, with funding ending early in April 1996. Because reauthorization was critical to the continued provision of vital HIV-related medical, mental health, and social services, advocates for HIV services were activated.

In congressional debate, legislators acknowledged the different faces of AIDS and emphasized that AIDS is the leading cause of death among men and women ages twenty-five to forty-four (Dunlap, 1995; Seelye, 1995). "Not everybody who has AIDS gets it from sex or drug needles. But . . . more to the point, gay people who have AIDS are still our sons, our brothers, our cousins, our citizens. They're Americans, too. They're obeying the law and working hard. They are entitled to be treated like everybody else," asserted President Bill Clinton while speaking at Georgetown University (Seelye, 1995).

But opposition emerged. During the legislative process, several issues came to the fore:

- *AIDS-related allocations versus those for other illnesses.* "At the federal level, until recently the overlap between groups advocating for health care services for people with HIV/AIDS and groups advocating on general health care finance and insurance issues has been a null set" (Westmoreland, 1995, 273). Some leaders, however, have sought to capitalize on competition for limited dollars. Sen. Jesse Helms (R-NC) placed a "hold" on the reauthorization bill, saying that AIDS receives too much money in comparison to cancer and heart disease and maintaining that "we've got to have some common sense about a disease transmitted by people deliberately engaging in unnatural acts" (Seelye, 1995). In response, reauthorization supporters were quick to note that U.S. Public Health Service figures documented total annual federal funding for AIDS at $6 billion, far less than the $36.3 billion in outlays for heart disease and the $16.9 billion for cancer. Helms's opposition was viewed as a continuation of his homophobic opposition to HIV funding and his vested interests in heart disease.
- *Mandatory testing of newborns.* In the House of Representatives, reauthorization was stalled by a move to require mandatory HIV testing of newborns for states desiring C.A.R.E. Act funds. A positive test on the newborn would always reveal the HIV status of the mother. This was opposed by many public health officials and women's and feminist organizations, as well as by many people living with HIV and by AIDS advocates.

### *Politics in the AIDS Community: Alive and Well*

Many observers would assume that AIDS advocates and health and human service professionals would unite as a powerful, political voice to facilitate reauthorization, but this has not been entirely true. The politics of limited resources, diverse needs, and coalition work, coupled with power imbalances, has served at times to splinter advocacy around Ryan White.

The CAEAR (Cities Advocating Emergency AIDS Relief) Coalition, a national alliance comprising localities and states that receive Ryan White monies, proved to be the ground where significant disagreement over AIDS policy and reauthorization strategy emerged. The group's original goals focused on increasing annual C.A.R.E. Act allocations in the first five years of the legislation. During this period new cities qualified for more or additional funds, further complicating the group's consensus decision-making process.

Individual localities, for example, disagreed about whether to pursue joint allocations for cities and states or to retain the 1990 legislation's practice of providing individual streams to qualified localities and states. Single appropriation, some argued, would merge the resources of cities and states, yielding a robust, unified voice for future congressional appropriations debates. Funded states, some of which lacked funded localities, feared profound neglect. Another dispute emerged around using something called the Medicare Wage Index within the funding formula as a means for adjusting allocations on the basis of regional service costs, which some states felt favored areas with higher costs.

As usual, difficult times serve as opportunities to query the goals, methods, and membership of advocacy organizations, as inconvenient as it usually seems. The members of the CAEAR Coalition found themselves struggling with several additional issues, such as retention of its single-focus mission statement as well as methods to resolve disagreements about operating principles, which favored consensus and restricted individual members' autonomy. Call it an inability to address these difficult issues, or an appropriate focus on reauthorization; either way, the coalition postponed addressing these issues until after reauthorization. The most obvious fallout of this dissension was that multiple points of view were expressed by AIDS advocates on Capitol Hill during the congressional debates. A divided constituency is more easily thwarted.

The CAEAR Coalition was not the only national voice driving reauthorization. The Human Rights Campaign Fund (HRCF) commissioned a public opinion poll to study voter attitudes toward AIDS funding. HRCF hired the Terrance Group, a respected Republican polling firm, and Lake Research, a well-known Democratic pollster, to study Americans' attitudes regarding government support of HIV/AIDS care, research, and prevention. In spring 1995, HRCF reported that broad nationwide support for AIDS funding exists among Democratic, Republican, and independent voters — 77 percent wanted to maintain or increase federal funding, with deep support in every region of the country and among all religious subgroups. Seventy-eight percent of those polled said that this is no time to retreat on the AIDS crisis, 56 percent said that they would be less inclined to vote for a member of Congress who voted against continued federal funding for AIDS care, and 45 percent said they believe the government is doing too little to respond to AIDS, including a plurality of the people who voted for Ross Perot in the 1992 presidential election (Human Rights Campaign Fund, Lake Research, & Terrance Group, 1995).

### *C.A.R.E. Act Reauthorization*

Despite the fractionated AIDS advocacy, in 1996 the U.S. Congress passed the reauthorization of the Ryan White legislation that expired in September 1995. Given that Ryan White is discretionary spending (categorical grant funding for nonentitlement programs) and that discretionary spending has been under an overall cap since the Budget Act of 1990 (any new money must come from cuts to other existing programs), it is a small miracle that Congress and the President were able to agree on the expenditures that provide additional funding for Ryan White's drug assistance program, ADAP.

## *Medicaid*

The Social Security Act Amendments of 1965 established the Medicaid program to provide health care to public assistance recipients and other qualified individuals. As an entitlement program, Medicaid benefits are available to any person who meets statutory eligibility criteria. The entitlement mechanism was originally created to reduce the disparities in medical care provided to the poor that existed among states and to distribute fairly the financial burden of such medical care.

The federal government has established mandatory services that must be covered by Medicaid and optional services that may be covered by Medicaid. Some states, such as New York, provide a comprehensive Medicaid program that includes medical services that extend well beyond the minimum mandatory level.

## *Cost Shifting and Cost Containment*

The 1980s produced significant federal cutbacks for most public welfare services at the same time that need escalated and the number of individual billionaires increased conspicuously (Fabricant & Burghardt, 1992). As a result, states were forced to reduce services, restrict eligibility, find ways of shifting expenses to other entities, or undertake some combination of these. Many states succeeded in decreasing their financial responsibility by shifting mental health expenditures to the federal government and to localities by converting services to Medicaid reimbursement. These arrangements parceled the largest financial responsibility for mental health services to the federal government (50–80 percent), then to the states (25–10 percent) and, last, to local communities (25–0 percent).

Despite the Medicaidization of mental health services, many states' fiscal responsibilities continued to grow as total expenditures grew. In New York, for example, total mental health expenditures increased from $2.7 billion in 1986 ($1 billion Medicaid) to roughly $4 billion ($2 billion Medicaid) by the end of 1993 (New York State Office of Mental Health, 1993). Consequently, many states engaged in a set of cost-containment practices, including:

- *Utilization reviews:* States set regulatory standards for record keeping and services. Payment is withheld if an agency fails to meet standards.
- *Medicaid utilization threshold systems:* States impose an annual limit on outpatient mental health services. In 1993 New York set a limit of forty visits and sought to reduce the threshold to thirty visits a year later. Agencies must submit paperwork to secure authorization for additional reimbursable visits.
- *Diagnostic related groups (DRGs):* Using groupings of specific "health" conditions, a standard maximum number of visits/services or maximum payment is predetermined. Providers, namely hospitals, can make money if they decrease the number of visits or the length of stay while collecting the standard payment. While psychiatry is excluded, this cost containment measure can create significant psychosocial issues related to premature or poor discharge planning.
- *Uniform case records:* States create recordkeeping requirements, including progress and contact notes, which can be reviewed to determine inappropriate or overextended services.
- *Certificates of need:* To operate new (and sometimes expanded) programming, states require agencies to file lengthy proposals and secure certificates of need. The state limits funding for new certificates, thereby limiting development of new programs.

## *The Future of Cost Containment: Medicaid Managed Care*

Now into the second decade of the AIDS pandemic, many states have filed federal Medicaid waivers to convert traditional Medicaid fee-for-service systems into state-run managed-care programs. The individual state programs have the potential to alter dramatically the health and the mental health care systems for persons living with HIV and AIDS.

The term *managed care* refers to a variety of arrangements between the state and private corporations that manage an array of services. Most state plans recognize some combination of the following categories of managed-care models:

- *Full-risk capitation:* Organizations receive a per-patient (per capita, or capitation) payment to provide a comprehensive set of benefits to enrollees and assume full financial risk. Enrollees select one of the organization's affiliated physicians as their primary care doctor, and all specialist services (mental health, substance abuse), hospital admissions, and other services must be approved by this provider/gatekeeper. Since the primary care provider's group pays, out of its capitation income, for most specialty services, providers or organization "gatekeepers" may be reluctant to make or approve the referral.
- *Partial-risk capitation:* A group of physicians agrees to provide a limited set of primary-care services to the enrollees in exchange for a monthly capitation payment. As with full-risk capitation, the patient selects a doctor to serve as a primary care provider, and that physician must approve all referral services and hospital admissions. Unlike the situation with full-risk capitation, however, the group of primary-care physicians bears no financial risk for the cost of services it does not provide directly. This model usually asks primary-care physicians to manage special care services but does not put them at financial risk for the cost of these services.
- *Enhanced fee-for-services:* An individual physician agrees to serve as primary-care provider and as case manager for referral services but assumes no financial risk. Instead, the physician is paid under a fee-for-service schedule that includes additional payment for the responsibility for managing special care services.

It should be emphasized that the documented cost-savings benefits of managed care as described in the literature are based almost exclusively on experience with full-risk capitation plans (Freund et al., 1989; Langwell, 1990; Luft, 1978, 1981).

*Potential Benefits of Full-Risk Capitation Plans*

From a client perspective, managed care promises greater access to health care and greater continuity of care, because a single physician or a small group is available to provide primary care and to coordinate other services. Theoretically, the patient has a clearly identified and readily available source of care when a problem arises. He or she is not obliged to seek out an appropriate specialist or clinic (and pay out-of-pocket) or forced to utilize emergency rooms because of a lack of relationship with a regular provider. In addition, there is evidence that members of capitation plans are more likely to receive preventive services such as immunizations, checkups, and periodic screening than are patients in fee-for-service relationships. This is related to the financial incentives built into capitated systems, which focus on preventing disease, thereby avoiding costly hospitalizations.

The principal drawback, from a client's perspective, is the requirement that initial contacts be restricted to a primary-care physician selected from the plan's "preferred physicians" network. This restriction on freedom of choice is typically redressed in two ways. First, patients are given a choice of plans and of physicians within plans. Second, patients who are dissatisfied with their chosen physicians may be reassigned to another physician within the plan or may disenroll from that plan and opt for another.

Equally important are the benefits that managed care promises taxpayers — those who pay for medical and mental health care covered by Medicaid. Numerous studies have demonstrated that full-risk capitation plans provide health care of competitive quality and at a significantly lower cost. The cost savings estimates are generally in the range of 20 to 40 percent. The savings are achieved in two basic ways. First, and most significant, is a much lower rate of acute hospitalization and shortened average lengths of stay. Second, these plans conserve resources by limiting use of referral specialists and emergency rooms. Hospital inpatient and emergency room use (most costly services) by the Medicaid population, for example, is higher in New York City than the national average. To the extent managed care shifts health care away from inpatient units and emergency rooms, it may be possible to save money.

## *A Critical Analysis*

State managed-care plans represent blueprints for a monumental restructuring of the mental health and AIDS primary-care systems, with the most relevant application to the health maintenance organization (HMO) industry (full-risk capitation) as differentiated from other managed-care models.

Some state plans exclude certain populations, such as the psychiatrically disabled (persons with major mental illness who receive SSI disability benefits) from managed-care plans. Persons diagnosed with major mental illness often represent the vast majority of recipients of mental health services and create the vast majority of mental health expenditures. Most state plans, however, bestow blank-check authority on the HMO industry to treat the health and the mental health needs of people living with HIV/AIDS, receiving Aid to Families with Dependent Children (AFDC) or Home Relief (local aid to mostly single poor adults, which some localities require to be repaid). Often states mandate that all incidental behavioral managed-care services (mental health and substance abuse) be included within the HMO capitated rate. Interestingly enough, some states have suggested that "incidental use" be defined as less than thirty out-patient visits and sixty inpatient days within a one-year period. This position has no clinical foundation. Most states, under pressure from the nonprofit provider groups and AIDS advocates, have more appropriately defined "incidental use."

Nationally, the majority of persons living with HIV/AIDS, families receiving AFDC, and adults receiving Home Relief grants who also receive mental health services are served by voluntary nonprofit mental health clinics in their own communities. These clinics would be most severely affected by a state's managed-care plans. While collaboration with the HMO industry to develop managed-care and special-care (mental health, substance use, mental retardation, AIDS/HIV) service delivery models is appropriate, often the terms laid out in state plans appear to provide the HMO industry carte blanche, without significant state oversight. Further analysis yields what I consider to be significantly inadequate public policy with real potential to overwhelm people's lives, foster significant underutilization, and increase long-term overall costs.

Often state plans fall significantly short of satisfying their managed-care policy objectives. When governors and legislatures set out to develop and implement statewide Medicaid managed-care programs, they often base their agenda on five specific goals:

— *Goal 1: To ensure that managed-care programs offer Medicaid recipients as wide a choice of primary care and other medical service providers as possible.*
For Medicaid recipients, the choice of a managed care provider will be based largely on an individual's primary needs at the time of enrollment — medical needs, most likely. Mental health needs, however, may develop or become apparent after the individual has enrolled in a plan, long after the opportunity to assess his or her unique needs in making a provider choice. For mental health services, this situation will result in little or no choice at all — a result of serious consequence. For Medicaid recipients with mental health needs (especially HIV-related), there are many unique aspects of treatment affecting choice of provider, including cultural competence and the availability of service in an individual's own community. Many plans are silent on or have completely ignored these issues.

— *Goal 2: To promote more rational patterns of medical and health service utilization by Medicaid recipients.*
Rational patterns for mental health service utilization are very different from what would be considered rational utilization patterns for medical and health services. Unlike other health care, psychiatric diagnosis is not a reliable predictor for length, frequency and intensity of treatment. Assessment and treatment of mental health disorders is not linear; many factors (as expressed by an integrated biopsychosocial/spiritual model for treatment of mental health disorders) affect the scope, length, frequency, and success of treatment, often leading to unpredictable and uneven patterns of usage. While many psychiatric disorders have a biochemical basis, their onset, course, and prognosis are uniquely affected by social, economic, and individual psychological factors. Also, to nonmental health care professionals, psychosocial, psychological, psychiatric, and medical conditions are often confused, even unrecognized. It is precisely for this reason that, when Medicare and Medicaid established diagnostic related groups to implement prospective payment systems for inpatient care, psychiatric conditions were exempted.

In addition, unlike the traditional medical model where consumers are often passive recipients of service, effective mental health treatment requires the consumer to take an interactive and dynamic role. To address unique issues and special needs, the community-based mental health system has devoted itself for many years to developing a specialized service delivery system that includes the many elements that seek to ensure quality care. Those elements include state licensing of providers, regulatory requirements for mental health service, quality assurance, treatment documentation and utilization review, procedural and substantive standards for mental health treatment planning and ongoing treatment plan updating, networks to enhance continuity of care, and innovative program models. State Medicaid managed-care plans propose delivery systems for mental health services that are largely un- or underregulated or that simply omit many of these critical elements.

— *Goal 3: To ensure quality of care within managed-care programs.* First, the managed-care industry's knowledge base and experience is grounded in the delivery of general medical services, not in comprehensive HIV/AIDS or mental health services. Second, the population it has historically served is the white middle class, not the Medicaid population. The mental health needs of individuals who have relatively stable employment, work environments with often generous benefits, and social supports are vastly different from those of the Medicaid population. Third, the managed-care treatment model is based on the delivery of service through narrowly defined channels, is often of a short-term nature, and does not integrate multiple systems. The mental health needs of the Medicaid population, especially those living with HIV/AIDS, dictate integration and coordination among a whole array of service delivery systems to address needs such as assistance with housing, entitlements, family interventions, crime/victimization, and protective or permanency planning services. Over many years, the community-based mental health system has been uniquely designed to address these needs. Why do states and the federal government assume that the managed-care industry would supply the same quality service as the community-based mental health system? Certainly, experience has not led to this assumption. Health care reform initiatives implemented by 1993 show that no state has a demonstrated model for successfully incorporating AIDS health and mental health issues into its managed-care program.

— *Goal 4: To enhance access to and availability of mainstream medical care and services by Medicaid recipients.*

Issues regarding how to provide enhanced access for primary health care are very different from the issues that must be addressed in order to enhance access to mental health care. Most state plans do in fact attempt to address access to health care for the Medicaid population, although most ignore issues of access to mental health care and substance abuse treatment and the added stressors associated with HIV/AIDS. Persons seeking mental health treatment in the general health care system often face stigma and discrimination, lack of coordination with other systems, and geographic, racial, and cultural isolation. Non-full-capitation models would offer equal access to health care without gerrymandering the entire mental health system and potentially jeopardizing access to mental health care. A health-care-only managed-care model would also achieve this goal. Yet many states refuse to explore models other than full capitation.

— *Goal 5: To establish cost-effective managed care programs.*
Some state plans have facilitated cost-effective managed-care programs by integrating medical and mental health care within one program. Other programs' cost savings may be attributed to limited mental health service delivery motivated by the financial incentive to underserve and/or failure to provide mental health services due to unrecognized need. Furthermore, many plans fail to address factors that may neutralize anticipated cost savings. Do state plans, for example, take into account the nature of the Medicaid population's utilization patterns, the fluidity of acute episodes of crisis, the likelihood that this population will move in and out of enrollment, and the probability that the Medicaid population may not change the way it has traditionally accessed mental health services? Whatever the reasons for anticipated cost savings, this mystery remains: Why do states overwhelmingly select full capitation to address the goal of cost savings? Why aren't new and innovative services, split capitation, global budgeting, or other cost-controlling mechanisms discussed with the existing nonprofit mental health sector before undertaking massive restructuring that benefits profit-making enterprises?

In sum, this analysis suggests that many managed care plans fall short of meeting the goals I have enumerated. In fact, the issue of competition among HMOs may further impede attainment of these goals by creating an environment where health rates are quoted so low in order to secure a contract that ultimately payments for special care, such as psychiatric and psychological services, will be used to offset health cost overruns.

Are we sure of the efficacy and validity of the HMO model, or are we experimenting with the mental health needs of people with HIV, poor people, and persons of color? This experimentation risks the potential collapse of the existing nonprofit community-based mental health system. This analysis suggests that managed-care planning often has very little to do with providing the special-care services that are needed for the Medicaid population and everything to do with accommodating reimbursement systems, creating profit incentives to underserve, and political expediency.

## *Federal Block Grants: A New Fiscal Reality*

Finally, it seems probable that federal block grants will be debated for some time, threatening a shift of federal health dollars to states to spend as they see fit in terms of who will receive what services.

Traditionally defined, block grants merge multiple federal funding streams (encompassing a wide array of services) into one funding stream that is less than the fiscal sum of its individual parts. They are administered by states, rather than by federal agencies, permitting great discretion and flexibility with minimal oversight.

Block grants differ from entitlement and categorical programs in several ways. Unlike entitlement programs, block grants are capped funding streams (that is, a maximum amount of money is dictated) that do not reflect changes in population need. Moreover, federal programs funded through block grants have broader programmatic objectives with fewer specifics than entitlement and categorical programs, and they eliminate federal minimum eligibility, service, and provider choice requirements.

The general rationale behind block grants is a desire to decrease the number of unfunded mandates on states and localities and to increase local programmatic flexibility. Despite this underlying policy rationale, block grants often require localities to meet complex programmatic requirements and to finance programs without increased federal assistance. While block grants have been an integral part of federal aid for the last twenty years, the current scope of block grant discussions represents a fundamental shift in the fiscal relationship among the federal, state, and local governments.

The effect of block grants on HIV/AIDS mental health funding may look something like this: An agency sensitive to community needs, such as the need for additional HIV/AIDS mental health care, may currently seek money from several federal funding streams, thereby piecing together a package of care that responds to the special needs of its patients. If a Medicaid block grant system is enacted, those various federal funding streams will not be available to tap. In fact, state legislators and administrators may dictate usage of the pooled money, likely not responding to the needs of special Medicaid populations.

## *Tools for Advocacy*

By now the careful reader has realized that policy-making in Washington and in state capitals significantly affects mental health practice and client care. The following suggests several responses:

- *It is not sufficient just to practice. At minimum, you must keep informed about HIV and about mental health policy issues.*

  You should also be involved in policy-making. Otherwise you run the risk of having the service delivery system, which includes your practice, reshaped or redirected without your participation. Public policy affects your practice and your client's care.

  — Push your professional organizations to represent your needs in Washington and at state capitals.
  — Engage (I didn't say lead) in grass-roots community organization and advocacy.

- *Don't negate the involvement of your clients in advocacy because you fear an inappropriate use of your professional power or interference with the therapeutic relationship.*

  Staff and supervisors must resolve this dilemma. When in doubt, why not ask your clients? It is fundamental that all helping relationships foster client empowerment. This requires knowledge and information sharing (forms of power) to promote the client's self-voice.
- *Do not wait for requests for funding proposals (RFPs) to land on your desk.*

  You should be involved in the process so that you can shape the RFPs. The optimal method is by having a continuing good relationship with agencies that affect your work. In this relationship, project officers and others will tell you what is occurring within the agency and will help you lobby for funding for your projects. If you do not have that relationship yet, then learn how agencies that affect you develop funding priorities. Then, when the priority-creation process is about to start, visit the decision makers and tell them what your clients need.

- *In the realm of practitioner accommodations, clinicians must become proficient with a world of short-term, cognitive-behavioral, and outcome-based modalities.*

  This does not mean you must forgo long-term therapies. However, you need to become knowledgeable and skillful in using short-term interventions to meet specified goals. You must also learn to live with HMOs' case managers, who are likely to try to get the most bang for very little buck.

  Clinicians must also prepare for "case management" that focuses on moving the client to less intensive services and demonstrating outcomes, rather than case management that focuses on getting customized services for clients.

- *Agencies need to assess their ability to compete in the managed-care environment.*

  Materials are readily available for such assessments. Consult, for example, the Center for Substance Abuse Treatment's (1994) *Managed Healthcare Organizational Readiness Guide and Checklist.*

  Agencies that offer only one service or a lot of that one service (horizontal integration) are not attractive to managed-care companies unless they represent a niche or serve a cultural/ethnic/linguistic or other identified special population. HMOs are interested in multilayer services that are in place and intensive enough to prevent hospitalization (one-stop shopping).

  - Agencies should reach out to HMOs or other networks seeking contracts.
  - Agencies must study their management information systems to determine their ability to gather and report data concurrently (real time, this week/month), not retrospectively. Consequently, infrastructure is critical, and agencies will need to build, buy, or lease it.

## *Conclusion*

People living with HIV/AIDS already face incredible obstacles in accessing medical care, maintaining quality of life, and often simply surviving. While many politicians on the left and the right agree on the need to enact positive reforms, proposals to dismantle the Medicaid system are of grave concern to people living with AIDS, their care partners, friends and families, health and mental health providers, and, ultimately, local communities and state governments.

### REFERENCES

Center for Substance Abuse Treatment (1994). *Managed healthcare organizational readiness guide and checklist.* Washington, DC: U.S. Department of Health & Human Services.

Decker, J. E., & Stubblebine, J. M. (1972). Crisis intervention and prevention of psychiatric disability: A follow-up study. *American Journal of Psychiatry, 129,* 725–729.

Dunlap, D. W. (1995, July 8). Different faces of AIDS are conjured up by politicians. *New York Times,* 7.

Fabricant, M., & Burghardt, S. (1992). *Welfare state crisis and the transformation of social service work.* New York: Sharpe.

Freund, D., Rossiter, L., Fox, P., Meyer, J., Hurley, R., Carey, T., & Paul, J. (1989). Evaluation of the Medicaid competition demonstrations. *Health Care Financing Review, 11(2),* 81–97.

Human Rights Campaign Fund, Lake Research, & Terrance Group (1995). *AIDS funding and voter attitudes.* Washington, DC: Author.

Langwell, K. (1990). Structure and performance of health maintenance organizations: A review. *Health Care Financing Review, 12,* 71–79.

Luft, H. S. (1978). How do health maintenance organizations achieve their "savings"? *New England Journal of Medicine, 298,* 1336–1343.

Luft, H. (1981). *Health maintenance organizations: Dimensions of performance.* New York: Wiley.

New York State Office of Mental Health (1993). *Statewide comprehensive plan for mental health services 1994–1998.* Albany, NY: Author.

Parad, H., & Parad, L. (1990). *Crisis intervention: The practitioner's sourcebook for brief therapy.* Milwaukee, WI: Family Service America.

Reid, W., & Shyne, A. (1969). *Brief and extended casework.* New York: Columbia University Press.

Seelye, K. (1995, June 30). Helms puts the brakes to a bill financing AIDS treatment. *New York Times,* A-12.

Warren, N., Fullwood, P., Lee, J., & Salitan, D. (Eds.) (1995). *Making a difference in a lot of ways: An assessment of Ryan White Title I outreach services in New York City.* New York: Hunter College Center on AIDS, Drugs, and Community Health.

Westmoreland, T. (1995). AIDS and politics: Death and taxes. *Perspectives in HIV Care — Bulletin of the New York Academy of Medicine, 72 (Summer Suppl.),* 273–282.

# Afterword: New Treatments, New Hopes, and New Uncertainties

*Mark G. Winiarski*

In 1996 something extraordinary occurred in the clinical care of persons with HIV/AIDS, which had stagnated after years of only moderate biomedical gains through the use of zidovudine (ZDV, AZT, Retrovir) and many disappointing clinical trials: The testing and licensing of new kinds of antiretroviral drugs, and the use of new combinations of drugs, began to suggest that improved and longer lives were possible, and there were hints that sometime in the near future the virus could be eradicated.

It seemed that everyone knew someone whose life had been renewed by use of a newly licensed drug or a combination of drugs that included newly licensed antiretrovirals. Newspapers were reporting miraculous recoveries from debilitation caused by HIV/AIDS. Some persons with AIDS, using new combination therapies, gained weight, found new energy and improved health, and decided to go back to work after months or years of disability. Viatical services, which paid AIDS patients for their life insurance policies on the bet that they would die relatively soon, had to rethink their positions.

A new mood was everywhere. A Bronx physician, who works with HIV-positive patients in a methadone program, reported that people who had shunned zidovudine were intrigued by the combination therapies, and that medical providers were enthusiastic about the new drugs after years of prescribing zidovudine.

Yet virtually all knowledgeable persons modulated their hopes and expressed skepticism or plain reluctance to become disappointed again. Very close to the surface of the optimistic reports is a very complicated reality, freighted with remarkable psychosocial and spiritual considerations that will comprise a large component of mental health care for persons affected by HIV/AIDS in the next decade.

"I'm very skeptical about the new class of drugs. Perhaps this is a defense mechanism so I don't get disappointed," said one HIV-positive man, an advocate for improved HIV/AIDS care. When interviewed, he was taking a protease inhibitor and reported moderate side effects. He told me, "Even if I get better in the next three years, the protease inhibitor is not a cure. I'm not thinking about my retirement plans or the house I'll be buying when I'm sixty. For me the psychological aspect of all this is a balance between my knowledge, fears, and hopes. Others less knowledgable than me may grab onto the headlines. Their sense of hope is based on a lot of advertising."

This man expressed the disconcerting uncertainty that most felt in reaction to the new drugs. From the beginning of the HIV/AIDS epidemic, many would seek to move from uncertainty to a psychological state of knowing, typically saying something like this: "I am glad now that I have been diagnosed with AIDS; the other shoe has fallen. Now I know what to expect." Later in the epidemic, "knowing" was too often expressed by way of quoting group statistics: *x* percentage number of infected people will have symptoms by year *a; y* percentage will be dead by year *b*. Those group-based numbers, which did not pertain to any specific individual, seemed to offer certainty.

Psychologically, the new therapies return persons affected by HIV/AIDS to uncertain times. The new therapies, rushed to market after limited testing, offer great uncertainties in exchange for the hope: It is unclear whether side effects will force discontinuation. It is unknown how long positive effects will last; prospects of continued improvement can be shattered overnight with side effects, dropoffs in efficacy, and unforeseen consequences. Clients may embrace the new therapies, but always echoing in the psyche is the question, "Who knows?"

Other psychosocial repercussions of the new therapies are noteworthy:

- Will everyone have access to these therapies, or will some people be excluded? The cost of a year's therapy in mid-1996 was estimated to range from $15,000 to $20,000. Will pharmaceutical companies reduce prices? Will insurance companies and other payors, such as Medicaid, decide not to pay, leaving these drugs only to the wealthy and those in clinical trials?

- The new regimens have rules that are difficult to follow. Combination therapies require many pills to be taken on a very strict schedule, and some with meals and some between meals. Scientists are concerned that poor adherence to regimens may increase the possibilities of viral mutations, leading to drug-resistant strains of HIV, as occurred with tuberculosis.
- Will some classes of individuals be automatically excluded because of problems following drug protocols? The author of an op-ed piece in the *New York Times* has suggested that the risk of creating drug-resistant mutated strains of HIV may justify withholding these drugs from "those who have demonstrated an inability to take medications consistently" (G. Rotello, The risk in a "cure" for AIDS, July 14, 1996, sec. 4, 17). If persons are excluded from available therapies, they are likely to be the powerless and those already oppressed and deprived of too many resources. As one physician said, "If that happens, they have every right to be pissed."
- These drugs have side effects. What will be the psychological response of someone who has to stop these medications because of side effects?
- The long-term effects of these treatments are still unknown.

Some point out social repercussions: That the new combination treatments may lull society into thinking that HIV/AIDS has been adequately addressed, thus eliminating funding for alternative strategies. As dangerous may be the belief by some HIV-positive persons treated with the new therapies that their HIV has disappeared and they can return to unsafe sexual practices.

## *Professional Practice in the Next Decade*

Each of these issues, and many more, will be in the hearts and on the minds of HIV-affected clients who seek mental health care, including psychotherapy, in the years ahead. The advent of these therapies and the psychosocial and spiritual implications underline the need to be not only compassionate but competent, utilizing the techniques and adapting models of care described in this book: Conceptualizing HIV/AIDS using a biopsychosocial model; becoming knowledgeable about the medical aspects of care; employing a "bending the frame" style of care that combines psychotherapy with other aspects of needed care, including support of adherence to the new therapies; attention to clients' spiritual aspects; applying new models of care that respond to clients' needs, and competently evaluating those models and clinical practices to determine what works and why.

Practitioners will need to keep current with the pace of new scientific developments. One practical tool for maintaining knowledge is the web site of the National AIDS Clearinghouse. With a computer, modem, and web access, it can be reached by typing http://www.cdcnac.org. This bulletin board has links to many sources of information, and one can search several databases using its gopher. (See also Appendix B.)

## *Tools for Clinical Practice*

Skillful providers will respond to the new therapies by considering the following:

- *As with all aspects of HIV/AIDS care, the skillful practitioner should know his or her opinions and feelings related to the psychosocial aspects of the new therapies—feelings regarding quality versus quantity of life, hope versus skepticism, among other aspects—but will refrain from influencing the client.*

  One example may indicate how a client may be injured by a therapist's attitudes. Let's say that the therapist is a believer that life should have quality rather than quantity, and that the therapist is fairly clear what quality entails. The client facing this therapist is unfamiliar with quality of life as the therapist conceptualizes it. The client may want to live long simply because that is a tenet of his or her religion. The client may want to live, in the hope of a cure, despite being a chronic drug user. The client may want to live to see children grow older, even if his or her existence seems marginal. If the therapist were to engage in a debate over the client's quality of life, or suggest in some subtle way that the client's life is subpar, it could be experienced—accurately—as an attack. The reverse may also be true: A client's life may appear to the therapist to have quality, but may seem poor to the client.

The skillful therapist knows that attitudes and opinions about issues such as quality of life are personally and idiosyncratically derived, and that therapy is not about foisting one's opinions onto clients.

- *The client may need help with his or her cost-benefit analysis. The therapist should ensure that psychosocial/spiritual variables are included.*

  Everyone makes a cost/benefit analysis, or tries to sidestep one. The therapist's delicate task is to assist the client in weighing all of his or her unique variables, and not to tilt the scales unfairly.

  In response to headlines and marketing, clients may want to rush, unthinking, into use of new therapies. Or, alternatively, some may say they can't make a decision, which is a decision, of sorts, in itself. If the new therapies are available to a particular client, the therapist should raise the issue if it doesn't surface. Then, therapeutic tasks may include:

— Exploration of taking a new therapy in the context of the larger question of the client's philosophy regarding quality of life versus quantity of life. This can lead to very rich discussion. It surely is appropriate for the therapist to ask such thought-provoking questions as, "What do you value, above all things?" or "With your partner dead, you seemed not to have much motivation to continue living. Does that influence your decision to bypass the new therapy?"

— Discussion regarding the client's attitudes specific to the new therapies. Is the client suspicious, as many were regarding AZT? What are the client's motivations regarding participation or nonparticipation? Does the client really want to take these medications or is he or she responding to external pressures? What are those pressures?

— Does the client have accurate information upon which to base a decision?

— Is the decision affected or delayed by a mood disorder or continuing substance abuse that requires attention?

— Is the client sufficiently motivated for a difficult protocol? Can the client enlist support from family, friends, and others in maintaining motivation?

— Can the therapist, or the agency, create support groups or other activities to assist clients with difficult drug regimens?

— What is the client's spiritual interpretation of the availability of the new treatments? Is the availability of the new therapy seen as a new opportunity for spiritual work?

- *The therapist must help the client balance hope and new uncertainties created by the new therapies.*

  The new therapies offer hope, which may be perceived by some as a day at a time and by others as two or three years of renewed life. But many clients mix skepticism with their hopes. This balancing act is stressful. One admits that control is relinquished to factors unknown. One takes a leap into the unknown. Psychotherapy can provide great assistance in this process, providing a medium for discussing and creating the balance, and supporting the client when the emotional balance is upset.

  This assistance with balance should also extend to a client's family and friends. They too are balancing, and their feelings are shifting. A therapist tells the story of a mother who readied her children for her death, but then began a new drug and improved markedly.

- *Mental health practitioners should assist clients who choose these therapies to adhere to their complicated drug treatment protocols.*

  Patients find it difficult to retain complicated information. Many clients will need assistance to understand their complicated therapies and to adhere to the protocols. Medical practitioners are finding that it is insufficient to explain the regimens just once. The client often has to hear about the different aspects many times. Psychosocial practitioners can assist with this.

  Therapists should become active helpers of their clients' adherence to new therapies. Those who work in medical settings, such as that described in chapter 13, may want to work with primary care providers to create systems that support adherence. For example, at Montefiore Medical Center, the medical director of a primary care program in the Substance Abuse Treatment Program and a psychologist are making plans to support patients in taking protease inhibitors, and the patients are responsive. Mental health practitioners should consider the following supportive strategies:

— Creation of therapy adherence support groups.

— Creation of buddy systems, in which two or more people can telephone each other continually to remind each other to take

medication and to provide support to one another when energy flags.
- Creation of family-oriented support, in which partners, spouses, siblings, and others are enlisted to assist adherence.
- Assistance with creation of reminder systems, such as refrigerator and medicine cabinet charts and use of items such as pill boxes with alarms.
- Brainstorming and focus group sessions with clients may provide useful suggestions regarding support. One colleague suggested enlisting the assistance of *bodega* shopkeepers in the Bronx, who would be urged to ask their customers, "Did you take your medication?"

• *If clients are excluded from therapies, they will be enraged. The therapist will be a lighting rod for that rage.*

The clients likely to be excluded from new therapies are likely to be those excluded from many resources and opportunities. These are the poor, those of minority races and cultures, people who have come to this country without adequate documentation, and persons who have addictions. The rage of the disadvantaged is all around us, and majority-culture individuals would notice if we were to drop our defenses.

The HIV/AIDS client excluded from new therapies will be rageful, having experienced yet another assault. The therapist must absorb the client's rage and never negate it. The therapist cannot excuse or defend the realities of our society and definitely should not dismiss the client with a statement such as, "Maybe next time."

• *Clients who improve with the combination therapies will face issues long put off.*

Many HIV-infected individuals, facing what to them was a certain death, opted out of many routine and troublesome aspects of life. Some exceeded their credit card limits and failed to pay bills. Others did not pay income taxes. Many isolated themselves from family members, acquaintances, and friends. And some detached themselves from their spiritual leanings. Then, they found that the new therapies renewed their bodies, and they are now concerned about renewing their psychological, social, and spiritual lives as well.

Psychotherapy issues may include:

- Financial matters such as debts, including lack of payment to medical providers, and taxes. Many areas have credit counseling services which mediate between clients and creditors, and a referral may be appropriate. Regarding taxes, a client may want to consult a tax attorney. Those unable to pay for a consultation may seek tax advice through legal-aid-type organizations.
- Psychological issues such as continuing substance abuse, untreated or otherwise ignored disorders such as depression, self-neglect in nutrition, and home environment.
- Social issues such as family members' feelings regarding the new health status. If family and friends were relating to the client as if he or she were imminently departing, with a variety of possibly mixed feelings, the social circle will have to adjust to a relatively healthier family member or friend. The healthier person may demand more power in the family system, thereby destabilizing it. Old roles, abdicated due to poor health, may have to be fought for. And, of course, if the new treatments fail, family and social systems will be destabilized once more, with the client possibly blamed for the continuing upset.
- Spiritual issues such as neglect of one's sense of immanence, feelings of despair as someone overlooked by the creator, rage and dismissal of God, and self-hate based on religious teachings. As noted in chapter 4, intractable spiritually based problems may require a referral to an empathic clergy person.

• *Those who have a renewed life may want to plan again.*

Perhaps many of us would welcome an opportunity to reenter life, taking the opportunity to do it in new ways — with less fear, with more love for self and more regard for others. While most of us, including some clients, would like to believe that the extended life offers a chance for a psychological "makeover," it is more likely that individuals will return to old patterns. Nevertheless, opportunities for adjustment are available, and the renewal should include the possibilities. The therapist may explore these areas, being certain that the client is not perceiving a demand:

- Ask the client what his or her ideal self is and who, or how, he or she would rather be, even over a short time. Explore barriers to desired improvement. Help the client identify just one small area of improvement that he or she wishes to tackle. Make this small improvement an early therapeutic goal.

- If the client believes relationships need attention, the client will need to evaluate his or her available emotional resources that can be allocated to repair, as well as barriers to hoped-for changes. One possible barrier may be that the other person is not capable of a relationship.

  Moreover, the therapist should be aware of his or her own fantasies regarding reunions and not make them the client's.

- Allow the client to do some concrete planning that may involve financial matters, scheduling of important events, remaining or moving, working or not. In all cases, exploration of the feelings and motivations are key.

- *The belief of some who have found renewed lives is that they have been "saved" by God. This opens a door for exploration of their spiritual lives.*

  As Sister Pascal Conforti notes in her essay on spirituality (chapter 4), the therapist's task is not to make judgments about the client's expressions of spirituality but to appreciate the client's revelation of something deeply personal. The therapist should listen and be open to the expressions. With the door of conversation about spirituality open, much can be discussed, including the client's spiritual history and how he or she wants to live spiritually in the extended life.

  The therapist should anticipate a crucial issue if the client interprets positive medical results as divine intervention: Will negative medical effects also be interpreted as divine intervention? And what will that mean to the client? Will it mean that God is displeased and punishing him or her?

- *Until more is known, clients should be counseled to use safer sex techniques regardless of their viral load measurements.*

  "My viral load test indicated no measurable HIV. So why should I use a condom?" That is a question likely to be raised countless times.

  There are two approaches, which ultimately converge, to this question. The first is an exploration of all the issues the client experiences around safer sex practices. As indicated in chapters 8 and 11, these issues are complicated and important. The client should understand why he or she wants to dispense with safer sex practices. The second approach involves a concrete response: Until the time when scientists are certain that HIV can be eradicated from the body, infected persons must continue to use safer sex techiques. While measurable HIV may not be found in the blood, scientists believe it nevertheless is still present in the body. I tend to think that clients know the concrete response, but that psychodynamic issues propel them into unsafe areas.

These are just a few of the issues that are already being discussed as we enter the epidemic's new era of hope coupled with uncertainty. If these issues and others discussed in this book have intrigued you or moved you, if your heart has found its place in HIV/AIDS-related mental health practice, then I invite you to join the many compassionate and skillful practitioners in this field.

# Appendix A: Medical Primer

## *What Is a Virus?*

A virus is a "nucleic acid molecule that can invade cells and replicate within them" (Joklik, 1988, 1). Joklik's text notes that viruses are considered to have some attributes of life, but terms such as *organism* and *living* are inapplicable. "Isolated virus particles are arrangements of nucleic and protein molecules with no metabolism of their own; they are no more alive than isolated chromosomes. Within cells, however, virus particles are capable of reproducing their own kind abundantly" (Joklik, 1988, 1). For a popular discussion of viruses, see Radetsky's *The Invisible Invaders* (1991).

## *What Is the Human Immunodeficiency Virus (HIV)?*

The virus we call HIV, HIV-1 being the most common, belongs to a group of viruses called retroviruses. Retroviruses are composed of two strands of single-stranded ribonucleic acid (RNA) surrounded by a fatty envelope. HIV's envelope and its surface proteins help it enter other cells. Although HIV is believed to attack many kinds of cells by attaching itself at receptors, or "docks," its infection of T-helper cells has received the most attention. T-helper cells are also called CD4 or CD4+ T-lymphocytes, so named for the specific surface molecule (Cluster Designation 4) that serves as the "dock" for HIV. After docking, HIV fuses with a protein on the T-helper cell. Once fused, the contents of the virus enter the T-helper cell. One of these contents, a viral enzyme called reverse transcriptase, produces from the viral RNA first a single strand and then a double strand of deoxyribonucleic acid (DNA). This DNA is called provirus and is integrated in the host cell's genetic code. From this incorporated provirus, new viral RNA is transcribed. Viral proteins follow, and new complete virus particles begin to bud off from the host cell. Ultimately, the T cell playing host to such viral replications is destroyed.

## *How Does Someone Get HIV?*

HIV exists in bodily fluids. Infection can occur when the bodily fluids of an HIV-infected person are put in another's body. This happens in the following ways:

- *During sex.* Also, there have been reported cases of HIV transmitted by artificial insemination with infected semen.
- *Through injection drug use.* Risk occurs when an HIV-infected person uses a syringe to shoot up and leaves some infected blood in it, and another person then uses the same syringe, thereby injecting infected blood along with the drugs.
- *From the infected mother to the fetus.* Because of the presence of the mother's anti-HIV antibodies, all babies born of HIV-infected mothers test HIV-positive immediately after birth. The mother's antibodies gradually disappear and from 13 to 30 percent of the babies subsequently develop their own antibodies and are found to be truly HIV-infected. A major study has shown that if pregnant women take zidovudine during the pregnancy and childbirth, and if the baby takes it during its first weeks of life, the risk of the baby's becoming HIV-positive itself is substantially reduced (Centers for Disease Control, 1995).
- *Through breast-feeding from the infected mother to the baby.*
- *By way of receipt of blood and blood products that have not been screened for the presence of HIV.* Routine testing in the United States has decreased this risk to negligible size. To avoid even that risk, surgeons who plan procedures suggest that patients stock

their own blood for transfusion, a procedure known as autologous transfusions. There have been reports from other countries that companies have failed to test blood products, thus endangering recipients.

## *What Is the HIV Test?*

Commonly used HIV tests screen not for the virus but for the antibody to the virus. Thus, those who test positive are sometimes referred to as HIV antibody-positive.

When routine testing is done, blood is taken from the individual. Then an enzyme immunoassay (EIA) or enzyme-linked immunosorbent assay (ELISA) is conducted. When antibodies to HIV are detected, another test is used to confirm the result. The second test is either a Western blot (WB) or immunofluorescence assay (IFA). When this second test confirms a positive result, the individual is told that he or she is HIV-positive.

When done competently, these tests are very accurate. In a study of EIA and WB testing of 630,190 units of blood from 290,110 donors, the rate of obtaining a result that falsely indicated someone was HIV-positive was 0.0006 (MacDonald et al. 1989).

Individuals can purchase a test kit and then send a specimen to a laboratory with a code, subsequently learning their results by phone. Proponents of home testing argue that this test will allow more individuals to know their HIV status. Critics say that emotional support in the event of a positive result, as well as prevention counseling, will be unavailable or less effective.

All tests for antibodies are limited by the necessity for the antibodies to be present. A person infected with HIV may take up to six months to produce antibodies. An antibody test during this period may indicate, falsely, that the person is HIV-negative.

## *Is There Any Direct Measure of HIV in a Person's Blood?*

Scientists have been asking why a person with a low T-helper cell count may do better physically than someone with more T-helper cells. It has been suggested that the amount of HIV in a person's body — called "viral load" — may have more to do with health, at least for some individuals. While their role in clinical practice is not yet established, tests of viral load are likely to play an increasingly important role in the next few years.

## *What Is Acquired Immune Deficiency Syndrome (AIDS)?*

AIDS is "the most severe manifestation of infection" with HIV, according to the federal AIDS Treatment Information Service (1995, 1).

The Centers for Disease Control and Prevention in 1993 revised the diagnostic criteria for AIDS in adults and adolescents. Persons who have HIV, no symptoms but a T-helper cell count below 200 have AIDS (Centers for Disease Control, 1992). In addition, an HIV-infected person with one of twenty-six AIDS-defining illnesses also would be diagnosed with AIDS. These twenty-six conditions include pulmonary tuberculosis, recurrent pneumonia and invasive cervical cancer, HIV wasting syndrome, Kaposi's sarcoma, *pneumocystis carinii* pneumonia, and toxoplasmosis of the brain.

## *What Are T Cells, and What Is Their Importance in HIV/AIDS?*

T cells are white blood cells that are involved in immune reactions. There are three categories of these cells: helper, killer, and suppressor.

Those concerned with HIV/AIDS have paid most attention to the T-helper cell. This cell helps orchestrate the immune response and serves as a biomedical marker of immune functioning. The HIV docks on the T-helper cells, takes them over, and subsequently kills them. With the death of these cells comes a decrease in immune functioning.

## *How Do Medical Staff Monitor Immune Functioning?*

The T-helper, or CD4, count, is a widely accepted — although not ideal — marker of immune function, and the diminishment of T-helper cells is viewed as an important sign of disease progression. Normally a person has in excess of 800 T-helper cells per cubic millimeter of blood. (When someone says, "I have 200 T-helper cells," he or she means 200 cells per cubic millimeter of blood.) Over the course of infection, the number of T-helper cells decreases as the cells are killed. When the count drops to fewer than 200 cells/cubic millimeter, an infected person is classified as having AIDS.

In addition to the absolute number of T-helper cells, which can vary from test to test for many reasons, including presence of other infections, medical staff also monitor the percentage of T-helper to total T cells. Total T cell levels remain relatively stable, although T-helper cells may die.

## *What Are Opportunistic Infections?*

Opportunistic infections are infections "that cause disease with increased frequency and/or of increased severity among HIV-infected persons, presumably because of immunosuppression" (Kaplan, Masur, Holmes, McNeil et al., 1995, p. S1). The authors list more than 100 organisms that cause opportunistic infections, including viruses, bacteria, fungi, and protozoa.

Common opportunistic infections in persons with AIDS include *pneumocystis carinii* pneumonia, caused by an organism that is genetically a fungus but is regarded as a parasite; retinitis, caused by cytomegalovirus; candidiasis, caused by fungus; and toxoplasmosis, caused by a protozoan parasite. The cause of Kaposi's sarcoma, another OI, is hotly debated; although it is a cancer, there seems to be a viral contribution to its causes. Persons with AIDS also get malignancies at a rate that far exceeds that in the normal population. Invasive cervical cancer and lymphoma are two malignancies seen in persons with AIDS.

## *What Are the Treatments for Opportunistic Infections?*

Most OIs have a specific treatment. And with improvements and new discoveries, these change often. Depending on medical circumstances, there are any number of protocols for treatment of *pneumocystis carinii* pneumonia alone. This area is very complex and ever changing, and it is suggested that mental health providers discuss their questions regarding medical treatment with trusted medical providers.

## *What Is AZT?*

AZT was the first major drug discovered to have an effect against HIV. It is also now commonly called zidovudine (ZDV) or Retrovir. It is in a class of drugs called reverse transcriptase inhibitors, which also now includes ddI and ddC. Originally used alone, it is credited with extending the longevity of many persons with AIDS. It is now studied and more widely used in combination with other drugs. Some individuals do not tolerate zidovudine, complaining of nausea, fatigue, malaise and insomnia. Most if not all patients treated with zidovudine for a long time develop some resistance to it, although the clinical significance of this is not always clear. Zidovudine has side effects, including a reduction in white and/or red blood cell counts.

## *What Are Protease Inhibitors?*

Protease inhibitors are a newer class of drugs that attack HIV at a different point in the reproduction process than does zidovudine. Typically, a protease inhibitor is prescribed along with other drugs to create a many-pronged attack on the virus. This results in drug regimens requiring fifteen or more pills daily. At least initially, protease inhibitors were priced at thousands of dollars for a year's supply.

## *What Is the Typical Medical Treatment for an HIV-Infected Person Who Has No Symptoms?*

The typical treatment strategy has two components. The first is an attack on the virus's replication process; the second is prevention of opportunistic infections.

The attack on viral replication is typically accomplished through combination therapies — simultaneous use of different types of drugs to disrupt replication at various stages of the process.

The U.S. Public Health Service and the Infectious Diseases Society of America have issued extensive guidelines for prevention of opportunistic infections. These guidelines appeared in *Clinical Infectious Diseases,* and reprints are available from the National AIDS Clearinghouse (Kaplan, Masur, Holmes, McNeil et al., 1995; Kaplan, Masur, Holmes, Wilfert et al., 1995; USPHS/IDSA Prevention of Opportunistic Infections Working Group, 1995). Standard-of-care recommendations include medications to prevent the opportunistic infections *pneumocystis carinii, toxoplasma gondii,* and tuberculosis, and often *mycobacterium avium* complex as well (Kaplan, Masur, Holmes, Wilfert, et al., 1995).

## *How Long Does It Take for a Person to Get AIDS after HIV Infection?*

The time from infection with HIV until the emergence of AIDS is called the incubation period. Our understandings of incubation periods as well as of survival times after the first opportunistic infection occurs are based on statistical analyses of groups of infected individuals. For any specific person the time course of the disease is unknowable.

Osmond (1994a) notes that "rates of progression to AIDS are very low in the first two years after infection and increase thereafter" (p. 1.7–

4). Bacchetti and Moss (1989), using San Francisco data, indicate that progression rates increase for seven years, when the estimated probability of developing AIDS is 8.2 percent, after which they drop slightly.

Many factors may affect an individual's incubation period. Some of these factors (called cofactors) proposed by scientists include other viruses, such as cytomegalovirus and Epstein-Barr virus, bacterial infections, and severe malnutrition. Others have suggested that emotional welfare and hope can play a part. Osmond (1994a) notes that "some persons have not manifested AIDS or progressive immunosuppression after more than a decade of infection, and their eventual fate is unknown" (p. 1.7–1).

### *How Long Will a Person Live after His or Her First Opportunistic Infection?*

Again, statistical analyses of group information do not describe or predict any single individual's experience. AIDS often led to death in less than one year early in the epidemic. Now, due to the availability of zidovudine, combination therapies, and pneumocystis prophylaxis, longevity has increased dramatically. Osmond (1994b), writing before protease inhibitors were licensed, noted that after the first opportunistic infection and with toleration of zidovudine therapy, the median (half of the studied group is below the median, and half above) survival time is from fifteen months to two years.

## REFERENCES

AIDS Treatment Information Service (1995, June). *Glossary of HIV/AIDS-related terms.* Rockville, MD: Author.

Bacchetti, P., & Moss, A. R. (1989). Incubation period of AIDS in San Francisco. *Nature, 338,* 251–253.

Centers for Disease Control (1992). 1993 revised classification system for HIV infection and expanded surveillance case definition for AIDS among adolescents and adults. *Morbidity and Mortality Weekly Report, 41(RR-17),* 1–19.

Centers for Disease Control and Prevention (1995). U.S. Public Health Service recommendations for human immunodeficiency virus counseling and voluntary testing for pregnant women. *Morbidity and Mortality Weekly Report, 44(RR-7),* 1–14.

Cohen, P. T., Sande, M. A., & Volberding, P. A. (Eds.) (1994). *The AIDS knowledge base* (2d ed.). Boston: Little, Brown.

Elbeik, T., & Feinberg, M. B. (1994). HIV isolation and quantitative methods. In P. T. Cohen, M. A. Sande, & P. A. Volberding (Eds.), *The AIDS knowledge base* (2d ed.) (2.4–1-2.4–19). Boston: Little, Brown.

Joklik, W. K. (1988). The nature, isolation, and measurement of animal viruses. In W. K. Joklik (Ed.), *Virology* (3d ed.) (1–7). Norwalk, CT: Appleton & Lange.

Kaplan, J. E., Masur, H., Holmes, K. K., McNeil, M. M., Schonberger, L. B., Navin, T. R., Hanson, D. B., Gross, P. A., Jaffe, H. W., & the USPHS/IDSA Prevention of Opportunistic Infections Working Group (1995). USPHS/IDSA guidelines for the prevention of opportunistic infections in persons infected with Human Immunodeficiency Virus: Introduction. *Clinical Infectious Diseases, 21(Suppl. 1),* S1-S11.

Kaplan, J. E., Masur, H., Holmes, K. K., Wilfert, C. M., Sperling, R., Baker, S. A., Trapnell, C. B., Freedberg, K. A., Cotton, D., Powderly, W. G., Jaffe, H. W., and the USPHS/IDSA Prevention of Opportunistic Infections Working Group (1995). USPHS/IDSA guidelines for the prevention of opportunistic infections in persons infected with Human Immunodeficiency Virus: An overview. *Clinical Infectious Diseases, 21(Suppl. 1),* S12-S31.

MacDonald, K. L., Jackson, J. B., Bowman, R. J., Polesky, H. F., Rhame, F. S., Balfour, H. H., Jr., & Osterholm, M. T. (1989). Performance characteristics of serologic tests for Human Immunodeficiency Virus type I (HIV-1) antibody among Minnesota blood donors. Public health and clinical implications. *Annals of Internal Medicine, 110,* 617–621.

Osmond, D. H. (1994a). HIV disease progression from infection to CDC-defined AIDS: Incubation period, cofactors, and laboratory markers. In P. T. Cohen, M. A. Sande, & P. A. Volberding (Eds.), *The AIDS knowledge base* (2d ed.) (1.7–1-1.7–19). Boston: Little, Brown.

Osmond, D. H. (1994b). Trends in HIV disease survival time. In P. T. Cohen, M. A. Sande, & P. A. Volberding (Eds.), *The AIDS knowledge base* (2d ed.) (1.3–1-1.3–7). Boston: Little, Brown.

Rabson, A. R. (1995). Enumeration of T-cell subsets in patients with HIV infection. *AIDS Clinical Care, 7,* 1–3.

Radetsky, P. (1991) *The invisible invaders.* Boston: Little, Brown.

USPHS/IDSA Prevention of Opportunistic Infections Working Group (1995). USPHS/IDSA guidelines for the prevention of opportunistic infections in persons infected with the Human Immunodeficiency Virus: Disease-specific recommendations. *Clinical Infectious Diseases, 21(Suppl. 1),* S32-S43.

Vella, S. (1995). Immunological and virological markers in HIV infection. *AIDS Clinical Care, 7,* 37–40.

# Appendix B: Resources — Obtaining HIV/AIDS Information Fast

HIV/AIDS information is so easily and inexpensively obtained that there is no excuse for having insufficient information. The best resource is a helpful librarian, who can show you what on-line and off-line data bases are available to you, as well as direct you to books, reports, and journals. If you do not have easy entry to a medical library, your librarian can likely arrange for guest privileges. Also, do not forget the availability of interlibrary loan arrangements. The following are sources of information, with special emphasis on fast retrieval through computers or fax services.

## *CDC National AIDS Clearinghouse*

The clearinghouse is the foremost repository of HIV/AIDS-related information. For starters, request the *Catalog of HIV and AIDS Education and Prevention Materials* and the *Guide to Selected HIV/AIDS-Related Internet Resources.* Information can be obtained in several ways:

Phone order for mail delivery of documents and for information about HIV/AIDS-related issues, such as service agencies and organizations and funding: (800) 458–5231. You can then talk to a representative.

Phone order for fax delivery: Call (800) 458-5231 and go through the telephone tree until you get to the fax service. You'll then have two options. The first is to request a fax of available documents. The second allows you to request documents by code number. In each case, you have to punch in your fax number. The response can be almost immediate.

E-mail order for mail delivery: aidsinfo@cdcnac.aspensys.com.

Information via a website: The CDC National AIDS Clearinghouse Internet Website is an impressive doorway to HIV/AIDS information and can be accessed by keying http://www.cdcnac.org. Its file transfer protocol site provides access to surveillance reports, clinical care guidelines, resource guides, and other information. Its gopher gives access to the AIDS Daily Summary, AIDS-related articles in government publications, statistics, funding, and other information.

The website will link you to many other web and gopher sites, including those of the CDC Division of HIV/AIDS Prevention, Centers for Disease Control and Prevention, Computerized AIDS Ministries, Food and Drug Administration, HIV/AIDS Ministries Network, the National Foundation for Infectious Diseases, the National Library of Medicine, and the Yahoo Page of AIDS Information Sites, where even more information can be found. The CDC NAC website is where I'd start any information search.

CDC National AIDS Clearinghouse Online, a computerized information network that allows you to obtain computerized access to the clearinghouse and bulletin board services: Set computer software to data bits, 8; parity, none; stop bits, 1, hardware flow control, On; Software flow control, Off; Terminal emulation, VT100 and dial (800) 851–7245. First-time users will get a series of prompts. You can also receive the service's quick reference guide through the Fax service (code 1006).

## *Other Websites*

The *Journal of the American Medical Association* has created an Internet site devoted to AIDS/HIV news, including clinical updates and journal article information. Its address: http://www.ama-assn.org/special/hiv/.

The Center for AIDS Prevention Studies at the University of California at San Francisco has an Internet home page with prevention information: http://www.caps.ucsf.edu/capsweb/

## *HIV/AIDS Treatment Information Service*

This free telephone service for providers and others provides information about the latest federally approved treatment options and research findings. Call (800)-HIV-0440. TTY is (800) 243-7012. Or you can send an e-mail information request to atis@cdcnac.aspensys.com.

Information regarding clinical trials of drugs can be obtained by calling (800)-TRIALS A.

## *Various HIV/AIDS-Related Electronic Bulletin Boards*

Using your computer and modem, you can also receive a wealth of information from electronic bulletin board services (known as BBSs). Note that some, like HandsNet, charge a subscription fee. Others, while free to subscribers, may entail long-distance phone charges. A list of bulletin board services can be obtained by fax from the NAC Fax service by requesting publication 2000.

HandsNet is subscribed to by the editor of this book. It is a gathering of several health and welfare bulletin boards, on topics including AIDS/HIV, substance abuse, legal services, rural issues, health issues, housing/community development, and children, youth, and families. With a subscription, you can modem in and select information from any of the boards. The software is very friendly and allows for key-word searches. The AIDS/HIV bulletin board is weak in reporting breaking news—I find I learn more, faster from the *New York Times*. But the health issues board and others give me access to much useful and timely information. Because a subscription is costly, you should urge your graduate program or library to subscribe. Contact: HandsNet, 20195 Stevens Creek Blvd., Suite 120, Cupertino, CA 95014. Phone (408) 257-4500.

Computerized AIDS Ministries Resource Network is sponsored by the Health and Welfare Ministries Program, General Board of Global Ministries, United Methodist Church. Content is primarily religious. Data line is (212) 222-2135.

HNS HIV-Net is sponsored by Home Nutrition Services and provides information for health care professionals. To register, modem to (800) 788-4118.

In addition, there are several regional bulletin boards and a network of BBSs called the AIDS Education and Global Information Service, which has many affiliate BBSs in the United States and Canada. For additional information, order the *Guide to Selected HIV/AIDS-Related Electronic Bulletin Boards* from the CDC National AIDS Clearinghouse.

## *Online Databases*

The National Library of Medicine has HIV/AIDS databases that can be accessed by computer, or a caller can speak to a representative. The computer costs are approximately $18 per hour of use. Purchase of Grateful Med software is recommended. For more information on how to access these and other NLM databases, call (800) 638-8480:

- AIDSLINE, with more than 100,000 references to books, journals, newsletters, audiovisuals, and abstracts of papers from scientific meetings.
- AIDSTRIALS and AIDSDRUGS, two databases with information on clinical trials of drugs and vaccines. Information from these databases can be obtained from a person by calling (800) TRIALS-A.
- HSTAT (Health Services and Technology Assesment Text) contains texts of official government clinical practice guidelines and other documents useful in health care decision making. This information can be obtained without computer by calling the HIV/AIDS Treatment Information Service, (800) HIV-0440.
- DIRLINE is an annotated directory listing 17,000 organizations, including 2,300 that provide nonclinical HIV/AIDS-related services.

## *Offline Databases*

Your academic library may have some of the following databases on CD-ROM:

*AIDS Compact Library,* by MacMillan New Media, which has full-text HIV/AIDS articles from a variety of journals, citations and abstracts from several databases, and two useful newsletters, *AIDS Clinical Care* and *AIDS Newsletter.*

*Compact Library: AIDS,* by the Medical Publishing Group, contains the text of *AIDS Knowledge Base,* a very helpful source of medical information; 4,000 full-text articles; and the AIDS subset of Medline, a National Library of Medicine database.

# Contributors

*David D. Barney, M.S.W.,* is the research and evaluation specialist at the National Native American AIDS Prevention Center, Oklahoma City, Oklahoma. He received his master's in social work from San Diego State University and is studying public health at the University of California, Berkeley.

*Robert L. Barret, Ph.D.,* is professor of counselor education at the University of North Carolina at Charlotte. Active in HIV-related psychotherapy for eleven years, he is a member of the senior faculty of the American Psychological Association's Project HOPE, a federally funded train-the-trainer program for HIV mental health services. He has a private practice in Charlotte and is the coauthor of *Gay Fathers.*

*Rebecca Bathon, M.S.W.,* is the coordinator of the Helena Hatch Special Care Center for women with HIV in the St. Louis, Missouri, metropolitan area. She is a former Ryan White C.A.R.E. Act services coordinator.

*G. Stephen Bowen, M.D., M.P.H.,* retired from government service in 1996 after serving most recently as director of the Bureau of Health Resources Development and associate administrator for AIDS of the Health Resources and Services Administration. He was an assistant surgeon general. Until his retirement, the Ryan White C.A.R.E. Act was administered under his leadership.

*Martha Ann Carey, Ph.D., R.N.,* is an evaluation specialist with the Center for Mental Health Services, Substance Abuse and Mental Health Services Administration, U.S. Public Health Service. In addition to HIV and mental health, her research interests include the development of research methodology for social science programs. She is currently the program director for the Employment Intervention Demonstration Program for persons with severe mental illness.

*Pascal Conforti, O.S.U., M.A.,* is director of pastoral services at the Spellman Center, a division of St. Clare's Hospital and Health Center, New

York, New York. She works directly with HIV-infected patients and their loved ones as well as with professional and volunteer caregivers in the areas of self-care, spirituality, pastoral education, and care of the terminally ill and dying. An Ursuline sister, she is a certified member of the National Association of Catholic Chaplains.

*Betty E. S. Duran, M.S.W.,* is director of the Direct Client Services Division of the National Native American AIDS Prevention Center in Oklahoma City. She is a tribal member of Pojoaque Pueblo in northern New Mexico and was the first female appointed to an all-male pueblo tribal council, in which she retains lifetime membership. Tribal offices held by Ms. Duran include tribal secretary, treasurer, and governor of Pojoaque Pueblo. She has a master's degree in social work from the University of Kansas.

*Noel Elia, M.S.W.,* is a social worker with the AIDS Mental Health and Primary Care Integration Project, Montefiore Medical Center, Bronx, New York. She also is a lecturer and trainer regarding substance abuse, AIDS, and grief and loss.

*Thomas Eversole, M.S.,* serves as training director for the American Psychological Association's Office on AIDS. He is an active trainer and curriculum developer in the areas of mental health services for HIV/AIDS, substance abuse, sexual minority youth, and cultural diversity, and works with the Community Mobilization for HIV/Substance Abuse Prevention.

*Dennee Frey, Pharm.D.,* was project director of AIDS Psychiatric Homecare at the Visiting Nurse Association of Los Angeles, Inc. She currently is coinvestigator of a Vanderbilt University project titled "Improving Pharmacotherapy in Home Health Patients."

*Barbara C. Kwasnik, M.S.W.,* is manager of psychiatric outpatient services at St. Joseph's Hospital and Medical Center, Paterson, New Jersey. Her professional experience includes program planning, administration, and thirteen years of clinical work in the emergency room and at a mental health clinic where she worked with inner-city children, adults, and families with multiple problems, including HIV, chronic illness, sexual abuse, posttraumatic stress disorder, and the dual diagnosis of mental illness and chemical abuse.

*Karen Meredith, M.P.H., R.N.,* is an instructor in medicine at the Washington University School of Medicine and director of the Helena Hatch Special Care Center for women with HIV/AIDS in the St. Louis, Missouri, metropolitan area. She has been involved in local and national HIV prevention and care efforts since the beginning of the epidemic.

*Rosemary T. Moynihan, S.C., Ph.D.,* is supervisor of the mental health program of the Comprehensive Care Center for HIV at St. Joseph's Hospital and Medical Center, Paterson, New Jersey. She has thirty-six years' experience working with adults, children, and families around issues of chronic fatal illness, including cancer and HIV, and with people who are multiply diagnosed with emotional disturbance, chemical addiction, and catastrophic illness. She has a master's in social work from Columbia University and a Ph.D. in clinical social work from New York University.

*Michael Mulvihill, Dr.P.H.,* is the director of the Research Division, Department of Family Medicine, Albert Einstein College of Medicine/Montefiore Medical Center, Bronx, New York. His doctorate in public health with a concentration in epidemiology is from Columbia University, and he is an expert in health services research.

*Michele Killough Nelson, Ph.D.,* is a clinical psychologist and director of the Mini Mental Health Clinic for HIV-infected and -affected individuals at the Medical College of Virginia/Virginia Commonwealth University in Richmond, Virginia. She is an assistant professor of psychiatry and teaches courses on working with dying individuals, AIDS Dementia Complex, psychological assessment, and borderline personality disorder. She writes on these topics and on working with transplant patients.

*Karen Oman, S.W.,* was project coordinator of AIDS Psychiatric Homecare at the Visiting Nurse Association of Los Angeles, Inc. She currently is bereavement coordinator for the association's Hospice Program.

*Kathy Parish, Ph.D.,* is a psychologist and site principal investigator of the Hemophilia Behavioral Intervention Evaluation Project at Huntington Memorial Hospital, Pasadena, California, in a cooperative agreement with the U.S. Centers for Disease Control and Prevention. She also has a private consulting practice.

*Marjorie H. Royle, Ph.D.,* is the research and evaluation coordinator for the Department of Psychiatry at St. Joseph's Hospital and Medical Center, Paterson, New Jersey. She received her Ph.D. in applied social psychology from Claremont Graduate School, Claremont, California, and has done evaluation research for the U.S. Navy and the United Church of Christ.

*Ariel Shidlo, Ph.D.,* is a clinical/community psychologist and program director for TalkSafe, a peer counseling program for HIV-negative gay and bisexual men at St. Vincent's Hospital and Medical Center, New York City. He is also on staff as a psychologist at the Columbia Center for Lesbian, Gay & Bisexual Mental Health, New York City.

*I. Michael Shuff, Ph.D.,* is associate professor of counseling psychology at Indiana State University, Terre Haute. He is director of the Heartland Care Center, a state-supported HIV/AIDS care center located on the university campus, which serves a five-county area in western Indiana. His professional experience with HIV/AIDS spans the past decade.

*Karina K. Uldall, M.D., M.P.H.,* is a psychiatrist at the University of Washington, Seattle, and principal investigator for the Special Projects of National Significance project "Management of Delirium in HIV/AIDS Patients," which educates providers and families about neuropsychiatric aspects of HIV/AIDS. She also worked on an earlier SPNS project at the Department of Public Health, Seattle, that facilitated integration of psychiatry into primary care practice at Harborview's Madison Clinic.

*William R. Wagner, M.S.W.,* has been a field social worker for the Visiting Nurse Association of Los Angeles Hospice Program.

*Dottie Ward-Wimmer, R.N.,* is a pediatric nurse and director of the children's program at the St. Francis Center, Washington, D.C. She helped establish the Immunology Service at Children's National Medical Center, Washington, D.C., and has published and taught about issues of loss, life-threatening illness, transition, violence, and abuse. She has testified before two presidential commissions on the impact of HIV/AIDS on children. She also is a certified professional counselor and a registered play therapist and has a private practice.

*Mark G. Winiarski, Ph.D.,* is the clinical director of the AIDS Mental Health and Primary Care Integration Project at Montefiore Medical Center, Bronx, New York. He also is principal investigator for an AIDS Mental Health Training Project funded by the Ittleson Foundation and the van Ameringen Foundation. He is an assistant professor of family medicine and psychiatry at the Albert Einstein College of Medicine, Bronx, New York, and was a senior faculty member of the American Psychological Association's Project HOPE. He is the author of *AIDS-Related Psychotherapy.*

*Douglas A. Wirth, M.S.W.,* is senior public policy analyst, community organizer, AIDS mental health coordinator, and director of government relations for the Coalition of Voluntary Mental Health Agencies of New York City. He recently coordinated the Community Mental Health Reinvestment campaign for major mental health reform in New York State. Mr. Wirth served as senior faculty with the American Psychological Association's Project HOPE and as associate director of Tamanawit Unlimited, a consulting firm in Seattle, Washington.

# Index

www.ingramcontent.com/pod-product-compliance
Lightning Source LLC
Chambersburg PA
CBHW022132020426
42334CB00015B/859

*9780814793114*